# Nanomedicine and Drug Delivery

# Nanomedicine and Drug Delivery

Edited by **Oscar Watson**

**S**YRAWOOD
PUBLISHING HOUSE

New York

Published by Syrawood Publishing House,
750 Third Avenue, 9th Floor,
New York, NY 10017, USA
www.syrawoodpublishinghouse.com

**Nanomedicine and Drug Delivery**
Edited by Oscar Watson

International Standard Book Number: 978-1-68286-100-4 (Hardback)

Printed in the United States of America.

# Contents

# Preface

Nanomedicine is a rapidly progressing field which has proven significant in the past few decades. Many successful clinical trials and the development of drugs for many diseases has been possible due to the progress in nanomedicine. This book on nanomedicine and drug delivery aims to equip the readers with in-depth knowledge of significant concepts such as nanotechnology based drugs, biological molecules, scanning probe microscopy, biological microelectromechanical systems, molecular interactions, biomedical imaging, etc. Compiled by an eminent panel of internationally renowned scientists and scholars, the case studies included in this book will prove to be immensely beneficial for students of biotechnology, nanotechnology and associated disciplines.

This book has been the outcome of endless efforts put in by authors and researchers on various issues and topics within the field. The book is a comprehensive collection of significant researches that are addressed in a variety of chapters. It will surely enhance the knowledge of the field among readers across the globe.

It gives us an immense pleasure to thank our researchers and authors for their efforts to submit their piece of writing before the deadlines. Finally in the end, I would like to thank my family and colleagues who have been a great source of inspiration and support.

**Editor**

# PapMV nanoparticles improve mucosal immune responses to the trivalent inactivated flu vaccine

Gervais Rioux[1†], Claudia Mathieu[1†], Alexis Russell[1], Marilène Bolduc[1], Marie-Eve Laliberté-Gagné[1], Pierre Savard[2] and Denis Leclerc[1*]

## Abstract

**Background:** Trivalent inactivated flu vaccines (TIV) are currently the best means to prevent influenza infections. However, the protection provided by TIV is partial (about 50%) and it is needed to improve the efficacy of protection. Since the respiratory tract is the main site of influenza replications, a vaccine that triggers mucosal immunity in this region can potentially improve protection against this disease. Recently, PapMV nanoparticles used as an adjuvant in a formulation with TIV administered by the subcutaneous route have shown improving the immune response directed to the TIV and protection against an influenza challenge.

**Findings:** In the present study, we showed that intranasal instillation with a formulation containing TIV and PapMV nanoparticles significantly increase the amount of IgG, IgG2a and IgA in lungs of vaccinated mice as compared to mice that received TIV only. Instillation with the adjuvanted formulation leads to a more robust protection against an influenza infection with a strain that is lethal to mice vaccinated with the TIV.

**Conclusions:** We demonstrate for the first time that PapMV nanoparticles are an effective and potent mucosal adjuvant for vaccination.

**Keywords:** PapMV nanoparticles, Adjuvant, Mucosal vaccine, Influenza, Trivalent inactivated flu vaccine, TIV, Seasonal flu vaccine, Mucosal immunity

## Background

Vaccination with trivalent inactivated flu vaccines (TIV) remains the most affordable and efficient way to control diseases caused by influenza virus. The TIV is reformulated on the recommendation of WHO at the beginning of every year based on the circulating strains of the virus in the population. From that point, the manufacture process takes up to 8 months before the release the vaccine [1]. During this period, strains change through antigenic drift and shift and consequently, contribute to the decrease of vaccine effectiveness.

The TIV are currently administered by the intramuscular route, which is not optimal for protection to an influenza infection that occurs in the respiratory tract. The favored route of vaccination to trigger mucosal immunity in the respiratory tract is the intranasal route [2,3]. However, the TIV was previously showed to be less immunogenic by the intranasal route [4,5]. The amount of antigen needed to trigger IgA production by this route must be increased by two fold which, directly impact the number of available doses [4,5]. Therefore, changes in the vaccine formulation to improve TIV efficacy in the respiratory tracts and increase the number of doses are needed [6].

Development of mucosal adjuvants that can improve both, the immune response to TIV in lungs and dose sparing became a priority [5,7,8]. Current available adjuvants are ineffective in inducing mucosal immunity because they cannot be administered by the intranasal route due to their biophysical properties. As an example, aluminium hydroxide, the most commonly used adjuvant in vaccines, is inefficient with TIV and cannot be used by the mucosal route [9]. New safe and potent adjuvants are therefore needed.

* Correspondence: denis.leclerc@crchudequebec.ulaval.ca
†Equal contributors
[1]Department of Microbiology, Infectiology and Immunology, 'Centre de recherche en Infectiologie', Laval University, 2705 boul. Laurier, Quebec City, PQ G1V 4G2, Canada
Full list of author information is available at the end of the article

In this study, we evaluated the potential of papaya mosaic virus (PapMV) nanoparticles to be used as a mucosal adjuvant. This hypothesis is supported by a previous report by our group showing that PapMV nanoparticles can trigger innate immunity in lungs of mice [10]. Instillation with PapMV nanoparticles triggered pro-inflammatory cytokines and chemokines secretion and immune cells recruitment shortly after treatment [10]. PapMV nanoparticles were also showed to be a TLR7 ligand, a receptor that activates innate immunity [11]. Furthermore, PapMV nanoparticles administered by the subcutaneous route were previously shown to improve and broaden the immune response to TIV in mouse and ferret animal models [7].

The objective of this study was to demonstrate that PapMV nanoparticles are able to induce mucosal immunity against TIV when administered by the intranasal route, in order to show its potential as a mucosal adjuvant. This route of administration was compared with subcutaneous injections as previously reported by our group [7].

## Methods

### PapMV nanoparticles production

PapMV nanoparticles were kindly provided by Folia Biotech Inc. (lot # L-5728, Quebec City, Canada). Those PapMV nanoparticles are comparable to a lot used in previous studies [10]. In brief, PapMV nanoparticles are constituted of PapMV coat proteins and assemble *in vitro* around an RNA transcript. The *Limulus Amebocyte* lysate (LAL) assay (Lonza, Walkersville, Maryland, USA) was used to evaluate the levels of LPS contaminants that were found to be below the detection limit. PapMV nanoparticles were characterized by electron microscopy and dynamic light scattering as described previously [12]. In brief, nanoparticles sizes were recorded with a ZetaSizer Nano ZS (Malvern, Worcestershire, United Kingdom) at 0.1 mg/ml in 10 mM Tris–HCl pH 8.0. Water diluted PapMV nanoparticles were stained with 3% acetate-uranyl on carbon-formvar grids then observed with a FEI-TECNAI-Spirit transmission electron microscope (FEI, Hillsboro, Oregon, USA).

### Vaccination protocol

Mice, 6 to 8-week-old BALB/c (10/group), were immunized twice at 14-day interval by the intranasal (i.n.) or subcutaneous (s.c.) routes with 50 µl of a formulation containing 2.1 µg of each hemagglutinin (HA) (TIV 2009–2010 (A/Brisbane/59/2007 (H1N1), A/Brisbane/10/2007 (H3N2), B/Brisbane/60/2008), cat #9815, GlaxoSmithKline) alone or adjuvanted by 21 µg of PapMV nanoparticles. Bleedings were performed at day 0 and 28 and bronchoalveolar lavages (BAL), at day 28 post-immunization.

### Antibody response quantification

BALs were performed using 700 µl of phosphate buffered saline and cells were purged from the samples by centrifugation. Blood sample were collected and centrifuged in BD Microtainer blood collection tubes (BD, Mississauga, Ontario, Canada) for 2 minutes at 10 000 × g. The harvested serums and BAL fluids were assayed for total IgG, IgG2a serotype and IgA against TIV or IgG2a against GST-NP by enzyme-linked immunosorbent assay (ELISA) as described elsewhere [7,13]. GST-NP is a C-terminal fusion of the influenza nucleoprotein to a glutathione S-transferase (GST) protein [7]. ELISAs were conducted by serial dilutions by two-fold steps starting at 1 in 50. Results are expressed as an antibody endpoint titer greater than threefold the background optical density values consisting of preimmune sera or control BAL fluids.

### Mice challenge with influenza virus

Mice were challenged 2 weeks after the last immunization with 250 plaque-forming units (pfu) of A/WSN/33(H1N1) influenza virus by 50 µl intranasal instillation. Weight losses and symptoms were monitored for 14 days post-infection. Symptoms are rated from 0 to 4 (no symptoms (0), lightly spiked fur and curved back [1], spiked fur and curved back [2], difficulty to move and light dehydration [3], severe dehydration, lack of reflex and ocular secretion [4]), where 4 is the highest score and mice are euthanized. Mice that lost more than 20% of their initial weight are also euthanized.

### Statistical analysis

Data from ELISA and challenge (day 8 weight losses and symptoms) were analyzed with a parametric ANOVA test. Tukey's post tests were used to compare differences among groups of mice. Kaplan-Meier survival curves were analysed by the log rank test. Values of $^*p < 0.05$, $^{**}p < 0.001$ and $^{***}p < 0.0001$ were considered statistically significant. Statistical analyses were performed using GraphPad PRISM 5.01.

### Ethics statement

All the work with animals has been done with institution approved ethics protocol by the "Comité de Protection des Animaux - CHUQ (CPA-CHUQ)". The approval of this project is found under the authorization number 2010–148.

## Results and discussion

PapMV nanoparticles are composed of the recombinant coat proteins of PapMV purified from *E. coli* and self-assembled around a single-stranded RNA. Transmission electron microscopy revealed that PapMV nanoparticles have a filamentous rod shape structure (Figure 1A) and

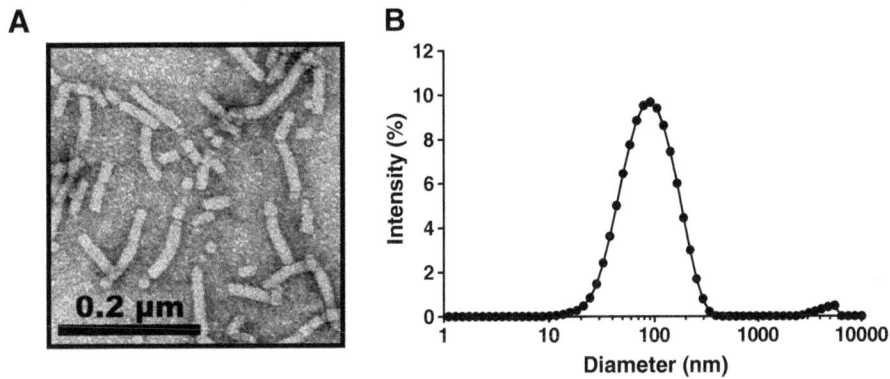

**Figure 1 Structure of the PapMV nanoparticles.** PapMV nanoparticles were observed with a transmission electron microscope and by dynamic light scattering. PapMV nanoparticles have a filamentous rod-shape structure **(A)** with an average length of 100 nm as shown by dynamic light scattering **(B)**.

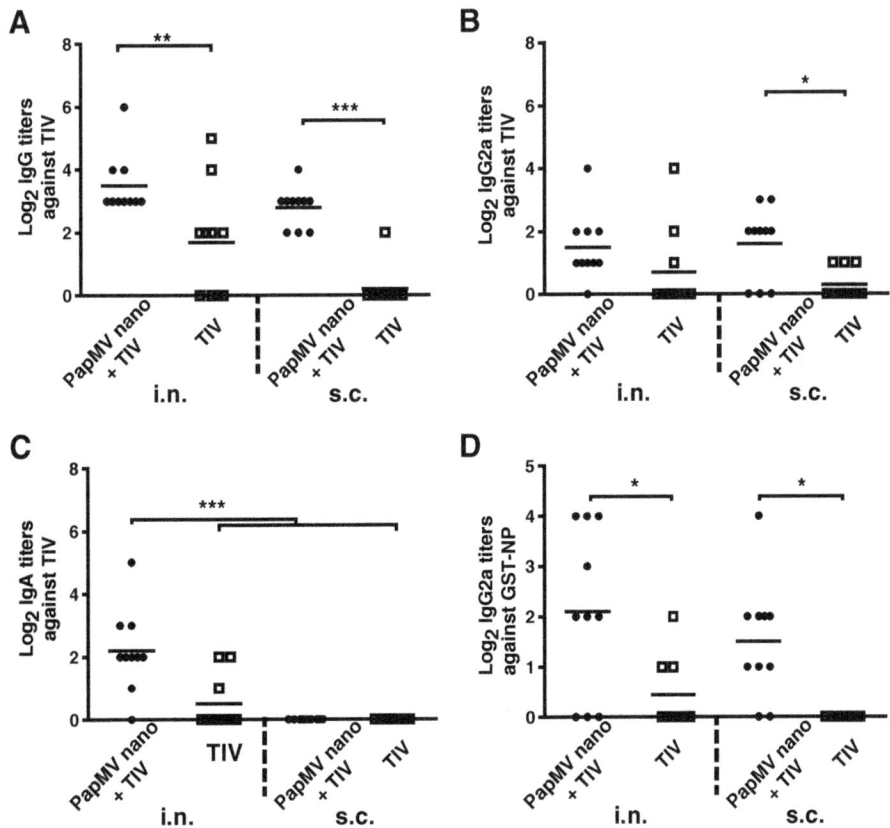

**Figure 2 PapMV nanoparticles improve the mucosal antibody response against TIV and NP in the lungs.** Balb/C mice (10/group) were vaccinated twice at a 14-day interval with TIV alone or adjuvanted by PapMV nanoparticles by intranasal (i.n.) or subcutaneous (s.c.) routes. Bronchoalveolar lavages were performed at day 28 and ELISA were conducted to evaluate the levels of total IgG **(A)**, IgG2a **(B)** or IgA **(C)** against TIV and IgG2a against NP **(D)**. Titers against TIV or GST-NP were not detected in the blood or BAL of PapMV nanoparticles or buffer vaccinated mice. *P < 0.05, **P < 0.01 and ***P < 0.001.

an average length of 100 nm, as confirmed by dynamic light scattering (Figure 1B).

To evaluate the potential of PapMV nanoparticles as a mucosal adjuvant, mice were immunized twice at 14 days interval by either the i.n. or s.c. routes with TIV alone or adjuvanted with PapMV nanoparticles. Antibodies levels against TIV in the BAL (Figure 2) and in the blood (Figure 3) were measured by ELISA at day 28. We showed that TIV adjuvanted with PapMV nanoparticles administered either by the i.n. or s.c. improved and potentiate the TIV as observed by the levels of total IgG titers directed against TIV (Figure 2A). IgG2a titers in the BAL showed significant higher levels in the aduvanted group only when administered by the s.c. route (Figure 2B). Interestingly, the group showing the highest IgA titers in the BAL was the adjuvanted TIV administered by the i.n. route (Figure 2C) showing clearly the effectiveness of PapMV nanoparticles to improve the mucosal antibody response in the lung. The ELISA also revealed that the adjuvanted vaccine broaden the immune

response to the TIV antigens through a significant increased in the lungs of the IgG2a titers directed to the influenza NP (Figure 2D), a highly conserved protein through all the strains of influenza often used in experimental influenza vaccines [7,14,15]. NP has also been identified as a key antigen to trigger cross-protection to influenza viruses [8,16-18]. It is therefore a good strategy to increase the immune response directed to this antigen using PapMV nanoparticles to broaden and improve protection to this virus. Through the course of the experiment, we have not notice any sign of toxicity associated with the use of PapMV nanoparticles.

In the blood, the levels of total IgG or IgG2a were higher than in the BAL with either route of immunization (Figure 3). We also showed that the titers in total IgG or IgG2a directed to TIV or GST-NP were similar when the adjuvanted formulation was administered by the i.n. or the s.c. route (Figure 3A-B, D). As expected, only the adjuvanted vaccine administered by the i.n. route could trigger in the blood a significant amount of

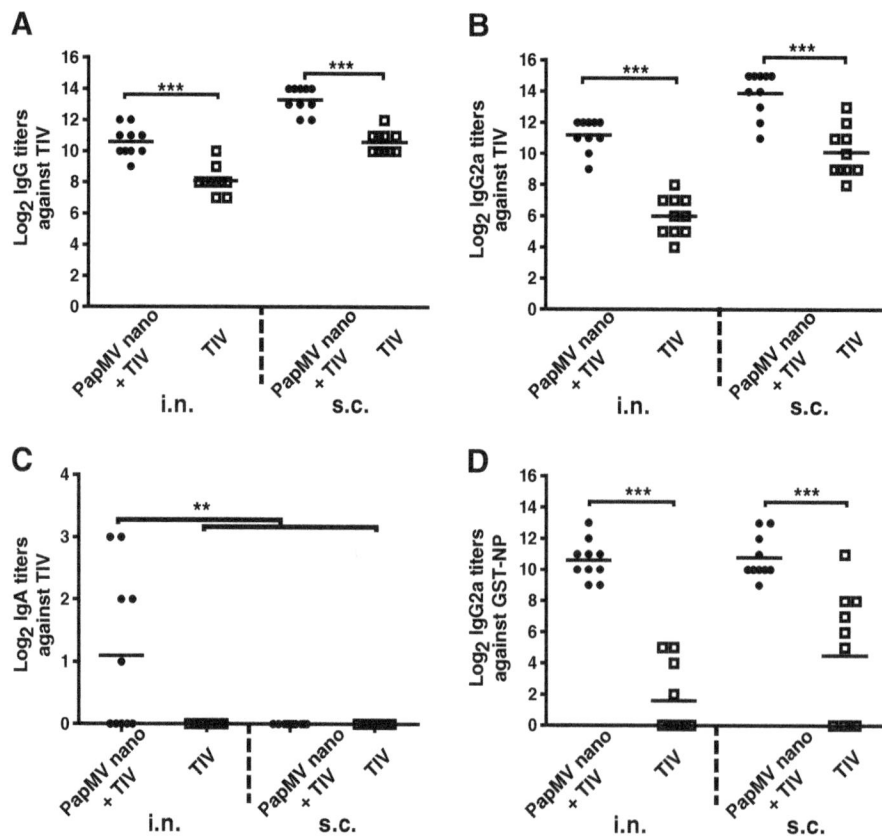

**Figure 3 PapMV nanoparticles improve the systemic antibody response against TIV and NP.** Balb/C mice (10/group) were vaccinated twice at a 14-day interval with TIV alone or adjuvanted with PapMV nanoparticles by intranasal (i.n.) or subcutaneous (s.c.) routes. Bleedings were performed at day 28 and ELISA were conducted to evaluate the levels of total IgG (A), IgG2a (B) or IgA (C) against TIV and IgG2a against NP (D). Titers against TIV or GST-NP were not detected in the blood or BAL of PapMV nanoparticles or buffer vaccinated mice. *P < 0.05, **P < 0.01 and ***P < 0.001.

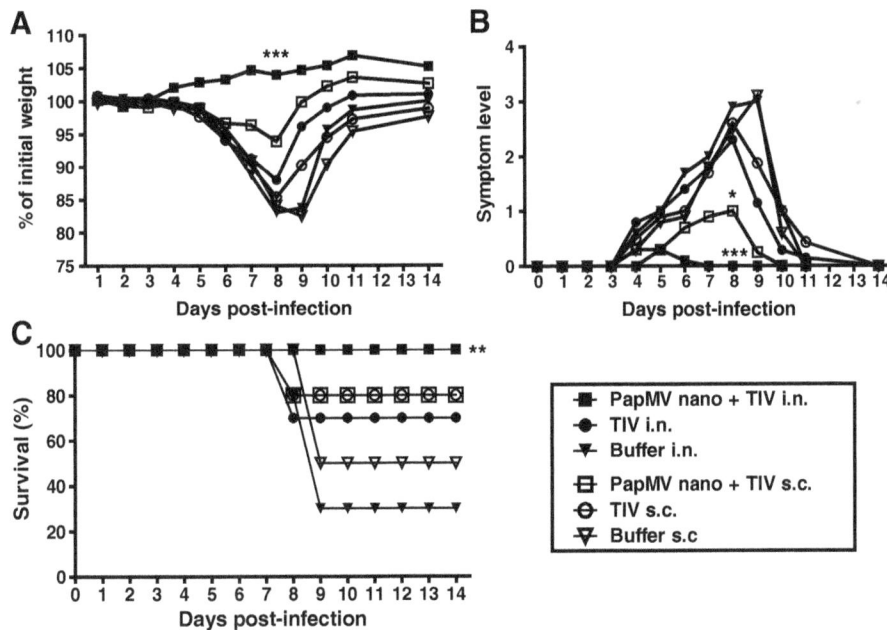

**Figure 4** Mice vaccinated with PapMV nanoparticles adjuvanted TIV showed an increased protection to an influenza challenge with influenza strain normally lethal to TIV vaccinated mice. Mice vaccinated twice with TIV adjuvanted or not by PapMV nanoparticles by intranasal (i.n.) or subcutaneous (s.c.) routes were challenged with 250 pfu of A/WSN/1933 (H1N1) influenza virus. Mice were monitored for weight loss (A), symptoms levels (B) and survival (C) for 14 days. Statistical analysis is applied between groups of the same immunization ways. *P < 0.05, **P < 0.01 and ***P < 0.001.

IgA directed to TIV (Figure 3C). Titers against TIV or GST-NP were not detected in the blood or BAL of PapMV nanoparticles or buffer vaccinated mice.

We previously showed that mice immunized s.c. with the TIV adjuvanted with PapMV nanoparticles induced protection against an strain of influenza that overcome the protection induced by the TIV [8]. In this study, we wish to validate that the adjuvanted TIV with PapMV nanoparticles administered by the intranasal route can also elicit this kind of protection. Therefore, we challenged vaccinated mice with A/WSN/33(H1N1), a strain of influenza that was previously showed to overcome the protection induced by the TIV. As expected, mice vaccinated with TIV by either route of immunization were not protected and showed major weight losses (more than 15%) (Figure 4A) and strong symptoms (Figure 4B); while mice immunized by the i.n. route with the PapMV adjuvanted TIV showed a weight increased (Figure 4A) without any symptoms during infection (Figure 4B). Mice immunized with the same formulation by the s.c. route lost 7% of their initial weight and showed mild symptoms at the infection peak (day 8) (Figure 4A,B). Finally, only mice immunized by the i.n. route with the adjuvanted TIV formulation showed 100% survival (Figure 4C). The PapMV adjuvanted i.n. vaccine generated a robust protection to the infection by an influenza strain normally lethal to TIV vaccinated mice.

PapMV nanoparticles is therefore an efficient mucosal adjuvant with strong potential for its used in human.

## Conclusions

In conclusion, we demonstrate for the first time that PapMV nanoparticle is an effective and potent mucosal adjuvant for vaccination against a respiratory disease. This technology fulfills an important medical need for a safe mucosal adjuvant that broadens the protection of the TIV.

**Abbreviations**

PapMV: Papaya mosaic virus; TIV: Trivalent inactivated flu vaccines; HA: Hemagglutinin; BAL: Bronchoalveolar lavage; ELISA: Enzyme-linked immunosorbent assay; NP: Nucleoprotein; GST: Glutathione S-transferase; Pfu: Plaque-forming units; i.n: Intranasal; s.c: Subcutaneous.

**Competing interests**

Author Denis Leclerc and Pierre Savard are shareholder of the company FOLIA BIOTECH INC., a start-up company that has the mandate to exploit commercially this technology to improve and design new vaccines. This does not alter the authors' adherence to all the journal policies.

**Authors' contributions**

GR performed mice experiments and drafted the manuscript. CM performed mice experiments and immunoassays and helped to draft the manuscript. GR and CM are considered to have equally contributed to this article. AR performed mice experiments and helped to draft the manuscript. MB, MELG and PS engineered the nanoparticles. DL supervised the study and revised the manuscript. All authors read and approved the final manuscript.

**Acknowledgment**

We would like to thank the "Plateforme de bio-imagerie du centre de recherche en infectiologie" for letting us use the transmission electron microscope. This work was supported by a grant from the Canadian Institute of Health Research [185160] and FOLIA BIOTECH INC.

**Author details**

[1]Department of Microbiology, Infectiology and Immunology, 'Centre de recherche en Infectiologie', Laval University, 2705 boul. Laurier, Quebec City, PQ G1V 4G2, Canada. [2]Neurosciences, Laval University, Quebec City, PQ, Canada.

**References**

1. Barr IG, McCauley J, Cox N, Daniels R, Engelhardt OG, Fukuda K, Grohmann G, Hay A, Kelso A, Klimov A, Odagiri T, Smith D, Russell C, Tashiro M, Webby R, Wood J, Ye Z, Zhang W: **Epidemiological, antigenic and genetic characteristics of seasonal influenza A(H1N1), A(H3N2) and B influenza viruses: basis for the WHO recommendation on the composition of influenza vaccines for use in the 2009–2010 Northern Hemisphere season.** *Vaccine* 2010, **28**(5):1156–1167.

2. Keitel WA, Cate TR, Nino D, Huggins LL, Six HR, Quarles JM, Couch RB: **Immunization against influenza: comparison of various topical and parenteral regimens containing inactivated and/or live attenuated vaccines in healthy adults.** *J Infect Dis* 2001, **183**(2):329–332.

3. Belyakov IM, Ahlers JD: **What role does the route of immunization play in the generation of protective immunity against mucosal pathogens?** *J Immunol* 2009, **183**(11):6883–6892.

4. Atmar RL, Keitel WA, Cate TR, Munoz FM, Ruben F, Couch RB: **A dose–response evaluation of inactivated influenza vaccine given intranasally and intramuscularly to healthy young adults.** *Vaccine* 2007, **25**(29):5367–5373.

5. Hong SH, Byun Y-H, Nguyen CT, Kim SY, Seong BL, Park S, Woo GJ, Yoon Y, Koh JT, Fujihashi K, Rhee JH, Lee SE: **Intranasal administration of a flagellin-adjuvanted inactivated influenza vaccine enhances mucosal immune responses to protect mice against lethal infection.** *Vaccine* 2012, **30**(2):466–474.

6. Woodrow KA, Bennett KM, Lo DD: **Mucosal vaccine design and delivery.** *Annu Rev Biomed Eng* 2012, **14**:17–46.

7. Savard C, Guérin A, Drouin K, Bolduc M, Laliberté-Gagné M-E, Dumas M-C, Majeau N, Leclerc D: **Improvement of the trivalent inactivated flu vaccine using PapMV nanoparticles.** *PLoS One* 2011, **6**(6):e21522.

8. Langley JM, Aoki F, Ward BJ, McGeer A, Angel JB, Stiver G, Gorfinkel I, Shu D, White L, Lasko B, Dzongowski P, Papp K, Alexander M, Boivin G, Fries L: **A nasally administered trivalent inactivated influenza vaccine is well tolerated, stimulates both mucosal and systemic immunity, and potentially protects against influenza illness.** *Vaccine* 2011, **29**(10):1921–1928.

9. Lawson LB, Norton EB, Clements JD: **Defending the mucosa: adjuvant and carrier formulations for mucosal immunity.** *Curr Opin Immunol Elsevier Ltd* 2011, **23**(3):414–420.

10. Mathieu C, Rioux G, Dumas M-C, Leclerc D: **Induction of innate immunity in lungs with virus-like nanoparticles leads to protection against influenza and Streptococcus pneumoniae challenge.** *Nanomedicine* 2013, **9**:839–848.

11. Lebel M-È, Daudelin J-F, Chartrand K, Tarrab E, Kalinke U, Savard P, Labrecque N, Leclerc D, Lamarre A: **Nanoparticle Adjuvant Sensing by TLR7 Enhances CD8+ T Cell-Mediated Protection from Listeria Monocytogenes Infection.** *J Immunol* 2014, **192**(3):1071–1078.

12. Rioux G, Majeau N, Leclerc D: **Mapping the surface-exposed regions of papaya mosaic virus nanoparticles.** *FEBS J* 2012, **279**(11):2004–2011.

13. Rioux G, Babin C, Majeau N, Leclerc D: **Engineering of papaya mosaic virus (PapMV) nanoparticles through fusion of the HA11 peptide to several putative surface-exposed sites.** *PLoS One* 2012, **7**(2):e31925.

14. Vemula SV, Ahi YS, Swaim A-M, Katz JM, Donis R, Sambhara S, Mital SK: **Broadly protective adenovirus-based multivalent vaccines against highly pathogenic avian influenza viruses for pandemic preparedness.** *PLoS One* 2013, **8**(4):e62496.

15. Wang W, Huang B, Jiang T, Wang X, Qi X, Gao Y, Yan W, Ruan L: **Robust immunity and heterologous protection against influenza in mice elicited by a novel recombinant NP-M2e fusion protein expressed in E. coli.** *PLoS One* 2012, **7**(12):e52488.

16. Carragher DM, Kaminski DA, Moquin A, Hartson L, Randall TD: **A novel role for non-neutralizing antibodies against nucleoprotein in facilitating resistance to influenza virus.** *J Immunol* 2008, **181**(6):4168–4176.

17. LaMere MW, Lam H-T, Moquin A, Haynes L, Lund FE, Randall TD, Kamiski DA: **Contributions of antinucleoprotein IgG to heterosubtypic immunity against influenza virus.** *J Immunol* 2011, **186**(7):4331–4339.

18. Lamere MW, Moquin A, Lee FE-H, Misra RS, Blair PJ, Haynes L, Lund FE, Kaminski DA: **Regulation of antinucleoprotein IgG by systemic vaccination and its effect on influenza virus clearance.** *J Virol* 2011, **85**(10):5027–5035.

# 2

# Enhancement of the killing effect of low-temperature plasma on *Streptococcus mutans* by combined treatment with gold nanoparticles

Sang Rye Park[1], Hyun Wook Lee[2], Jin Woo Hong[3], Hae June Lee[4], Ji Young Kim[1], Byul bo-ra Choi[5], Gyoo Cheon Kim[5*] and Young Chan Jeon[6*]

## Abstract

**Background:** Recently, non-thermal atmospheric pressure plasma sources have been used for biomedical applications such as sterilization, cancer treatment, blood coagulation, and wound healing. Gold nanoparticles (gNPs) have unique optical properties and are useful for biomedical applications. Although low-temperature plasma has been shown to be effective in killing oral bacteria on agar plates, its bactericidal effect is negligible on the tooth surface. Therefore, we used 30-nm gNPs to enhance the killing effect of low-temperature plasma on human teeth.

**Results:** We tested the sterilizing effect of low-temperature plasma on *Streptococcus mutans* (*S. mutans*) strains. The survival rate was assessed by bacterial viability stains and colony-forming unit counts. Low-temperature plasma treatment alone was effective in killing *S. mutans* on slide glasses, as shown by the 5-log decrease in viability. However, plasma treatment of bacteria spotted onto tooth surface exhibited a 3-log reduction in viability. After gNPs were added to *S. mutans*, plasma treatment caused a 5-log reduction in viability, while gNPs alone did not show any bactericidal effect. The morphological changes in *S. mutans* caused by plasma treatment were examined by transmission electron microscopy, which showed that plasma treatment only perforated the cell walls, while the combination treatment with plasma and gold nanoparticles caused significant cell rupture, causing loss of intracellular components from many cells.

**Conclusions:** This study demonstrates that low-temperature plasma treatment is effective in killing *S. mutans* and that its killing effect is further enhanced when used in combination with gNPs.

**Keywords:** Gold nanoparticle, Low-temperature plasma, *Streptococcus mutans*, Sterilization, Oral care

## Background

Dental caries is a chronic infection of worldwide prevalence, and it represents oral health problems associated with oral bacteria [1]. Although remarkable technical developments have been made in dental treatment, dental caries remains a major oral health problem in most countries [2]. Dental caries commonly occur on the occlusal and proximal surfaces of the tooth, particularly in its pits and fissures. These sites are structurally difficult to approach when treating a decayed tooth. In clinical management, a carious tooth is simply removed by

dental handpiece drilling, after which a restorative material is used to fill the empty space. During this process, a greater amount than necessary of healthy tooth tissue is often removed along with the decayed part. Furthermore, if the cavity is filled without completely removing bacteria, the remaining bacteria cause recurrence of dental caries. Therefore, a novel method that strongly inhibits the causative pathogens regardless of their spatial accessibility to hand-held tools and decreases the excessive removal of the healthy parts of the tooth is highly desirable.

Low-temperature atmospheric pressure plasma has been used for biomedical applications such as sterilization, cancer treatment, blood coagulation, and wound healing [3]. Since plasma generates high amounts of reactive oxygen species (ROS) and hydroxyl radicals

* Correspondence: ki91000m@pusan.ac.kr; jeonyc@paran.com
[5]Department of Oral Anatomy, School of Dentistry, Pusan National University, Yangsan 602-739, Rep. Korea
[6]Department of Dental Prosthetics, School of Dentistry, Pusan National University, Yangsan 602-739, Republic of Korea
Full list of author information is available at the end of the article

(•OH), it is highly effective in killing bacteria such as *Escherichia coli*, *Candida albicans* [4,5], *Pseudomonas aeruginosa* [6], and *Lactobacillus casei* [7]. The bactericidal property of non-thermal plasmas has been recently used against oral pathogens. Effective killing of *Enterococcus faecalis* has been reported using low-frequency air plasma and pulse-modulated He plasma needles [8]. A microwave plasma pencil has been reported to induce a high death rate of *Streptococcus mutans* with $H_2O_2$ [9]. However, plasma treatment alone needs a relatively long time for killing *S. mutans* [9,10].

*S. mutans*, a facultative anaerobic [11] and high acid-producing bacterium [12], has been identified as the principal cause of dental caries. Acidic substances produced by *S. mutans* destroy the dental enamel, leading to severe tooth decay. Plasma treatment has been reported to induce a high death rate of *S. mutans*. However, in those studies, the plasma temperature was too high for application to human tissues. [13,14]. Being gram-positive, *S. mutans* has a thick cell wall to protect it from the external environment. This thick cell wall makes it more difficult to kill gram-positive than gram-negative bacteria. Furthermore, the presence of gram-positive bacteria in very narrow crevices of a tooth limits their accessibility for various treatments. In this study, gold nanoparticles (gNPs) were used to enhance the killing effect of low-temperature plasma on *S. mutans*. Because of the high electric conductivity of gNPs, we assumed that they could be activated by plasma. Stimulated gNPs would then cause high levels of cellular

stress, which could lead to the death of the bacteria. The aim of this study was to enhance the killing effect of low-temperature plasma on *S. mutans* by means of gNPs for dental caries treatment.

## Results

### Enhancement of the killing effect of plasma by using gNPs

To investigate the killing effect of plasma, a cover glass was coated with 5 μL (~$10^8$ colony-forming units (CFUs)/mL) of a suspension of *S. mutans*. The survival curve showed a 5-log reduction in cell viability by plasma treatment for 300 s. Using gNPs attached to *S. mutans* cells in combination with plasma treatment yielded a 6-log reduction in viability (Figure 1). The killing effect of plasma on *S. mutans* cannot be due to a thermal effect because the plasma temperature did not exceed 37°C for longer than 5 min (Figure 2).

The killing effect of plasma on *S. mutans* cells was lower for cells spotted onto the surface of the tooth than for cells on a cover glass. To enhance the bactericidal effect, gNPs were employed. After the addition of gNPs to *S. mutans* for 1 h, plasma treatment significantly decreased the viability of *S. mutans* cells. Plasma-only treatment of *S. mutans* cells for 300 s showed a 3-log reduction, while cells treated with gNPs and plasma exhibited a 5-log decrease (Figure 3). The difference in the killing effect with plasma only and combination treatment with gNPs and plasma was statistically significant ($p < 0.05$).

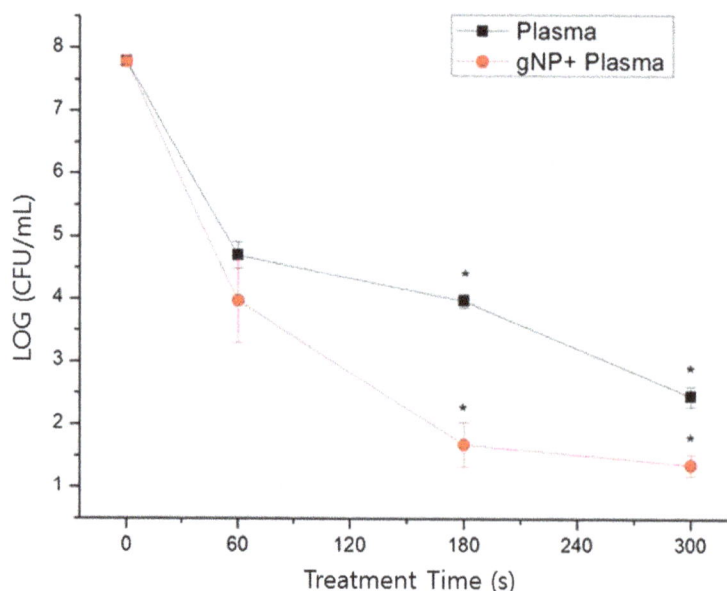

**Figure 1 Enhanced killing effect can be achieved using combined gold nanoparticle (gNP) and low-temperature plasma treatment for** *Streptococcus mutans* **cultured on a cover glass.** Bacterial viability was assessed by plate counting. The difference between the death rates for plasma-only and plasma plus gNPs was statistically significant ($p < 0.05$).

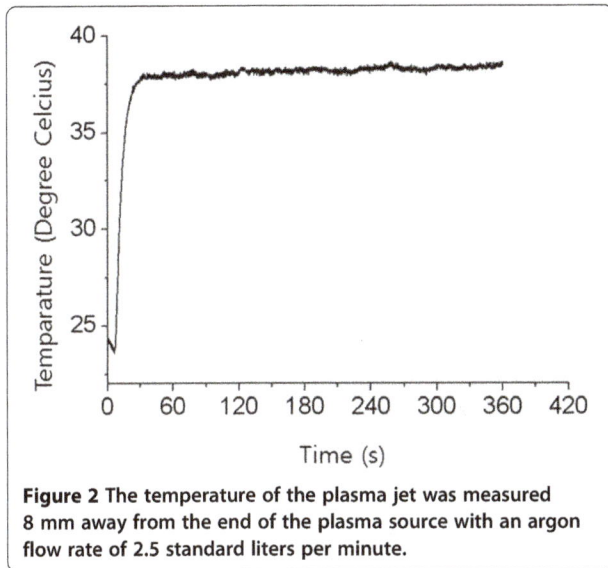

**Figure 2** The temperature of the plasma jet was measured 8 mm away from the end of the plasma source with an argon flow rate of 2.5 standard liters per minute.

### Viability staining of S. mutans cells

The viability of S. mutans was analyzed using fluorescence microscopy. S. mutans was stained with SYTO 9® and propidium iodide (PI). SYTO 9® (green fluorescence) can label all living bacteria in a population, whereas PI (red fluorescence) can only penetrate bacteria with damaged membranes, which causes a decrease in SYTO 9® fluorescence intensity. Control cells and bacteria treated only with gNPs showed green fluorescence (Figure 4A and B), while red fluorescence was detected in S. mutans cells treated with microwave plasma for 60 s (Figure 4C). The

combination treatment of plasma and gNPs showed only a few green fluorescent cells (live), which were detected among mostly red fluorescent cells (dead) (Figure 4D).

### Morphological examination of cell damage by transmission electron microscopy

Using transmission electron microscopy (TEM), we analyzed the morphological changes in S. mutans cells after plasma treatment. The cell membrane was smooth, and cell division was observed in the control experiment (Figure 5A). After plasma treatment, the cell membrane and cell wall were disrupted, but the cytosol was retained within the cell (Figure 5B). After addition of gNPs, which bind to the cell wall of S. mutans, the plasma treatment significantly ruptured the cell walls (Figure 5C) and led to the release of its cytoplasmic components (Figure 5D).

### Discussion

This study demonstrates that gNPs enhance the killing effect of low-temperature plasma on S. mutans. Conventionally, oral antiseptic agents have been widely used to reduce the number of oral bacteria. However, their usage for long periods might lead to side effects such as tooth staining, dry mouth, and taste disturbance [15]. Currently, lasers are being used in many fields of dentistry, including caries treatment [16]. A laser beam is an intense, coherent, and highly directional beam of light. These characteristics of lasers are of limited benefit for cavity treatment in a tooth with a curved surface and an irregular shape. For instance, in the case of periapical

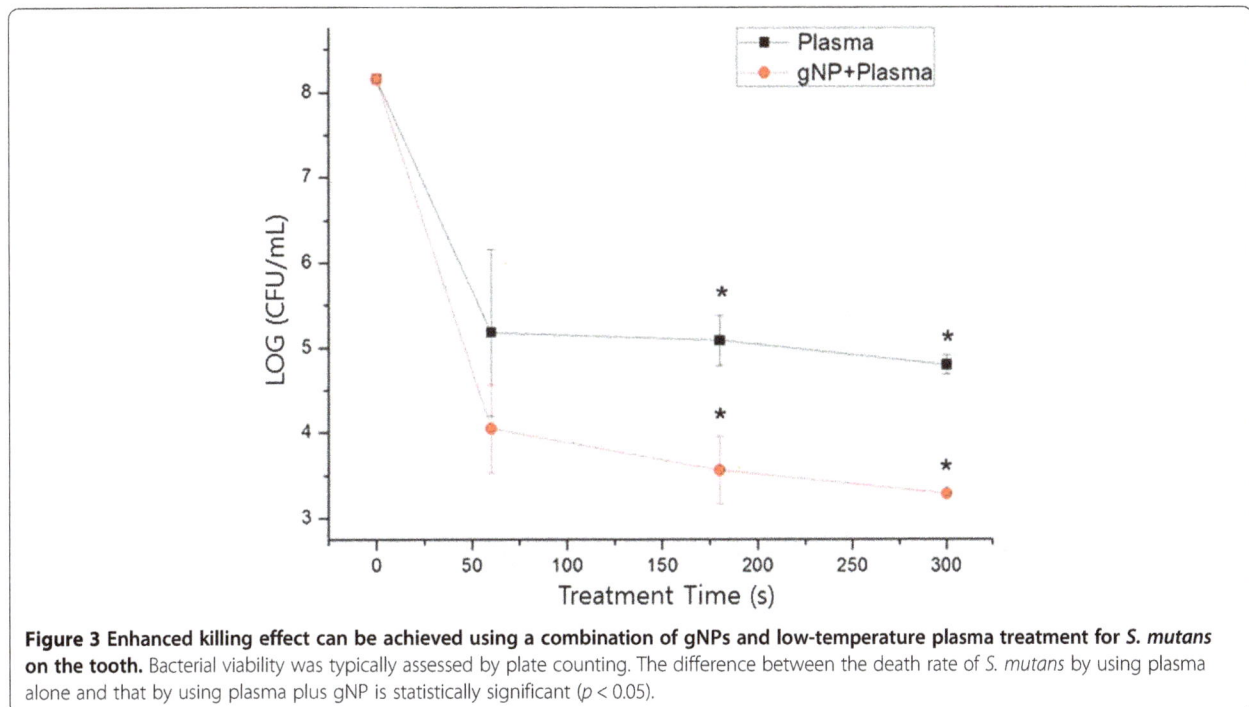

**Figure 3 Enhanced killing effect can be achieved using a combination of gNPs and low-temperature plasma treatment for S. mutans on the tooth.** Bacterial viability was typically assessed by plate counting. The difference between the death rate of S. mutans by using plasma alone and that by using plasma plus gNP is statistically significant ($p < 0.05$).

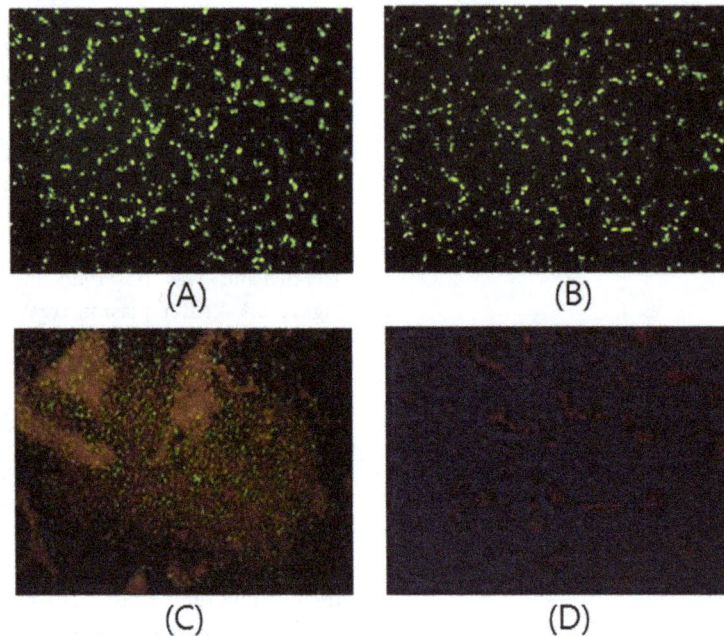

**Figure 4 Viability staining of *S. mutans* cells. (A)** Untreated control cells. **(B)** *S. mutans* cells treated with gNPs. **(C)** *S. mutans* cells treated with plasma only. **(D)** *S. mutans* cells treated with gNPs and plasma. All treatments were applied for 30 s, and cells were stained with SYTO 9 and propidium iodide. Images were observed under a fluorescence microscope (magnification, ×400).

infections, it is difficult to apply laser beams to the infection site. However, plasma is an ionizing gas, which results in high flexibility for application to various oral structures and for overcoming such spatial limitations. Thus, plasma can easily approach an infection site and effectively kill oral pathogens.

Although many studies have been carried out to determine the mechanism of killing by plasma, the exact mechanism is not yet clearly understood. This might be due to the multitude of plasma-generated components such as ROS, charged particles, and electrostatic and electromagnetic fields. Thus, it is possible that several components work together to produce a synergistic effect rather than a single component contributing to the sterilization. Plasma can produce a large amount of ROS when it passes through air, and in particular, high levels of •OH are generated when plasma reacts with water or tissue fluid. It is well known that •OH effectively kills

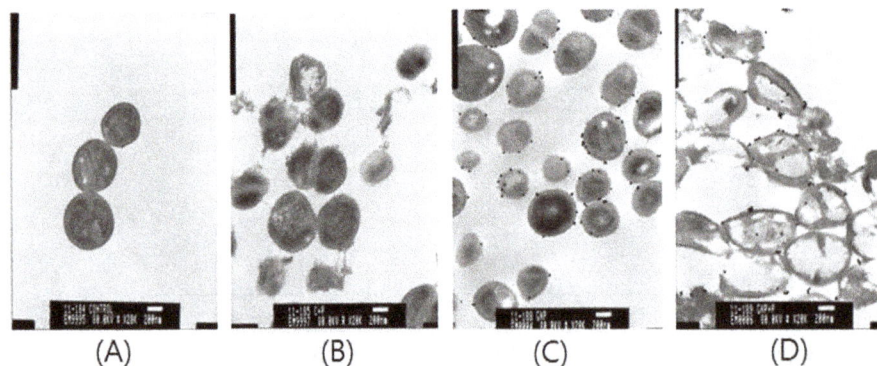

**Figure 5 Transmission electron microscopy images of *S. mutans* treated with low-temperature plasma and gNPs (×20,000). (A)** Control cells without any treatment. **(B)** *S. mutans* cells treated with plasma only. **(C)** *S. mutans* cells treated with gNPs only. **(D)** Morphological features of *S. mutans* cells after combined treatment with plasma and gNPs.

bacteria. Furthermore, the half-life of plasma-generated ROS is very short, and hence, its retention in the oral cavity is short and less likely to induce harmful effects on tissues. Although the plasma is called low-temperature plasma, plasma gas generates heat, which should not lead to thermal damage to tissues. In other articles reporting the killing effect of plasma, thermal damage could be observed owing to the high temperature of plasma [13,14]. Considering that temperatures higher than 42.5°C induce pulpal damage, the plasma temperature should be maintained below 40°C. As shown in Figure 2, the temperature of the plasma used in this experiment did not exceed 37°C for longer than 5 min. Thus, plasma-induced thermal damage to the oral tissues was unlikely.

In this study, plasma treatment showed a 5-log reduction in S. mutans cells on the cover glass. This significant bactericidal effect decreased to a 3-log reduction when S. mutans was grown on the tooth surface. Although a 3-log reduction of S. mutans obviously represents a high bactericidal effect, the residual bacteria could cause recurrent dental caries. Accordingly, as a new method to overcome this issue, we used gNPs in combination with low-temperature plasma to achieve a high level of effectiveness and rapid killing of S. mutans. In this study, we used 30-nm colloidal shaped gNPs. gNPs are well known for biosafety and uptake into the cell [17]. The shape and size of gNPs can be easily controlled [18], which has led to their widespread application in diagnostics [19], therapeutics, and drug delivery [20]. According to one study, the electric field at the adhesion point between gNPs and membrane was amplified when gNPs attached to the surface of a nuclear membrane were exposed to plasma [21]. In an earlier study by our group, we showed that gNPs stimulated by plasma induced selective cancer cell death in melanoma and oral squamous carcinoma cells [22,23]. In the current study, gNPs were bound to S. mutans cells walls, and no alterations were observed in the S. mutans cells. Plasma treatment of S. mutans was more effective against gNP-attached cells than against the gNP-free ones. TEM images showed severe cell wall damage with plasma treatment. Furthermore, the combination treatment of gNPs and plasma led to cell wall rupture, such that most intracellular components were released. This finding suggests that the plasma energy, which may have been amplified by gNPs, could induce severe stress to the S. mutans cell walls. The most likely mechanisms of the synergistic effect of the microwave plasma and gNPs might be enhanced electric field and local heating near the gNPs. High electric conductivity and the nano-size geometry of the gNPs lead to electric field concentration on gNPs [21-23]. The enhanced electric field near the gNPs might attract or repel charged particles. This could cause ion bombardment from the plasma [24] and

gathering of charged particles inside bacteria, leading to the rupture of the cell wall. Joule heating of the gNPs can be an important factor. An earlier study showed high thermal power dissipation of gold by a radio frequency electric field, and it increased as the size of gNPs decreased [25]. These suggestions can explain the severe damages to the bacteria cell walls.

Considering these data, the use of gNPs in combination with plasma has proven very effective in killing the bacteria hidden in the very small spaces of the tooth. Therefore, this technique can limit the number of bacteria remaining within the tooth structure and markedly decrease the recurrence of dental caries.

The microwave plasma jet has a resonator structure. Most of the microwave power is consumed for sustaining the plasma and is reflected at the open end of the microwave plasma source [26]. Only little microwave power can leak from the microwave plasma source. A low E-field has been found to exist near the open end, and the E-field intensity reduces exponentially as the distance increases [27]. This indicates that the effect of microwave leakage on patients is negligible.

## Conclusions

Low-temperature plasma can be applied to various tooth structures for therapy and preventive dentistry. Furthermore, plasma-stimulated gNPs attached to S. mutans significantly destroyed the cells walls, thereby promoting cell death. We suggest that the technique using plasma and gNPs could be a good method for dental caries treatment in dental clinics.

## Methods

### Plasma source

Microwave driven–atmospheric pressure plasma was employed for killing S. mutans. The plasma source was based on the coaxial transmission line resonator [26], and it generated a low-temperature plasma jet. It was operated by a palm-size power module [28] with a 2.5 W net input power. Argon gas was supplied to the plasma source through a flow meter (KOFLOC, Ar-05). We covered the end of the plasma source with an acrylic cap that had a smaller output area (diameter of output hole, 2 mm) than the plasma source. The stability of the plasma jet at the acrylic cap increased without change in the characteristics of the plasma (Figure 6).

### Temperature measurement

Generally, microwave-driven plasma has high temperatures. However, by using a very low operating power (2.5 W) and adjusting the gas flow, we could obtain low-temperature plasma. Under constant input power, the temperature of the plasma jet was dependent of the gas flow rate. The temperature of the plasma jet was

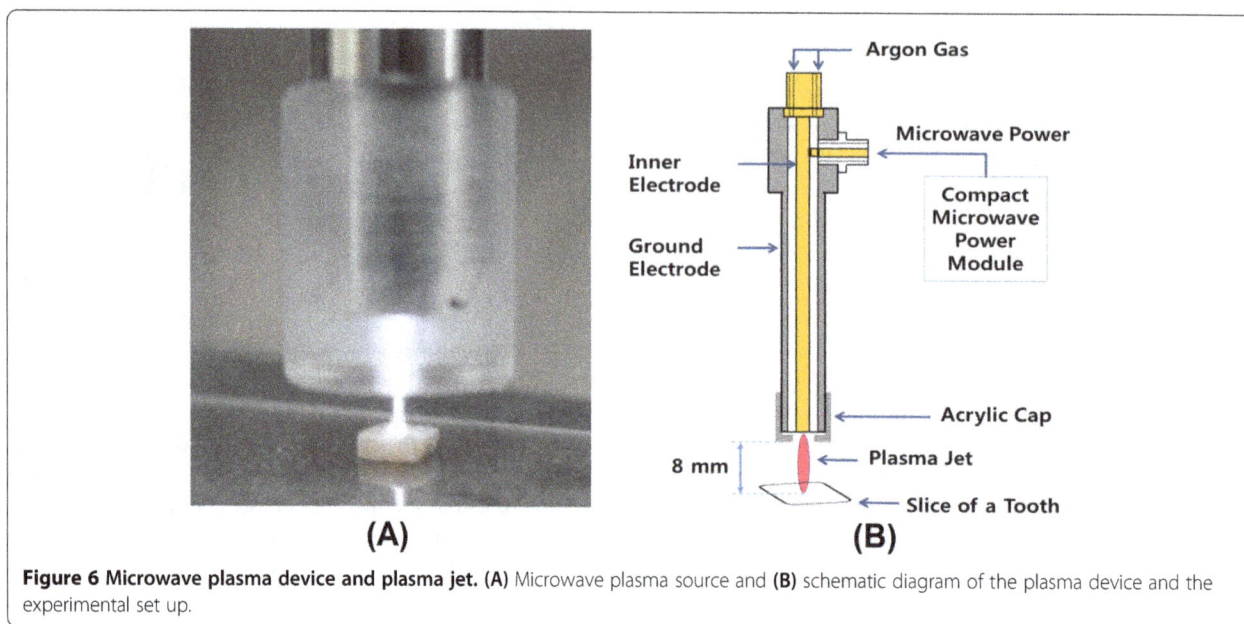

**Figure 6 Microwave plasma device and plasma jet. (A)** Microwave plasma source and **(B)** schematic diagram of the plasma device and the experimental set up.

measured using a The temperature of the plasma jet was measured using a thermometer with an optical fiber probe (FTI-10, FISO Technologies). The probe was located 8 mm away from the end of the plasma source, and the plasma jet contacted the probe. The location of the probe coincided with the location of the target tooth in the sterilization experiment. The maximum temperature reached was 41.1°C, and it decreased to 37°C in 5 min (Figure 2). The gas flow rate was set to 2.5 standard liters per minute. The length and diameter of the plasma jet were approximately 8 mm and 2 mm, respectively.

### Tooth slicing and sample preparation
Tooth slices of 2 mm thickness and approximately 3 mm diameter were cut from extracted human molars with a low-speed diamond saw (Struers, Copenhagen, Denmark). The exposed tooth surface was smoothened with Sic abrasive paper with grinding (grit P 120, 800, 1200). Subsequently, the tooth slices were cleaned for 10 min in the ultrasonic cleaner, autoclaved at 121°C for 15 min, and stored in phosphate-buffered saline (PBS). Five microliters of the *S. mutans* solution was spotted onto the tooth surface and allowed to dry out for 15 min at room temperature. The distance between the plasma jet and the tooth surface was 8 mm. The contamination on the tooth surface was plasma-treated for 60 s, 180 s, and 300 s. After plasma treatment, the tooth slices were vortexed for 30 s in 1 mL PBS, and 100 µL of these samples was inoculated onto agar plates in a 10-fold serial dilution. The agar plates were incubated at 37°C for 24 h before the colonies were counted (IRB No. 05-2012-023).

### Treatment of bacteria on cover glass
*S. mutans* on cover glass were treated with non-thermal plasma. All conditions were performed in the same manner as in experimental tooth slices.

### Bacterial strains and culture conditions
The strain of *S. mutans* (KCTC 3065/ATCC 25175) was grown in brain heart infusion (BHI) broth (Fluka, Switzerland). *S. mutans* was cultivated overnight in liquid media incubated at 37°C, and the cells were diluted with PBS to a final concentration of approximately $10^8$ CFUs/mL.

### Preparation of gNPs
Effective binding of *S. mutans* was achieved using 30-nm colloidal gNPs. *S. mutans* cells were cultured in BHI broth medium for 24 h at 37°C and harvested by centrifugation at 4,000 rpm for 5 min at 4°C. The supernatant was discarded, and 10 mM sodium bicarbonate (pH = 8.8) was added to the gNPs to resuspend them. *S. mutans* cells were added to the gNPs and incubated for 1 h at 37°C. Subsequently, they were centrifuged at 4°C for 5 min at 4,000 rpm. The supernatant was discarded, and sodium bicarbonate buffer was used for the final suspension solution.

### Bacterial viability staining
After the plasma treatment, *S. mutans* was stained with the nucleic acid stains SYTO 9® (Invitrogen-Molecular Probes, OR, USA) and PI (Sigma Aldrich, MO, USA) according to the manufacturer's instructions. Cells were

visualized and classified as live or dead by fluorescence microscopy (Axioskop; Zeiss, Germany).

## Transmission electron microscopy

Bacterial samples for TEM imaging were fixed with 2.5% glutaraldehyde for 2 h at 4°C and then incubated with 1% osmium tetroxide for 1 h at 4°C. After the cells were rinsed, dehydrated in ethanol, and infiltrated with propylene oxide, they were embedded in Epon. Ultrathin sections were stained with uranyl acetate and lead citrate and observed using TEM at Electron microscopy Facility, Department of Ophthalmology, Pusan National University Hospital (JEM 1200EX-II; JEOL, Japan).

## Statistical analysis

Statistical analysis was performed using SPSS (SPSS version 18 for Windows, SPSS Inc., USA). The logarithmic values of each bacterial plate count were calculated and analyzed using the Student's $t$-test. A $p$-value less than 0.05 was considered statistically significant.

### Abbreviations
BHI: Brain heart infusion; CFU: Colony-forming unit; gNP: Gold nanoparticle; PBS: Phosphate-buffered saline; PI: Propidium iodide; TEM: Transmission electron microscopy.

### Competing interests
The authors declare that they have no competing interests.

### Authors' contributions
HJL analyzed the data, and YCJ contributed in collecting tooth samples. SRP, HWL, and BRC carried out the laboratory experiments and analyzed the data. GCK provided technical input and devised the project idea. SRP and GCK wrote the manuscript. JYK contributed to interpretation of data. All authors read and approved the final manuscript.

### Acknowledgements
This study was supported by the Medical Research Institute Grant (2011–22), Pusan National University Hospital.

### Author details
[1]Department of Dental Hygiene, Kyungnam College of Information and Technology, Busan 617-701, Rep. Korea. [2]Department of Electrical Engineering, Pohang University of Science and Technology, Pohang 790-784, Rep. Korea. [3]Department of Korean Internal Medicine, School of Korean Medicine, Pusan National University, Yangsan 626-870, Korea. [4]Department of Electronics Engineering, Pusan National University, Busan 609-735, Rep. Korea. [5]Department of Oral Anatomy, School of Dentistry, Pusan National University, Yangsan 602-739, Rep. Korea. [6]Department of Dental Prosthetics, School of Dentistry, Pusan National University, Yangsan 602-739, Republic of Korea.

### References
1. Petersen PE, Bourgeois D, Ogawa H, Estupinan-Day S, Ndiaye C: The global burden of oral diseases and risks to oral health. *Bull World Health Organ* 2005, **83**:661–669.
2. Shinada K, Ueno M, Konishi C, Takehara S, Yokoyama S, Kawaguchi Y: A randomized double blind crossover placebo-controlled clinical trial to assess the effects of a mouthwash containing chlorine dioxide on oral malodor. *Trials* 2008, **9**:1–8.
3. Kalghatgi S, Kelly CM, Cerchar E, Torabi B, Aleksee O, Fridman A, Friedman G, Clifford JA: Effects of non-thermal plasma on mammalian cells. *PLoS ONE* 2011, **6**:1–11.
4. Koban I, Geisel MH, Holtfreter B, Jablonowski L, Hübner NO, Matthes R, Masur K, Weltmann KD, Kramer A, Kocher T: Synergistic effects of nonthermal plasma and disinfecting agents against dental biofilms in vitro. *ISRN Dentistry* 2013, **2013**:1–10.
5. Kvam E, Davis B, Mondello F, Gamer AL: Nonthermal atmospheric plasma rapidly disinfects multidrug-resistant microbes by inducing cell surface damage. *Antimicrob Agents Chemother* 2012, **56**:2028–2036.
6. Yang L, Chen J: Low temperature argon plasma sterilization effect on *Pseudomonas aeruginosa* and its mechanisms. *J Electrostatics* 2009, **67**:646–651.
7. Rupf S, Lehmann A, Hannig M, Schafer B, Schubert A, Feldmann U, Schindler A: Killing of adherent oral microbes by a non-thermal atmospheric plasma jet. *J Med Microbiol* 2010, **59**:206–212.
8. Pei X, Lu X, Liu J, Liu D, Yang Y, Ostrikov K, Chu PK, Pan Y: Inactivation of a 25.5 µm *Enterococcus faecalis* biofilm by a room-temperature, battery-operated, handheld air plasma jet. *J Phys D Appl Phys* 2012, **45**:1–5.
9. Lee HW, Lee HW, Kang SK, Kim HY, Won IH, Jeon SM, Lee JK: Synergistic sterilization effect of microwave-excited nonthermal Ar plasma, H2O2, H2O and TiO2, and a global modeling of the interactions. *Plasma Sources Sci Technol* 2013, **22**:1–11.
10. Molnar I, Papp J, Simon A, Anghel SD: Deactivation of *Streptococcus mutans* biofilms on a tooth surface using he dielectric barrier discharge at atmospheric pressure. *Plasma Sci Technol* 2013, **15**:535–541.
11. Hamada S, Masuda N, Kotani S: Isolation and serotyping of Streptococcus mutans from teeth and feces of children. *J Clin Microbiol* 1980, **11**:314–318.
12. Yang B, Chen J, Yu Q, Lin M, Mustapha A, Hong L, Wang Y: Oral bacterial deactivation using a low-temperature atmospheric argon plasma brush. *J Dent* 2011, **39**:48–56.
13. Vargo JJ: Clinical applications of the argon plasma coagulator. *Gastrointest Endosc* 2004, **59**:81–88.
14. Fridman G, Peddinghaus M, Ayan H, Fridman A, Balasubramanian M, Gutsol A, Brooks A, Fredman G: Blood coagulation and living tissue sterilization by floating-electrode dielectric barrier discharge in air. *Plasma Chem Plasma Process* 2006, **26**:425–442.
15. Tamura S: Effects of oral streptococci on biofilm formation by cariogenic bacteria in dual species cultures. *Kokubyo Gakkai Zasshi* 2008, **75**:38–48.
16. Ghadimi S, Chiniforush N, Bouraima SA, Johari M: Clinical approach of laser application in different aspects of pediatric dentistry. *J Lasers Med Sci* 2012, **3**:84–90.
17. Spivak YS, Bubnov RB, Yemets LM, Lazarenko LM, Tymoshok NO, Ulberg ZR: Gold nanoparticles - the theranostic challenge for PPPM: nanocardiology application. *EPMA J* 2013, **4**:1–17.
18. Kong MG, Keidar M, Ostrikov K: Plasmas meet nanoparticles-where synergies can advance the frontier of medicine. *J Phys D Appl Phys* 2011, **44**:174018.
19. Huang CJ, Chiu PH, Wang YH, Yang CF: Synthesis of the gold nanodumbbells by electrochemical method. *J Colloid Interface Sci* 2006, **303**:430–436.
20. Cheng J, Gu YJ, Cheng SH, Wong WT: Surface functionalized gold nanoparticles for drug delivery. *J Biomed Nanotechnol* 2013, **9**:1362–1369.
21. Tiwari PK, Kang SK, Kim GJ, Choi J, Mohamed AAH, Lee JK: Modeling of Nanoparticle-mediated electric field enhancement inside biological cells exposed to AC electric Fields. *Jpn J Appl Phys* 2009, **48**:087001–087007.
22. Kim GC, Kim GJ, Park SR, Jeon SM, Seo HJ, Iza F, Lee JK: Air plasma coupled with antibody-conjugated nanoparticles: a new weapon against cancer. *J Phys D Appl Phys* 2009, **42**:32005–32009.
23. Choi BB, Choi YS, Lee HJ, Lee JK, Kim UK, Kim GC: Nonthermal plasma-mediated cancer cell death; targeted cancer treatment. *J Therm Sci Tech* 2012, **7**:399–404.
24. Ostrikov K, Neyts EC, Meyyappan M: Plasma nanoscience: from nano-solids in plasmas to nano-plasmas in solids. *Adv Phys* 2013, **62**:1–110.
25. Moran CH, Wainerdi SM, Cherukuri TK, Kittrell C, Benjamin J, Wiley BJ, Nicholas NW, Curley SA, Kanzius JS, Paul Cherukuri P: Size-dependent joule heating of gold nanoparticles using capacitively coupled radiofrequency fields. *Nano Res* 2009, **2**:400–405.
26. Choi J, Iza F, Do HJ, Lee JK, Cho MH: Microwave-excited atmospheric-pressure micro plasmas based on a coaxial transmission line resonator. *Plasma Sources Sci Technol* 2009, **18**:1–8.
27. Lee HW, Kang SK, Won IH, Kim HY, Kwon HC, Sim JY, Lee JK: Distinctive plume formation in atmospheric Ar and He plasmas in microwave

frequency band and suitability for biomedical applications. *Phys Plasmas* 2013, **20**:1–13.

28. Park SJ, Choi J, Park GY, Lee SK, Cho YS, Yun JI, Jeon SM, Kim KT, Lee JK: Inactivation of S.mutans using an atmospheric plasma driven by a palm-size-integrated microwave power module. *IEEE Trans Plasma Sci* 2010, **38**:1956–1962.

# 3

# The role of lipid-based nano delivery systems on oral bioavailability enhancement of fenofibrate, a BCS II drug: comparison with fast-release formulations

Tengfei Weng[1,2], Jianping Qi[1*], Yi Lu[1], Kai Wang[1,2], Zhiqiang Tian[1], Kaili Hu[3], Zongning Yin[2] and Wei Wu[1]

## Abstract

The aim of this study was to compare various formulations solid dispersion pellets (SDP), nanostructured lipid carriers (NLCs) and a self-microemulsifying drug delivery system (SMEDDS) generally accepted to be the most efficient drug delivery systems for BCS II drugs using fenofibrate (FNB) as a model drug. The size and morphology of NLCs and SMEDDS was characterized by dynamic light scattering (DLS) and transmission electron microscopy (TEM). Their release behaviors were investigated in medium with or without pancreatic lipase. The oral bioavailability of the various formulations was compared in beagle dogs using commercial Lipanthyl® capsules (micronized formulation) as a reference. The release of FNB from SDP was much faster than that from NLCs and SMEDDS in medium without lipase, whereas the release rate from NLCs and SMEDDS was increased after adding pancreatic lipase into the release medium. However, NLCs and SMEDDS increased the bioavailability of FNB to 705.11% and 809.10%, respectively, in comparison with Lipanthyl® capsules, although the relative bioavailability of FNB was only 366.05% after administration of SDPs. Thus, lipid-based drug delivery systems (such as NLCs and SMEDDS) may have more advantages than immediate release systems (such as SDPs and Lipanthyl® capsules).

Keywords: Fenofibrate, Solid dispersion, Nanostructured lipid carrier, Self-microemulsifying drug delivery system, Bioavailability

## Background

According to the definition of the Biopharmaceutics Classification System (BCS) proposed by Amidon in 1995, both BCS II and IV drugs are poorly soluble in aqueous solution [1]. About 40% of new drug candidates identified by chemical screening are poorly soluble in water (BCS II or IV drugs), which greatly hinders their translation into the clinic [2]. However, the transmembrane permeation behavior of BCS II drugs is significantly different to that of BCS IV drugs. Generally, the apparent permeability coefficient ($Papp$) of BCS II drugs is greater than $10^{-6}$, whereas the $Papp$ of BCS IV drugs is lower than $10^{-8}$ owing to various barriers such as low dissolution rate, low transmembrane permeability, efflux by transporter in the gut wall and first pass effect by metabolic enzymes [3]. To improve the oral bioavailability of these drugs, novel formulation technologies or drug delivery systems have emerged, including solid dispersion [4,5], nanocrystals [6], cyclodextrin inclusion [7,8], nanoemulsions [9], polymeric and lipidic nanoparticles (e.g. PLGA nanoparticles, solid lipid nanoparticles and nanostructure lipid carriers) [10-12]. These formulations can enhance oral absorption of drug molecules by improving dissolution in the gastrointestinal tract (GIT) [6], facilitating adhesive interactions within the mucosa [13], increasing drug stability and improving lymphatic transport [14]. Nevertheless, different formulations have distinguishing features and facilitate absorption by distinct mechanisms. Solid dispersion and cyclodextrin inclusion improve the dissolution rate of poorly soluble drugs, but do not increase

* Correspondence: qijianping@fudan.edu.cn
[1]School of Pharmacy, Key Laboratory of Smart Drug Delivery of Ministry of Education, Fudan University, Shanghai 201203, PR China
Full list of author information is available at the end of the article

transmembrane permeability [15,16]. Nanocrystals are a fast-release system that has similar effects to those of solid dispersion and cyclodextrin inclusion [6], whereas nanoparticles can alter the permeability of the intestinal membrane by uptake of intact nanoparticles, facilitating adhesion and retention in the GIT and improving membrane fluidity, thus leading to increased absorption via the paracellular or transcellular route [17,18]. Furthermore, the fate of nanoparticles containing lipids in the GIT is different to to that of polymer nanoparticles. Digestion products of lipid nanoparticles can solubilize lipophilic drugs and the presence of endogenous bile salts may alter the intrinsic permeability of the intestinal membrane [19,20]. Although each drug delivery system may be recognized to improve oral bioavailability of poorly soluble drugs, we aimed to identify the optimal formulation technology for delivery of BCS II or IV drugs. Therefore, in this study, we first compared the bioavailability of different drug delivery systems loaded with the BCS II drug, fenofibrate (FNB).

FNB, a widely used hypolipidemic agent, is a typical BCS II drug. Due to its very low solubility in aqueous solution, the oral bioavailability is limited by slow dissolution [21]. In the clinic, micronized FNB (Lipanthyl® capsules) showed significantly improved dissolution and enhanced oral bioavailability. More recently, various oral carrier systems were developed to increase oral absorption of FNB, including solid dispersion [4], a self-microemulsifying drug delivery system [22], liposome containing bile salts [23], mesoporous carbon [24], nanocystals [21] and lipid-based formulations [25]. Although these systems successfully increase the oral bioavailability of FNB, the optimal formulation remains to be identified by comparing the oral bioavailability of FNB after administration of different formulations.

Herein, the oral bioavailability of FNB-loaded into the lipid-based delivery systems, SMEDDS and NLCs, was compared with that of fast-release FNB SDPs and micronized Lipanthyl® capsules in beagle dogs.

## Results and discussion
### Preparation and characterization of SDP, NLCs and SMEDDS

FNB-loaded SDP, NLCs and SMEDDS were prepared successfully. Since FNB-loaded SDPs and NLCs were prepared according to our previous study [25,26], the detailed characterization data are not shown in this report. The particle size of the obtained NLCs was $93.76 \pm 1.25$ nm (polydispersity index (PDI), $0.222 \pm 0.014$), the zeta potential was $-29.1 \pm 4.1$ mV and the entrapment efficiency was approximately $96.66 \pm 1.01\%$, which are similar to the values obtained in our previous study [25]. FNB-loaded SMEDDS were microemulsified in deionized water, pH 1.2 HCl

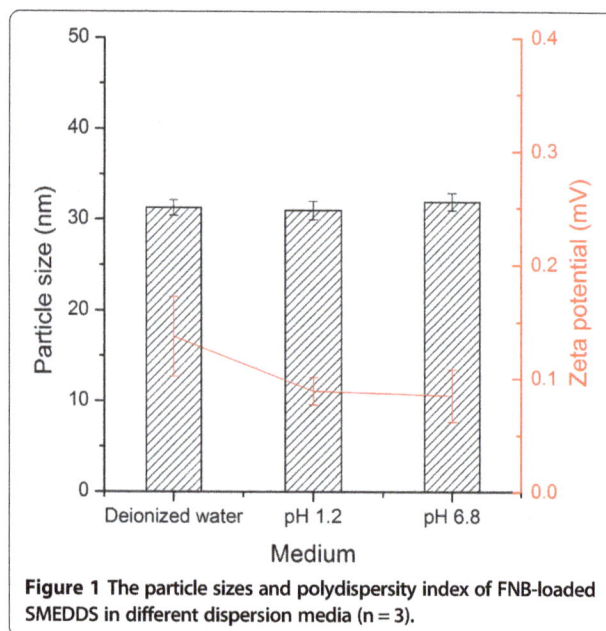

**Figure 1** The particle sizes and polydispersity index of FNB-loaded SMEDDS in different dispersion media (n = 3).

solution and pH 6.8 PBS immediately; the particle size and PDI are shown in Figure 1.

### Morphology

Transmission electron microscopy (TEM) was employed to observe the morphology of NLCs and microemulsions formed by SMEDDS; micrographs are presented in Figure 2. The NLCs (Figure 2A) were spherical in shape and approximately 100 nm in size. TEM showed that the SMEDDS were emulsified in deionized water to generate uniform spherical microemulsion droplets approximately 20 nm in size (Figure 2B).

### In vitro release

The profiles of FNB release from the three test formulations and the reference (commercial Lipanthyl® capsules containing micronized FNB) in the media with or without pancreatic lipase are shown in Figure 3. FNB was released rapidly from Lipanthyl® capsules and SDPs, with a cumulative release of more than 80% within 60 min. Only about 25% of the FNB was released from SMEDDS within 24 h and even less (about 12%) from the NLCs. However, pancreatic lipase changed the dissolution behavior of SMEDDS and NLCs. In release medium containing pancreatic lipase, the release of FNB from SDPs and Lipanthyl® capsules was not altered significantly compared with that in medium without lipase. Nevertheless, the release from SMEDDS and NLCs was evidently improved, with more than 60% and 40% of FNB released from SMEDDS and NLCs in 24 h, respectively. The similarity factor ($f_2$), which is recommended by FDA for evaluation of the similarity of release profiles [27], was

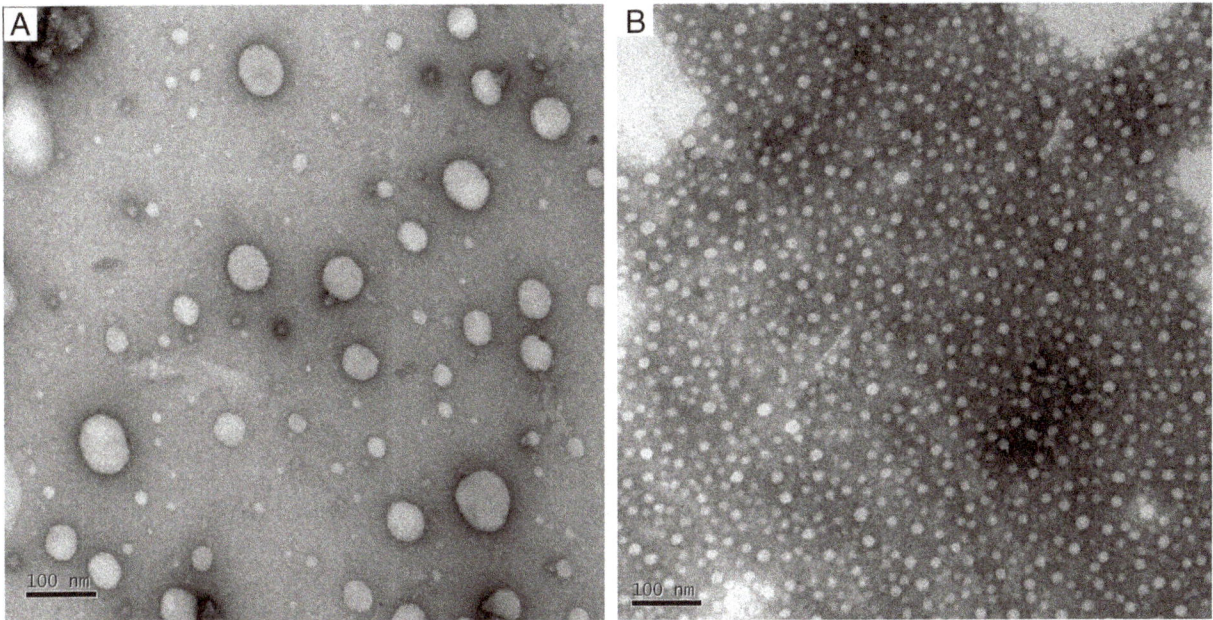

**Figure 2** Morphology of FNB-loaded NLCs (A) and microemulsions droplets formed by SMEDDS (B) observed by transmission electron microscopy.

employed to evaluate the influence of lipase on FNB release according to the following formula:

$$f_2 = 50 \times \lg\left(\sqrt{\left[1 + \left(\frac{1}{n}\right)\sum_{i=1}^{n}(x_{ti}-x_{ri})^2\right] \times 100}\right)$$

where $x_{ti}$ and $x_{ri}$ are the cumulative release of time interval "$i$" in release medium with and without pancreatic lipase,

respectively, and n is the time interval. When $f_2$ is between 50 and 100, the variation in every observation point between the two release profiles is not more than 10%, which is considered to represent similarity. If $f_2 < 50$, the two release profiles are considered to be dissimilar. The $f_2$ of the four formulations are displayed in Table 1. The release profiles of FNB from Lipanthyl® capsules and SDPs were not altered by the addition of lipase to the release medium, although the release profiles from SMEDDS and NLCs in two release media differed considerably, which indicates that intestinal lipase is important to the release of poorly

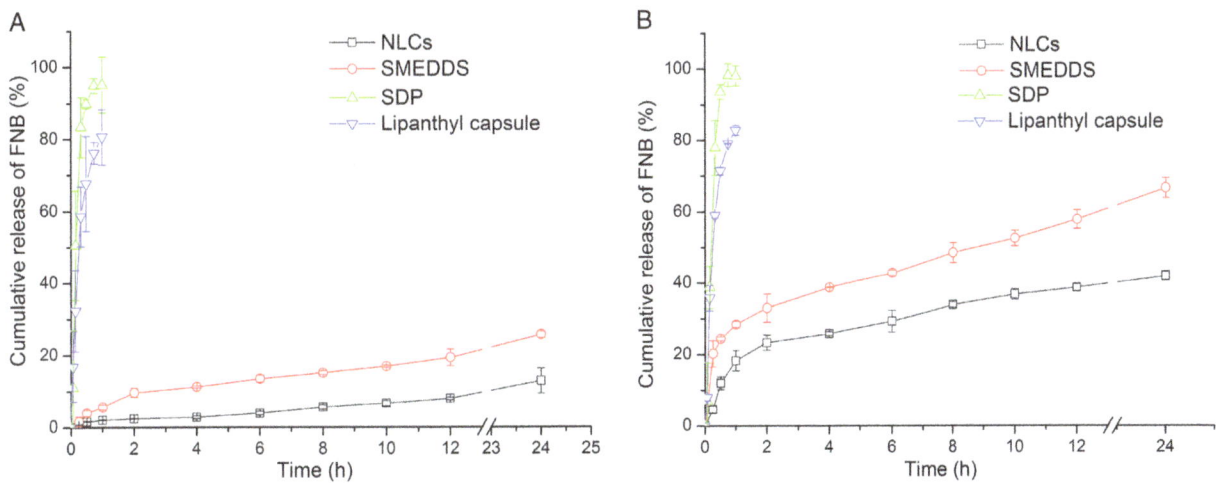

**Figure 3** *In vitro* release profiles of FNB from SDP, NLCs, SMEDDS and Lipanthyl® capsules in release media without (A) or with (B) pancreatic lipase (n = 3).

**Table 1 The $f_2$ values of release profiles of FNB in release media with or without pancreatic lipase**

| Formulations | Lipanthyl® capsules | SDP | SMEDDS | NLCs |
|---|---|---|---|---|
| $f_2$ | 67.1 | 60.7 | 36.5 | 42.4 |

soluble drugs from lipid-based drug delivery systems, such as SMEDDS and NLCs.

## Oral bioavailability

To illustrate the optimal formulation for BCS II drugs, oral bioavailability of FNB-loaded SDPs, NLCs and SMEDDS in beagle dogs were compared. The mean plasma FNB concentration versus time plots of the four formulations are shown in Figure 4 and the pharmacokinetic parameters obtained by analysis based on statistical moment theory are shown in Table 2.

After oral gavage administration of the three FNB formulations to beagle dogs, the $C_{max}$ and AUC of all of the formulations were improved compared with those of Lipanthyl® capsules. NLCs and SMEDDS in particular exhibited enhanced absorption compared with SDPs. The relative bioavailability of NLCs and SMEDDS were 705.11% and 809.10%, respectively, compared with Lipanthyl® capsules, while that of SDPs was only 366.05%. Compared with Lipanthyl® capsules, the $T_{max}$, MRT and $t_{1/2}$ of fenofibric acid showed no significant changes after oral administration of all three formulations.

Theoretically, the oral bioavailability of BCS II drugs is restricted mainly by poor dissolution in the GIT. Generally speaking, the oral bioavailability of BCS II drugs is improved greatly if the *in vitro* dissolution is enhanced [28]. Therefore, micronization, nanosuspension, solid dispersion and cyclodextrin inclusion are widely used to improve the oral bioavailability of BCS II drugs [28]. Previous *in vitro* and *in vivo* evaluations of the reference, Lipanthyl® capsules, which are a product of micronized FNB and nanosuspensions of FNB suggested the FNB is rapidly released from Lipanthyl® capsules, SDPs and nanosuspensions, and that SDPs or nanosuspensions improve the oral bioavailability of FNB compared with that of the Lipanthyl® capsules [29]. Similar dissolution does not lead to the same oral absorption, which may be due to the various influences of the GIT contents on dissolution of drugs from the different formulations.

Although FNB was released very slowly and in small amounts from lipid-based drug delivery systems, such as NLCs and SMEDDS, the cumulative release of FNB increased with introduction of lipase. Pancreatic lipase, bile salts and phospholipids are continuously secreted into the GIT. Lipid-based drug delivery systems are digested by pancreatic lipase to form secondary structures, such as mixed micelles, cubic or hexagonal nanoparticles and vesicular carriers [30]. Therefore, drugs can be solubilized in these secondary derivatives when lipid-based formulations are digested [31]. SDPs, nanosuspensions or micronized drugs significantly increase drug dissolution, but oral absorption is promoted only by the original absorption pathways of the drug itself. Nevertheless, lipid-based drug delivery systems may enhance the absorption of drugs through diverse pathways [32].

On the one hand, NLCs and SMEDDS can adhere to the gut wall to increase retention time in GIT. The particle sizes of NLCs and SMEDDS were below 100 nm, which endows them with a massive specific surface area and facilitates the adhesion of nanoparticles by the mucus layer [33,34]. On the other hand, many reports have suggested that the digestion of lipid-based drug delivery systems in the GIT is the most important factor required to enhance the absorption of poorly soluble drugs [35-37]. Exogenous lipids stimulate the secretion of biliary lipids (bile salts, phospholipids and cholesterol), which combine with lipid digestion products to generate a series of colloidal species, including micelles, mixed micelles, vesicles and emulsion droplets [38]. These colloidal species provide a reservoir of solubilized drug at the absorptive site and generate the concentration gradient required to drive improved absorption. Luminal amphiphiles, such as bile salts, may also enhance the solubilization of drugs by improving wetting at concentrations below the critical micellar concentration [39]. Thus, the drug concentration increases during the digestion process, which improves the transport across non-stirred water layers and then the bio-membranes. In addition, fatty acids and monoglycerides produced during digestion increase the fluidity and permeability of membranes due to their surface activity, which is also an important factor in enhancing drug absorption [40]. Furthermore, lymphatic transport can also increase the oral bioavailability

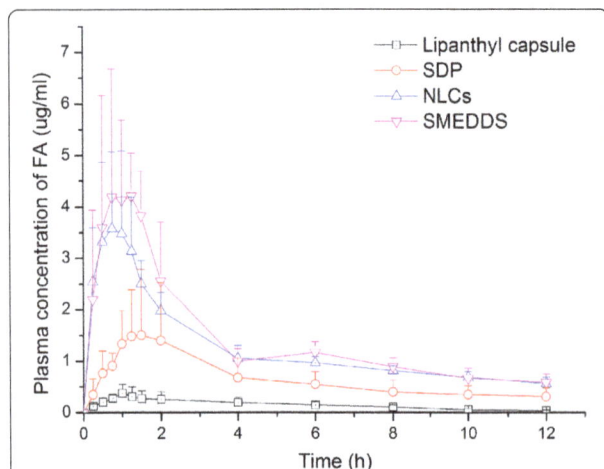

**Figure 4** Mean plasma concentration-time profiles of fenofibric acid in beagle dogs after oral administration of FNB-loaded SDP, NLCs, SMEDDS and Lipanthyl® capsules (n = 6).

**Table 2 The main pharmacokinetic parameters of fenofibric acid in beagle dogs after oral administration of FNB-loaded SDP, NLCs, SMEDDS and Lipanthyl® capsules (n = 6)**

| Parameters | Lipanthyl® capsules | SDP | NLCs | SMEDDS |
|---|---|---|---|---|
| $C_{max}$ (μg/mL) | 0.41 ± 0.17 | 1.82 ± 1.18* | 3.87 ± 1.40*# | 5.31 ± 1.18*#▲ |
| $T_{max}$ (h) | 1.04 ± 0.29 | 1.13 ± 0.59 | 0.92 ± 0.34 | 0.96 ± 0.43 |
| $t_{1/2}$ (h) | 3.40 ± 1.55 | 9.58 ± 7.64 | 8.09 ± 3.25* | 6.25 ± 2.15* |
| $MRT_{(0-t)}$(h) | 4.24 ± 0.24 | 4.45 ± 0.18 | 4.22 ± 0.42 | 4.00 ± 0.28 |
| $AUC_{(0-t)}$ (μg/mL*h) | 2.13 ± 0.69 | 7.81 ± 4.36* | 15.04 ± 2.34*# | 17.26 ± 3.43*# |
| $F_1$ (%) | — | 366.05 | 705.11 | 809.10 |
| $F_2$ (%) | — | — | 192.62 | 221.03 |
| $F_3$ (%) | — | — | — | 114.75 |

$F_1$, $F_2$ and $F_3$ are relative bioavailability of other formulations compared with Lipanthyl® capsules, SDP and NLCs, respectively.
*$P < 0.05$, compared with Lipanthyl® capsule.
#$P < 0.05$, compared with SDP.
▲$P < 0.05$, compared with NLCs.

of lipophilic drugs [41]. Lipid vehicles may enhance lymphatic transport of lipophilic compounds by simulating the production of chylomicrons. Lipophilic drugs enter the lymphatic system in association with the triglyceride core of the chylomicrons [42]. The digestibility of the vehicle is a prerequisite for the production of the fatty acids necessary to drive chylomicron production [43].

## Conclusion

FNB-loaded SDPs, NLCs and SMEDDS were prepared and their *in vitro* and *in vivo* properties were compared. SDPs significantly increased the release of FNB in medium with and without lipase, which is similar to the characteristics of Lipanthyl® capsules. Pancreatic lipase improved the release of FNB from NLCs and SMEDDS remarkably. However, the oral bioavailability of FNB after administration of NLCs and SMEDDS was significantly higher than that of SDP and Lipanthyl® capsules ($P < 0.05$). Therefore, lipid-based drug delivery systems (such as NLCs and SMEDDS) are more advantageous than the other drug delivery systems (solid dispersion or micronization) for BCS II drugs, due to the multiple absorption enhancement mechanisms. Lipid-based drug delivery systems may be an excellent candidate for oral formulation of insoluble drugs.

## Methods

### Materials

FNB was purchased from Nhwa Pharmaceutical Group (Xuzhou, China). Polyvinylpyrrolidone (PVP K30) was kindly gifted from China Division, ISP Chemicals Co. (Shanghai, China). Non-pareil pellets (Suglets® sugar spheres PF101, 710–850 μm in diameter) were provided by NP Pharm (Bazainville, France). Precirol ATO 5 and Captex 100 were kindly provided by Gattefossé Co. (Saint Priest, Cedex, France) and Abitec Co. (OH, USA), respectively. Polysorbate 80 (Tween-80) was supplied by Shenyu Pharmaceutical and Chemical Co., Ltd (Shanghai). Oleoyl

macrogolglycerides (Labrafil M® 1944 CS) and diethylene glycol monoethyl ether (Transcutol P®) were purchased from Gattefossé Co. Ethoxylated castor oil (Cremophor® EL) was obtained from BASF Corporation (Ludwigshafen, Germany). HPLC grade methanol and acetonitrile were purchased from Tedia (Carson City, NV, USA). Deionized water was prepared using a Milli-Q purification system (Millipore, Billerica, MA, USA). All other chemicals were of analytical grade and were used as received.

## Preparation of FNB-loaded delivery systems

### Preparation of solid dispersion pellets (SDP)

FNB-loaded SDPs were prepared using a Mini-Glatt fluid-bed coater (Wurster insert; Glatt GmbH, Binzen, Germany) based on previously established procedures [26]. FNB, PVP K30 and sodium dodecyl sulfate (SDS) (4:3:3, w/w/w) were dissolved in 90% ethanol. The resulting solution was sprayed through a nozzle (0.5 mm in diameter) onto the fluidized non-pareil pellets to obtain a coating weight gain of approximately 100%. The detailed operating conditions were as follows: product temperature, 35°C – 40°C; air flow rate, 97–103 m³/h; spray rate, 0.6 mL/minute; atomizing air pressure, 1.4–1.5 bar. The pellets were further dried for 15 min after coating completion.

### Preparation of nanostructured lipid carriers (NLCs)

The NLC suspension was prepared by the melting-emulsification method according to our previously described procedures [25]. Briefly, 1.14 g solid lipid phase (Precirol ATO 5) and 0.48 g liquid lipid phase (Captex 100) were melted at 80°C and mixed. Then 60 mg FNB was dissolved in the lipid mixture. The melted mixture was then dispersed in a hot (80°C) aqueous solution (30 mL) containing Tween-80 (2%, w/v) for 3 min at a rate of 8,000 rpm using a high-speed Ultra Turrax blender (QilinBeier, Jiangsu, China) to produce the coarse emulsion.

Subsequently, the coarse emulsion was homogenized using a high-pressure homogenizer (Microfluids, Nano DeBee, USA) for three cycles under 20,000 psi. The obtained hot NLC suspension was cooled to room temperature for use in further investigations.

### Preparation of self-microemulsifying drug delivery systems (SMEDDS)

The formulation of FNB-loaded SMEDDS was performed according to previously described methods with modifications [44]. Briefly, FNB, Labrafil M 1944 CS (oil phase), Cremophore EL (surfactant) and Transcutol P (co-surfactant) were mixed in ratio of 40/520/585/195 (w/w). The obtained SMEDDS was stored at 4°C before use.

### Measurement of particle size

Particle size was measured by Zetasizer Nano® (Malvern Instruments, Malvern, UK) equipped with a 4 mW He-Ne laser (633 nm) at 25°C. The NLC suspension was diluted 15-fold with deionized water before measurement. The particle size of SMEDDS was determined after microoemulsification in deionized water. Three measurements were conducted, and the number of runs in each measurement was automatically determined by the software.

### Transmission electron microscopy (TEM)

TEM was used to characterize the morphology of NLCs and SMEDDS. Prior to examination, microemulsion drops were obtained by emulsifying SMEDDS in deionized water. The NLCs suspension and microemulsion droplets were then placed on copper grids and negatively stained with 2% (w/v) phosphotungstic acid for 5 min at room temperature. Finally, the grids bearing NLCs and microoemulsion droplets were observed with a JEM-1230 transmission electron microscope (JEOL, Tokyo, Japan).

### Entrapment efficiency of NLCs

The entrapment efficiency of NLCs was determined by ultrafiltration. Briefly, 0.4 mL NLCs was added to an ultrafiltration tube (100 kD) and then centrifuged for 10 min at $4,000 \times g$. The concentrations of FNB in the filtrate ($C_{free}$) was determined by HPLC directly. The concentration of FNB original NLCs ($C_{total}$) were determined as following method. Briefly, 0.4 mL of NLCs suspension was dissolved in 100 mL methanol. The FNB released into methanol from NLCs rapidly with the help of ultrasound. After ultrasound treatment of 20 min, the mixed solution was centrifuged for 10 min under $10,000 \times g$. The supernatant was injected into HPLC to determine $C_{total}$. The entrapment efficiency (EE) was calculated according to the following equation.

$$EE = \frac{C_{total} - C_{free}}{C_{total}} \times 100\%$$

### Release test

The release test was performed in a ZRS-8G dissolution tester (Tianda Tianfa Technology Co. Ltd, Tianjin, China) according to the Chinese Pharmacopoeia (2010) Appendix Method III. To clarify the effect of lipase on the release of lipid formulations (NLCs or SMEDDS), we selected two different release media; phosphate balanced saline (pH 6.8) containing 2% Cremophor EL with or without pancreatic lipase (100 IU/mL). Four formulations (containing 3 mg FNB) were added into 100 mL release medium that was thermostatically maintained at $37 \pm 0.5°C$ and stirred at a revolution speed of 100 rpm. SDP was sealed into hard gelatin capsules. Samples of 0.5 mL were withdrawn at specific time intervals and immediately ultrafiltered (Millipore, 100 kD) at $4,000 \times g$ for 10 min. The ultrafiltrate was assayed for FNB by HPLC as described later in the text.

### Bioavailability study

The bioavailability of SDPs, NLCs and SMEDDS containing FNB was evaluated in beagle dogs using commercially available Lipanthyl® capsules (micronized FNB, Solvay Pharma) as a reference. Beagle dogs (adult males, $15.0 \pm 0.5$ kg) used in the experiments received care in compliance with the Principles of Laboratory Animal Care and the Guide for the Care and Use of Laboratory Animals. Experiments followed protocols approved by the Fudan University Institutional Animal Care and Use Committee.

Four formulations were administered to the dogs by oral gavage at an equivalent dose of 3 mg/kg FNB. Blood samples (1.5 mL) were then collected into heparinized tubes at designated time intervals: 0.25, 0.5, 0.75, 1, 1.25, 1.5, 2, 4, 6, 8, 10 and 12 h. Plasma was separated by centrifugation for 10 min at $4,000 \times g$ and frozen at -18°C for subsequent analysis. FNB, as a prodrug, is rapidly metabolized into its major active metabolite, fenofibric acid (FA), after absorption. Intact FNB cannot be detected in the plasma after oral administration; therefore, pharmacokinetic evaluation of FNB was based on the quantification of FA in the plasma [45]. FA in dog plasma was extracted by liquid-liquid extraction procedures established in our previous study and the concentration of FA was determined by HPLC [23].

Pharmacokinetic parameters were calculated by non-compartmental analysis based on statistical moment theory using DAS professional software version 2.0 (Anhui, China). The pharmacokinetic parameters, such as peak plasma concentration ($C_{max}$), the time to maximum plasma concentration $(T_{max})$, and the area under the concentration-time curve between 0 and 12 h $(AUC_{0-12})$ were determined.

## HPLC analysis

Both *in vitro* and *in vivo* samples were determined by HPLC system (Agilent 1260 series, California, USA) comprising an auto sampler, a pump, a column oven, and a tunable ultraviolet detector. The analytical column was a C18 column (Diamonsil®, 5 μm, 4.6 mm × 250 mm, Dikma, China) guarded with a refillable precolumn (C18, 2.0 mm × 20 mm, Alltech, USA). The flow rate was 1.0 mL/min. The UV-detector was set at a wavelength of 287 nm. The column temperature was set to 40°C. In terms of *in vitro* determination of FNB, the mobile phase consisted of methanol and deionized water mixed at a ratio of 90/10 (v/v). However, the mobile phase was composed of a mixture of methanol, water and 10% phosphoric acid (70/30/1, v/v/v) for *in vivo* determination of FA. Indomethacin (10 μg/mL) was used as an internal standard [23].

## Statistical analysis

All data were expressed as mean ± standard deviation (SD). One-way ANOVA followed by Tukey's test was performed to assess the statistical significance of differences. Results with $P < 0.05$ were considered statistically significant.

### Competing interests

The authors declare that they have no competing interests.

### Authors' contributions

TW performed the majority of the experiments and wrote the manuscript with JQ and WW. JQ, WW, YL and ZY designed the overall project and aided with data interpretations. KW and ZT assisted with the animal experiments. KH assisted to perform the transmission electron microscopy. All authors read and approved the final manuscript.

### Acknowledgements

We are grateful for the financial support from Shanghai Commission of Science and Technology (14JC1490300, 11 nm0506700). Dr. Wu would also want to thank Shanghai Commission of Education (10SG05) and Ministry of Education (NCET-11-0114) for personnel fostering support.

### Author details

[1]School of Pharmacy, Key Laboratory of Smart Drug Delivery of Ministry of Education, Fudan University, Shanghai 201203, PR China. [2]West China School of Pharmacy, Sichuan University, Chengdu, Sichuan 610041, PR China. [3]Murad Research Center for Modernized Chinese Medicine, Shanghai University of Traditional Chinese Medicine, Shanghai 201203, PR China.

## References

1. Amidon GL, Lennernas H, Shah VP, Crison JR: **A theoretical basis for a biopharmaceutic drug classification: the correlation of in vitro drug product dissolution and in vivo bioavailability.** *Pharm Res* 1995, 12:413–420.
2. Chen H, Khemtong C, Yang X, Chang X, Gao J: **Nanonization strategies for poorly water-soluble drugs.** *Drug Discov Today* 2011, 16:354–360.
3. Benet LZ: **The role of BCS (biopharmaceutics classification system) and BDDCS (biopharmaceutics drug disposition classification system) in drug development.** *J Pharm Sci* 2013, 102:34–42.
4. Kawakami K, Zhang S, Chauhan RS, Ishizuka N, Yamamoto M, Masaoka Y, Kataoka M, Yamashita S, Sakuma S: **Preparation of fenofibrate solid dispersion using electrospray deposition and improvement in oral absorption by instantaneous post-heating of the formulation.** *Int J Pharm* 2013, 450:123–128.
5. Chen Z, Xie Y, Guan P, Xu Y, Qi J, Lu Y, Wu W: **Enhanced oral bioavailability of all-trans-retinoic acid by 2-hydroxypropyl-β-cyclodextrin inclusion complex pellets prepared by fluid-bed coating technique.** *Asian J Pharm Sci* 2011, 6:202–207.
6. Ige PP, Baria RK, Gattani SG: **Fabrication of fenofibrate nanocrystals by probe sonication method for enhancement of dissolution rate and oral bioavailability.** *Colloids Surf B: Biointerfaces* 2013, 108:366–373.
7. Tokumura T, Muraoka A, Machida Y: **Improvement of oral bioavailability of flurbiprofen from flurbiprofen/beta-cyclodextrin inclusion complex by action of cinnarizine.** *Eur J Pharm Biopharm* 2009, 73:202–204.
8. Gao Y, Nishimura K, Hirayama F, Arima H, Uekama K, Schmid G, Terao K, Nakata D, Fukumi H: **Enhanced dissolution and oral bioavailability of coenzyme Q10 in dogs obtained by inclusion complexation with γ-cyclodextrin.** *Asian J Pharm Sci* 2006, 1:95–102.
9. Monteiro LM, Lione VF, Do Carmo FA, Do Amaral LH, Da Silva JH, Nasciutti LE, Rodrigues CR, Castro HC, De Sousa VP, Cabral LM: **Development and characterization of a new oral dapsone nanoemulsion system: permeability and in silico bioavailability studies.** *Int J Nanomedicine* 2012, 7:5175–5182.
10. Ling G, Zhang P, Zhang W, Sun J, Meng X, Qin Y, Deng Y, He Z: **Development of novel self-assembled DS-PLGA hybrid nanoparticles for improving oral bioavailability of vincristine sulfate by P-gp inhibition.** *J Control Release* 2010, 148:241–248.
11. Das S, Chaudhury A: **Recent advances in lipid nanoparticle formulations with solid matrix for oral drug delivery.** *AAPS PharmSciTech* 2011, 12:62–76.
12. Zhuang CY, Li N, Wang M, Zhang XN, Pan WS, Peng JJ, Pan YS, Tang X: **Preparation and characterization of vinpocetine loaded nanostructured lipid carriers (NLC) for improved oral bioavailability.** *Int J Pharm* 2010, 394:179–185.
13. Gupta PN, Khatri K, Goyal AK, Mishra N, Vyas SP: **M-cell targeted biodegradable PLGA nanoparticles for oral immunization against hepatitis B.** *J Drug Target* 2007, 15:701–713.
14. Beloqui A, Solinis MA, Delgado A, Evora C, Isla A, Rodriguez-Gascon A: **Fate of nanostructured lipid carriers (NLCs) following the oral route: design, pharmacokinetics and biodistribution.** *J Microencapsul* 2013, 31:1–8.
15. Sun N, Zhang X, Lu Y, Wu W: **In vitro evaluation and pharmacokinetics in dogs of solid dispersion pellets containing Silybum marianum extract prepared by fluid-bed coating.** *Planta Med* 2008, 74:126–132.
16. Chen Z, Lu Y, Qi J, Wu W: **Enhanced dissolution, stability and physicochemical characterization of ATRA/2-hydroxypropyl-beta-cyclodextrin inclusion complex pellets prepared by fluid-bed coating technique.** *Pharm Dev Technol* 2013, 18:130–136.
17. Shaikh J, Ankola DD, Beniwal V, Singh D, Kumar MN: **Nanoparticle encapsulation improves oral bioavailability of curcumin by at least 9-fold when compared to curcumin administered with piperine as absorption enhancer.** *Eur J Pharm Sci* 2009, 37:223–230.
18. Sonaje K, Lin KJ, Tseng MT, Wey SP, Su FY, Chuang EY, Hsu CW, Chen CT, Sung HW: **Effects of chitosan-nanoparticle-mediated tight junction opening on the oral absorption of endotoxins.** *Biomaterials* 2011, 32:8712–8721.
19. Porter CJ, Kaukonen AM, Taillardat-Bertschinger A, Boyd BJ, O'Connor JM, Edwards GA, Charman WN: **Use of in vitro lipid digestion data to explain the in vivo performance of triglyceride-based oral lipid formulations of poorly water-soluble drugs: studies with halofantrine.** *J Pharm Sci* 2004, 93:1110–1121.
20. Memvanga PB, Eloy P, Gaigneaux EM, Preat V: **In vitro lipolysis and intestinal transport of beta-arteether-loaded lipid-based drug delivery systems.** *Pharm Res* 2013, 30:2694–2705.
21. Zuo B, Sun Y, Li H, Liu X, Zhai Y, Sun J, He Z: **Preparation and in vitro/in vivo evaluation of fenofibrate nanocrystals.** *Int J Pharm* 2013, 455:267–275.

22. Patel AR, Vavia PR: Preparation and in vivo evaluation of SMEDDS (self-microemulsifying drug delivery system) containing fenofibrate. *AAPS J* 2007, **9**:E344–E352.

23. Chen Y, Lu Y, Chen J, Lai J, Sun J, Hu F, Wu W: Enhanced bioavailability of the poorly water-soluble drug fenofibrate by using liposomes containing a bile salt. *Int J Pharm* 2009, **376**:153–160.

24. Niu X, Wan L, Hou Z, Wang T, Sun C, Sun J, Zhao P, Jiang T, Wang S: Mesoporous carbon as a novel drug carrier of fenofibrate for enhancement of the dissolution and oral bioavailability. *Int J Pharm* 2013, **452**:382–389.

25. Tian Z, Yi Y, Yuan H, Han J, Zhang X, Xie Y, Lu Y, Qi J, Wu W: Solidification of nanostructured lipid carriers (NLCs) onto pellets by fluid-bed coating: preparation, in vitro characterization and bioavailability in dogs. *Powder Technol* 2013, **247**:120–127.

26. Tang N, Lai J, Chen YP, Lu Y, Wu W: Fenofibrate solid dispersion pellets prepared by fluid-bed coating: physical characterization, improved dissolution and oral bioavailability in beagle dogs. *J Chin Pharm Sci* 2009, **18**:156–161.

27. Fei Y, Kostewicz ES, Sheu MT, Dressman JB: Analysis of the enhanced oral bioavailability of fenofibrate lipid formulations in fasted humans using an in vitro-in silico-in vivo approach. *Eur J Pharm Biopharm* 2013, **85**:1274–1284.

28. Buckley ST, Frank KJ, Fricker G, Brandl M: Biopharmaceutical classification of poorly soluble drugs with respect to "enabling formulations". *Eur J Pharm Sci* 2013, **50**:8–16.

29. Weng TF, Qi J, Lu Y, Yin Z, Wu W: Preparation and bioavailability study in beagle dogs of fenofibrate nanosuspension. *Chin J Pharm* 2014, **45**:23–239.

30. Porter CJ, Pouton CW, Cuine JF, Charman WN: Enhancing intestinal drug solubilisation using lipid-based delivery systems. *Adv Drug Deliv Rev* 2008, **60**:673–691.

31. Porter CJ, Trevaskis NL, Charman WN: Lipids and lipid-based formulations: optimizing the oral delivery of lipophilic drugs. *Nat Rev Drug Discov* 2007, **6**:231–248.

32. Liu YO, Fan JM, Wang XQ, Zhang Q: Preparation of sorafenib self-microemulsifying drug delivery system and its relative bioavailability in rats. *J Chin Pharm Sci* 2011, **20**:164–170.

33. He C, Yin L, Tang C, Yin C: Size-dependent absorption mechanism of polymeric nanoparticles for oral delivery of protein drugs. *Biomaterials* 2012, **33**:8569–8578.

34. Wang S, Ye T, Zhang X, Yang R, Yi X: Myricetin loaded in microemulsion for oral drug delivery: formulation optimization, intestinal absorption in situ recirculation and in-vivo evaluation. *Asian J Pharm Sci* 2012, **7**:293–300.

35. Dahan A, Hoffman A: The effect of different lipid based formulations on the oral absorption of lipophilic drugs: the ability of in vitro lipolysis and consecutive ex vivo intestinal permeability data to predict in vivo bioavailability in rats. *Eur J Pharm Biopharm* 2007, **67**:96–105.

36. Dahan A, Hoffman A: Rationalizing the selection of oral lipid based drug delivery systems by an in vitro dynamic lipolysis model for improved oral bioavailability of poorly water soluble drugs. *J Control Release* 2008, **129**:1–10.

37. Porter CJ, Charman WN: In vitro assessment of oral lipid based formulations. *Adv Drug Deliv Rev* 2001, **50**(Suppl 1):S127–S147.

38. Kossena GA, Charman WN, Wilson CG, O'Mahony B, Lindsay B, Hempenstall JM, Davison CL, Crowley PJ, Porter CJ: Low dose lipid formulations: effects on gastric emptying and biliary secretion. *Pharm Res* 2007, **24**:2084–2096.

39. Luner PE, Vander Kamp D: Wetting behavior of bile salt-lipid dispersions and dissolution media patterned after intestinal fluids. *J Pharm Sci* 2001, **90**:348–359.

40. Pabla D, Akhlaghi F, Zia H: Intestinal permeability enhancement of levothyroxine sodium by straight chain fatty acids studied in MDCK epithelial cell line. *Eur J Pharm Sci* 2010, **40**:466–472.

41. Khoo SM, Shackleford DM, Porter CJ, Edwards GA, Charman WN: Intestinal lymphatic transport of halofantrine occurs after oral administration of a unit-dose lipid-based formulation to fasted dogs. *Pharm Res* 2003, **20**:1460–1465.

42. Gershkovich P, Hoffman A: Uptake of lipophilic drugs by plasma derived isolated chylomicrons: linear correlation with intestinal lymphatic bioavailability. *Eur J Pharm Sci* 2005, **26**:394–404.

43. Caliph SM, Charman WN, Porter CJ: Effect of short-, medium-, and long-chain fatty acid-based vehicles on the absolute oral bioavailability and intestinal lymphatic transport of halofantrine and assessment of mass balance in lymph-cannulated and non-cannulated rats. *J Pharm Sci* 2000, **89**:1073–1084.

44. Hu L, Wu H, Niu F, Yan C, Yang X, Jia Y: Design of fenofibrate microemulsion for improved bioavailability. *Int J Pharm* 2011, **420**:251–255.

45. Streel B, Hubert P, Ceccato A: Determination of fenofibric acid in human plasma using automated solid-phase extraction coupled to liquid chromatography. *J Chromatogr B Biomed Sci Appl* 2000, **742**:391–400.

# Folic acid conjugated cross-linked acrylic polymer (FA-CLAP) hydrogel for site specific delivery of hydrophobic drugs to cancer cells

Jisha Jayadevan Pillai[1], Arun Kumar Theralikattu Thulasidasan[2], Ruby John Anto[2], Devika Nandan Chithralekha[1], Ashwanikumar Narayanan[1] and Gopalakrishnapillai Sankaramangalam Vinod Kumar[1*]

## Abstract

**Background:** The hydrogel based system is found to be rarely reported for the delivery of hydrophobic drug due to the incompatibility of hydrophilicity of the polymer network and the hydrophobicity of drug. This problem can be solved by preparing semi-interpenetrating network of cross-linked polymer for tuning the hydrophilicity so as to entrap the hydrophobic drugs. The current study is to develop a folic acid conjugated cross-linked pH sensitive, biocompatible polymeric hydrogel to achieve a site specific drug delivery. For that, we have synthesized a folic acid conjugated PEG cross-linked acrylic polymer (FA-CLAP) hydrogel and investigated its loading and release of curcumin. The formed polymer hydrogel was then conjugated with folic acid for the site specific delivery of curcumin to cancer cells and then further characterized and conducted the cell uptake and cytotoxicity studies on human cervical cancer cell lines (HeLa).

**Results:** In this study, we synthesized folic acid conjugated cross-linked acrylic hydrogel for the delivery of hydrophobic drugs to the cancer site. Poly (ethyleneglycol) (PEG) diacrylate cross-linked acrylic polymer (PAA) was prepared via inverse emulsion polymerization technique and later conjugated it with folic acid (FA-CLAP). Hydrophobic drug curcumin is entrapped into it and investigated the entrapment efficiency. Characterization of synthesized hydogel was done by using Fourier Transform-Infrared spectroscopy (FT-IR), Transmission Electron Microscopy (TEM), Differential Scanning Calorimetry (DSC). Polymerization and folate conjugation was confirmed by FT-IR spectroscopy. The release kinetics of drug from the entrapped form was studied which showed initial burst release followed by sustained release due to swelling and increased cross-linking. In vitro cytotoxicity and cell uptake studies were conducted in human cervical cancer (HeLa) cell lines.

**Conclusions:** Results showed that curcumin entrapped folate conjugated cross-linked acrylic polymer (FA-CLAP) hydrogel showed higher cellular uptake than the non folate conjugated form. So this can be suggested as a better delivery system for site specific release of hydrophobic cancer drugs.

## Background

Hydrogels are polymeric networks having three-dimensional configuration capable of imbibing high amounts of water or biological fluids. Their water absorbing property is mainly attributed to the presence of hydrophilic groups such as –OH, –CONH–, –CONH$_2$–, and –SO$_3$H in the polymers. Due to the contribution of these groups and domains in the network, the polymer is thus hydrated to different degrees, depending on the aqueous environment and polymer composition [1]. These ionizable functional groups present in it affect its permeability mechanical stability and biocompatibility to a greater extends [2]. Along with that these structures have some common physical properties resembling that of the living tissues, which is attributed to their high water content, soft and rubbery consistency, and low interfacial tension with water or biological fluids [3-5]. The high water content make it soft and wet just like a biological material mimicking the extracellular matrix similar to macromolecular based compound in the human body [6,7].

* Correspondence: gsvinod@rgcb.res.in
[1]Chemical Biology, Rajiv Gandhi Centre for Biotechnology, Thiruvananthapuram-695 014, Poojappura, Kerala, India
Full list of author information is available at the end of the article

Hydrogel based drug delivery is a type of controlled delivery system were the gel swell resulting in release of drug from the polymer in a controlled manner. As water penetrate through the polymer chain the glass temperature of the polymer decreases and make the hydrogel rubbery [8]. These hydrogels have highly porous structure which helps incorporation of drug into it. The high water content and high porosity help them easy release of the drug within certain hours to days. The porosity of hydrogel can be tuned to the required size of the drug by the addition of cross linker to it. And thus it help in the controlled release of drug [9,10]. The polymer used for the preparation of hydrogel is of natural, synthetic and semi-synthetic origin. Even though natural polymers have good bioactive properties [11] they are found to have low mechanical strength so we make use of synthetic polymers because of their good mechanical strength and well-defined structure which can be modified to improve the biocompatibility and biodegradability [12,13].

Polyacrylic acid based polymers are one of such ideal candidates for the synthesis of hydrogel system for the controlled drug delivery because of the swelling behavior in aqueous environment [14]. It is a type of pH sensitive polymer [15,16] which shows swelling at higher pH due to the presence of ionizable carboxyl groups in it and can release the drug at neutral pH. The main drawback associated with PAA based drug delivery system is rapid release of drug from it which can be controlled by cross-linking. The cross-linking helps in slow drug release due to small mesh size which can be advantageous for controlled drug delivery applications. Cross-linking also improves the physical properties of the hydrogel including mechanical strength, degradability and diffusivity of drugs from the system. The solubility of polymer in the aqueous environment can also be prevented using cross-linking [17,18].

Curcumin, a naturally occurring yellow coloured polyphenol obtained from the rhizome of the perennial herb *Curcuma longa*, is found to have potent anticancer properties [19]. It inhibit proliferation and induces apoptosis in various cancer cell lines isolated from malignancies like leukemia, breast, lung, prostate and colon tumors [20-23]. Studies were also done in various tumerogenetic models [24-29] and some clinical trials were also done in patients which confirmed the potential of curcumin as a tool for cancer therapy. But its clinical application becomes limited due to poor water solubility, minimal systemic bioavailability, degradation in alkaline pH and photo degradation. So the therapeutic efficacy of curcumin can be increased by incorporating curcumin in a biocompatible polymer which enhances the solubility in aqueous solution and extends the release.

One of the main problems associated with cancer therapy is its unwanted side effect towards normal cells along with the cancer cells. An active targeting strategy can improve the therapeutic efficacy of drugs and reduces the side effects [30-34]. For that we have to modify the polymer nanoparticles with certain ligands that have its specific receptor on cancer cell surface. Folate receptor has been extensively investigated for targeting various tumor cells since it is normally expressed in various types of cancer cells [35-38]. So the cross-linked polymeric hydrogel nanoparticles which were structurally modified with folic acid can help in easy targeting and up taking of drugs by the cancer cells.

The hydrogel based system is found to be rarely reported for the delivery of hydrophobic drug due to the incompatibility of hydrophilicity of the polymer network and the hydrophobicity of drug. This problem can be solved by preparing semi-interpenetrating network of cross-linked polymer for tuning the hydrophilicity so as to entrap the hydrophobic drugs. The current study is to develop a folic acid conjugated cross-linked pH sensitive biocompatible polymeric hydrogel to achieve a site specific drug delivery. For that, we have synthesized a folic acid conjugated PEG cross-linked acrylic polymer (FA-CLAP) hydrogel and investigated its loading and release of curcumin. Here we used inverse emulsion polymerization technique proposed by Vanderhoff et al. for the polymerization of acrylic acid where an aqueous solution of hydrophilic monomer acrylic acid is dispersed in a continuous lipophilic phase with the aid of surfactants to promote the formation of water in oil (W/O) emulsion [39]. The formed polymer hydrogel was then conjugated with folic acid for the site specific delivery of curcumin to cancer cells and then further characterized and conducted the cell uptake and cytotoxicity studies on human cervical cancer cell lines (HeLa).

## Results and discussion
### Synthesis and characterization of FA-CLAP hydrogel
Curcumin loaded folic acid conjugated cross-linked acrylic polymer (FA-CLAP) hydrogel were synthesized successfully using inverse emulsion polymerization technique (Figure 1). Inverse emulsion polymerization is a controllable technique used for the preparation of well-defined nanoparticles. In the present study, we prepared acrylic polymer cross-linked with polyethylene glycol diacrylate by inverse micro emulsion polymerization method which is cross-linked with folic acid through ethylenediamine for targeted delivery of curcumin to cancer cells. Inverse polymerization helps in the easy facilitating of free radical polymerization of acrylic monomer with PEG diacrylate in presence of ammonium persulfate. PEG, a highly biocompatible and hydrophilic polymer with low Tg and polyacrylic acid in the system imparts pH sensitivity. The hydrogel that we prepared displays pH sensitive nature which can be exploited for site specific controlled drug delivery. Folic acid is also

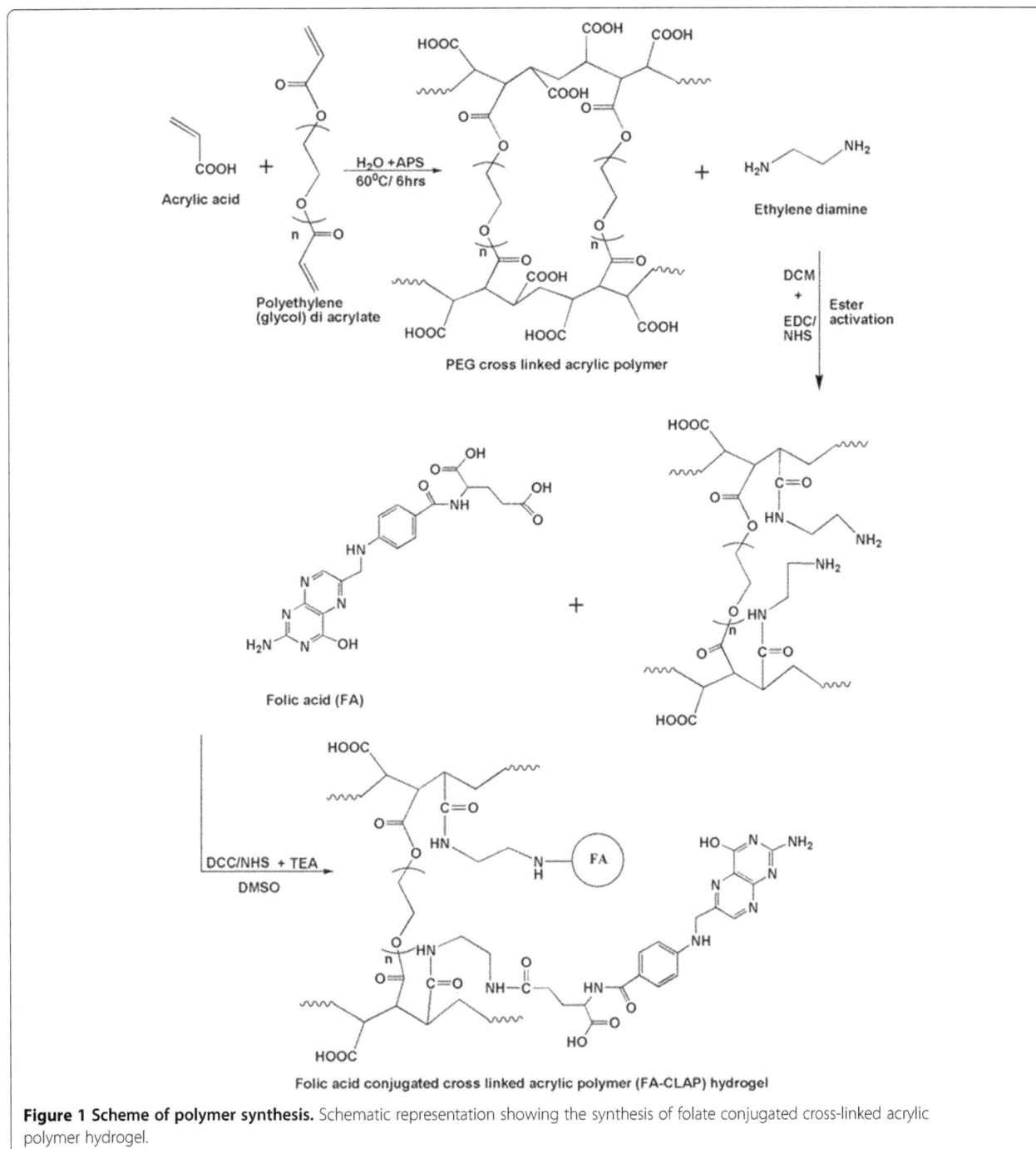

**Figure 1 Scheme of polymer synthesis.** Schematic representation showing the synthesis of folate conjugated cross-linked acrylic polymer hydrogel.

conjugated with the hydrogel that helps in the targeted delivery of the drug encapsulated hydrogel towards the cancer cells since many cancer cells are expressing folic acid on its surface and pH sensitivity helps in the swelling of the hydrogel in the required site with the sustained release of drug on that particular site. The percentage swelling in a pH dependant manner was analyzed and given in Additional file 1.

## Characterization
Morphology and the size of the particles were studied using Transmission electron microscopy. The nanoparticles obtained were of size range of 160–190 nm with narrow size distribution (Figure 2). The folic acid conjugated cross-linked polymer hydrogel particle shows a round morphology with nanometric size range. Particle size was found to increase with folic acid conjugation in it.

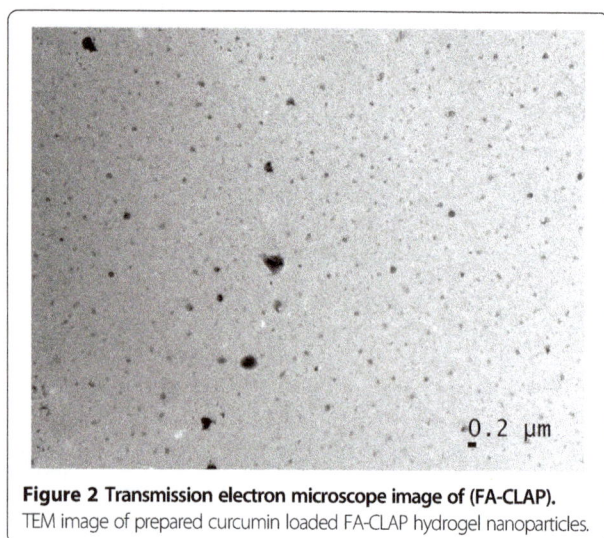

**Figure 2 Transmission electron microscope image of (FA-CLAP).** TEM image of prepared curcumin loaded FA-CLAP hydrogel nanoparticles.

Role of size in drug delivery is well known. Optimal size should be needed for a drug delivery particle so that it will not easily leak out of the capillaries and also not easily up taken by the macrophages. Here also we developed a particle which is having a size of about 190 nm that is optimal for the cellular uptake and the folic acid conjugation will help in the active targeted delivery of nanoparticle into the cancer site. Active targeting help in faster accumulation of nanoparticles in the cancer site and help in the release of drug to that particular site [12].

DSC was done to find the thermal behavior of the nanoparticles. DSC of folic acid conjugated cross-liked acrylic polymer and curcumin loaded folic acid conjugated cross-linked polymer were done as showed in Figure 3. Folic acid conjugated polymer shows an endothermic peak at 115°C which after loading with curcumin showed a decrease in value (endothermic peak at 85°C) and the nanogel was found to be stable up to 200°C.

The DSC of FA-CLAP hydrogel shows endothermic transition peak at 115°C which can be due to the loss of loose and bound water in the hydrogel [40]. The gel appeared to be thermally stable up to 200°C. Curcumin was loaded to the cross-linked acrylic polymer through physical adsorption by post loading method. And the DSC of curcumin loaded FA-CLAP hydrogel shows an endothermic peak at 85°C. Cross-linking using PEG diacrylate provides hydrophobicity to the acrylic hydrogel which enhances the uptake of curcumin, a hydrophobic drug. Swelling of the polymer occurs at a pH above the pKa of the carboxyl group of acrylic acid. Swelling increases with COO- groups and decreases with increasing cross-links.

The cross-linking and folate conjugation was confirmed by FTIR spectroscopy. FTIR spectroscopy clearly gives idea about cross-linking and conjugation of folic acid into the polymer (Figure 4). FTIR of cross-linked PAA with EDA (ethylenediamine) was shown in Figure 4(A) in which the peak at 3428.7 cm$^{-1}$ may be due to N-H stretching of free amino group in ethylenediamine and peak at 1633.6 cm$^{-1}$and 1566.7 cm$^{-1}$ may be of stretching of amide bond I and II that is formed between ethylenediamine and cross-linked PAA which indicates EDA conjugation with the polymer. Peak at 2950.9 cm$^{-1}$ may be due to aliphatic C-H stretching of poly acrylate. FTIR of FA-CLAP hydrogel was shown in Figure 4(B) in which the absorption band at 2929.6 cm$^{-1}$ is due to asymmetric C-H stretching vibration of folic acid. In addition to this other peaks like 1485.3 cm$^{-1}$ (–C = C- aromatic stretching of phenyl ring) and 1411.8 cm$^{-1}$ (OH deformation of phenyl skeleton) confirm the presence of folic acid in FA-CLAP [41]. Peaks at 1626.5 cm$^{-1}$ and 1574.9 cm$^{-1}$ are due to amide I and

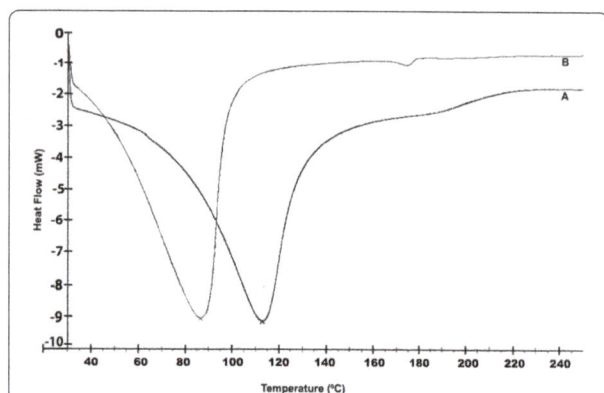

**Figure 3 Differential scanning calorimetry (DSC) of hydrogel.** DSC of samples **(A)** FA-CLAP hydrogel **(B)** Curcumin-entrapped FA-CLAP hydrogel.

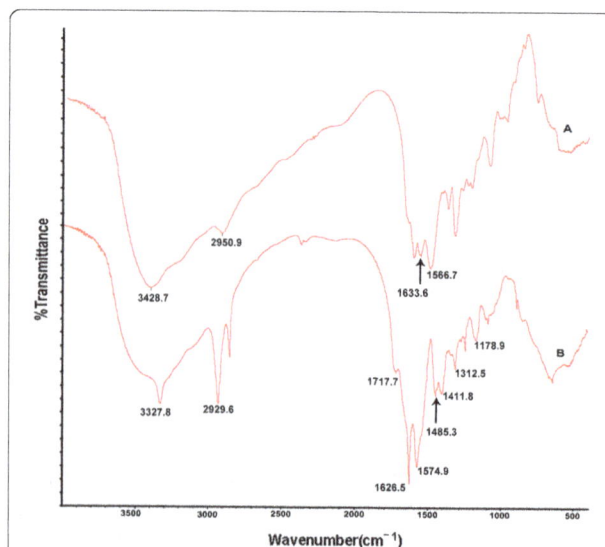

**Figure 4 Fourier transform infra red spectra.** FTIR of the synthesized co polymer: **(A)** Polyacrylic acid with ethylenediamine **(B)** FA-CLAP hydrogel.

amide II band present in FA-CLAP. Peak at 1312.5 cm$^{-1}$ may be due to C = N medium stretching in the pteridine ring of folic acid which all confirmed the folic acid conjugation with ethylenediamine conjugated cross-linked PAA. It shows peak at 1717.7 cm$^{-1}$ which may be due to the presence of free COOH groups in the prepared polymer.

### In-vitro drug release

Curcumin is found to be poorly soluble in water and it form flakes in it. So it is incorporated in a cross-linked polymer hydrogel for delivery to the cancer site. For making targeting more specific, folate conjugation was also done to it. This makes the release of the drug from hydrogel in a controlled manner by the swelling of the gel. Entrapment efficiency of folic acid conjugated cross-linked polymer was found to be 61.2 ± 1.2%. In vitro release profile of entrapped drug curcumin from FA-CLAP was done and is shown in (Figure 5). Here the polymer showed an initial release of 10% within 2 hrs and 20-40% release with in 24 hrs (Higuchi diffusion model [42]) because of swelling of hydrogel and thereafter the release occur in slow sustained manner which might be due to the decrease in the swelling because of increased cross-linking. The release was markedly noticeable from 120–200 hours were 50% of the increase in drug release was observed. After 200 hours almost 97% of the drug was released and a steady state was observed. Due to the presence of folic acid, targeted release of drug is possible. Controlled and targeted release of drug from the cross-linked polymer is a desirable property for most of drug delivery applications as it reduces the side effect and increases the bioavailability.

### Cell uptake studies
#### Curcumin entrapped FA-CLAP show better cellular uptake compared to free curcumin

We analyzed whether folic acid conjugation to PAA nanocurcumin surface can improve the drug delivery to cancer cells, since cancer cells over-express folate receptors. The internalization of curcumin to the cells was visualized by confocal microscopy and the results indicate that curcumin entrapped FA-CLAP hydrogel show better cell uptake than free curcumin dissolved in DMSO (Figure 6).

### MTT assay
#### Folic acid-conjugated PAA (FA-CLAP) nanocurcumin induce cytotoxicity in HeLa cells

We compared the efficacy of folic acid-conjugated PAA (FA-CLAP) nanocurcumin with its free counterpart in inducing cell death of HeLa cells. HeLa cells were exposed to free curcumin or folic acid-conjugated PAA nanocurcumin (5–50 µM) for 72 h. The nanoformulation imparts high cytotoxicity than free curcumin in dose dependent manner especially for 15 µM, 25 µM and 50 µM. The results indicate that the folic acid-conjugated PAA nanocurcumin (FA-CLAP) show comparatively better efficacy in inducing cytotoxicity of HeLa cells than free curcumin dissolved in DMSO (Figure 7).

### Acridine orange (AO)/ethidium bromide (EB) staining
#### Conjugation of Folic acid on PAA nanocurcumin slightly enhance the apoptotic effect induced by the latter in HeLa cells

Ability of curcumin in inducing apoptosis of HeLa cells were assessed by AO/EB staining. HeLa cells were exposed to free curcumin or folic acid-conjugated PAA (FA-CLAP) nanocurcumin (25 µM) for 24 h. When treated with AO/EB mixture the untreated cells showed bright green chromatin due to AO staining. The damaged membrane of the apoptotic cells allowed EB to get in, giving red color to the nucleus. In Figure 8 we can vividly observe more number of cells in the red colour (6 out of 16 cells, ~40%) than blank curcumin (2 out of 10 cells, ~20%).The results indicate that conjugation of folic acid on PAA nanocurcumin enhances its apoptotic activity in HeLa cells compared to the free curcumin dissolved in DMSO as assessed by increase in number of EB stained cells (Figure 8).

### Conclusions

Curcumin, which has many medicinal properties mainly, lacks its activity due to its low water solubility. So through this work the delivery of hydrophobic drug curcumin is done by incorporating the drug into cross-linked hydrogel matrix and the cell uptake which was another problem was further enhanced by introducing folic acid into the system. It was found that folic acid conjugated cross-linked hydrogel polymer (FA-CLAP) loaded with curcumin showed better cellular uptake compared to the non-folate hydrogel particles. So this

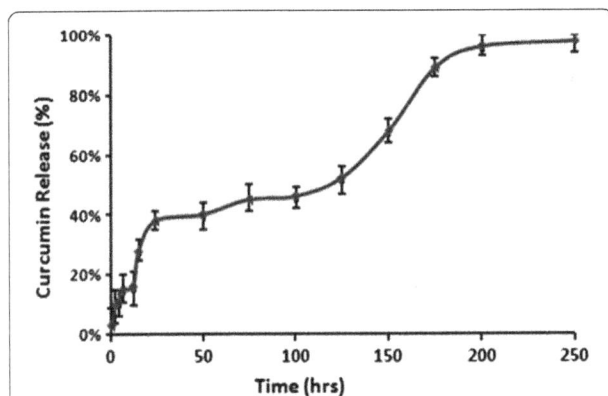

**Figure 5 In vitro release of curcumin.** Release kinetics of curcumin from FA-CLAP hydrogel.

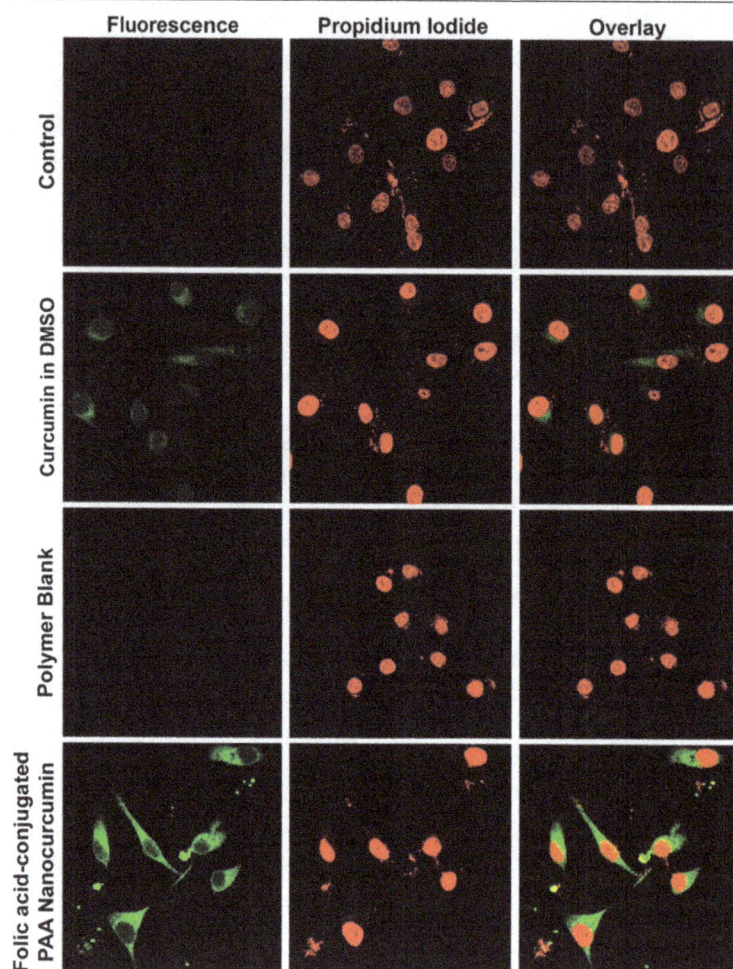

**Figure 6 Cellular uptake image.** Cell uptake of folic acid-conjugated PAA (FA-CLAP) nanocurcumin and free curcumin: HeLa cells were treated with curcumin formulations as mentioned in materials and methods and confocal images were taken in the FITC channel.

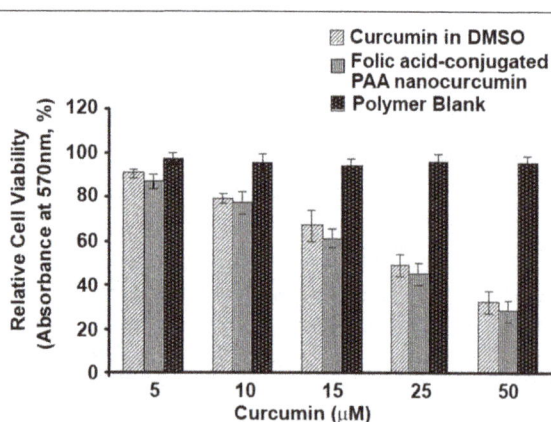

**Figure 7 Cytotoxic effect of folic acid-conjugated PAA nanocurcumin.** HeLa cells were treated with folic acid-conjugated PAA (FA-CLAP) nanocurcumin or curcumin in DMSO. Optical densities were measured and relative cell viability was plotted.

can be used as a better system for the site specific delivery of hydrophobic drugs.

## Methods

### Materials

Acrylic acid (Mw ~ 72), cross-linker poly (ethylene glycol) diacrylate (Mw ~ 238,), Curcumin, Ammonium persulphate (APS), Span 80 (Sorbitan monooleate), Tween 80 (Poly (ethyleneglycol) sorbitan monooleate), 3-(4,5-dimethylthiazol-2-yl)-2, 5-diphenyltetrazolium bromide (MTT), ethylenediamine and folic acid were purchased from Sigma-Aldrich, Germany. Acridine orange and ethidium bromide were purchased from Sigma Aldrich. DMEM was purchased from Life Technologies (Grand Island, NY, USA). MTT was purchased from Calbiochem, Germany and Propidium Iodide from Calbiochem, USA. All other reagents and chemicals were of

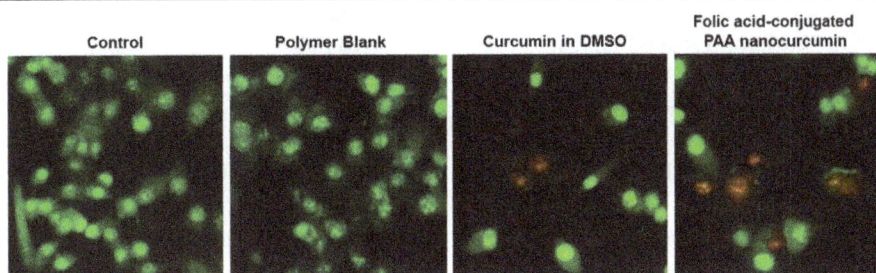

**Figure 8 Fluorescence images of HeLa cells treated by free curcumin or folic acid-conjugated PAA (FA-CLAP) nanocurcumin showing apoptosis.** HeLa cells were treated with different curcumin formulations for 24 h and were stained with acridine orange and ethidium bromide solutions as mentioned in materials and methods and fluorescence images were taken using an inverted fluorescent microscope.

analytical grade or above, and used without further purification.

## Preparation of folic acid conjugated cross-linked polymeric nanoparticles

### Preparation of cross-linked acrylic polymer

The cross-linked acrylic polymer (1%) was prepared by inverse emulsion polymerization technique. Emulsification was done by dispersing aqueous phase consisting of 10% acrylic acid, 5% sodium hydroxide and 15% water with continuous lipophilic phase consisting of liquid paraffin (68%), emulsifiers (2%), Span 80 and Tween 80 (75:25 ratio). For cross-linking, 1% of PEG diacrylate was added to the mixture followed by the addition of initiator, ammonium persulfate (APS). The temperature for polymerization was at 60°C for 6 hours. The cross-linked polymeric particles were isolated by centrifugation (10,000 rpm) for 30 min. The isolated polymeric particles were washed several times with hexane and stored for further structural modifications.

### Conjugation of folic acid to the prepared cross-linked polymeric particles (FA-CLAP)

For the conjugation of folic acid to the prepared cross-linked polymeric particles, first the cross-linked polymeric particle (850 mg. 1.2 eq) has to be treated with ethylenediamine (3.2 ml, 0.65 eq) through carbodiimide chemistry for the availability of free amine group for the binding of activated folic acid to it. Simultaneously folic acid (220 mg, 0.5 eq) has to be ester activated then it is allowed to react with ethylenediamine conjugated cross-linked acrylic hydrogel. A measured amount of this ethylenediamine conjugated cross-linked polymeric particles (550 mg) was dissolved in DMSO. The reaction mixture is kept overnight stirring, for the completion of folic acid conjugation; cross-linked polymeric particles were isolated by centrifugation (10,000 rpm) for 30 min. The isolated folic acid conjugated cross-linked polymeric hydrogel (FA-CLAP) was washed several times and then freeze dried to remove solvent and water. The freeze dried product was stored in vacuum. The polymerization of acrylic acid with PEG diacrylate cross-linking and folic acid conjugation was characterized using DSC and FT-IR spectroscopy. The amount of folic acid conjugated was also estimated (see Additional file 1).

## Drug loading

Loading of curcumin in folic acid conjugated cross-linked polymeric nanoparticles (FA-CLAP) was done by post-polymerization method. 100 mg of the lyophilized powder was dispersed in 10 mL distilled water. Curcumin was dissolved in chloroform and the drug solution in chloroform was added to the polymeric solution with constant vortexing and sonication. The curcumin loaded FA-CLAP hydrogel was then lyophilized to obtain dried powder.

## Characterization of prepared hydrogel nanoparticles

Morphological analysis of the free and curcumin loaded FA-CLAP nanoparticles were then characterized using transmission electron microscopy (TEM, JEOL 1011, and Japan). The samples of the nanoparticle suspension in water milli-Q at 25°C were dropped on to formvar-coated grids and measurements were taken only after the samples were completely dried.

Folic acid conjugation in the parent polymer was confirmed using FTIR spectroscopy. FTIR spectroscopy was performed on a Spectrum 65 (Perkin Elmer). Spectra were recorded between 4000 and 600 $cm^{-1}$ wave number range. Dried samples were mixed with KBr and further compressed in to pellets for making measurements.

Differential Scanning Calorimetry (DSC) was done to analyze the thermal behavior of the FA-CLAP and Curcumin loaded FA-CLAP hydrogel. DSC thermograms obtained were then analyzed using an automatic thermal analyzer system (Pyres 6 DSC, Perkin-Elmer, USA). Samples were placed in standard aluminum pans and heated from 20 to 250°C at a rate of 10°C/minute under constant purging of $N_2$ at 10 mL/minute. An empty pan, sealed in the same way as that of the sample, was used as a reference.

### Entrapment efficiency

A known amount of the curcumin loaded folic acid conjugated cross-linked polymer (FA-CLAP) hydrogel nanoparticles were dissolved in methanol and vigorously vortexed to get a clear solution and it is kept for 24 hours, and then filtered through 0.1 μM membrane filter. The absorbance of the filtrate was then taken at 420 nm by using UV absorbance (Perkin Elmer, USA). The entrapped amount of curcumin was then determined by actual entrapment ratio (AER), expressed in terms of amount of curcumin per weight of nanoparticles [43]. Entrapment efficiency can be calculated by the equation

$$\text{Entrapment Efficiency } (\%) = \text{AER} / \text{TER} \times 100$$

(AER = Measured drug wt/ Nanoparticle wt & TER = Initial drug wt/ drug wt & polymer wt). Where (AER) is Actual entrapment ratio and (TER) is Theoretical entrapment ratio. Nanogel wt means the weight of the nanogel with curcumin taken for calculating entrapment efficiency and Initial drug weight means drug initially taken for the entrapment.

### In vitro release kinetics

For *in vitro* release study, a known amount of curcumin loaded FA-CLAP were dispersed in 10 mL of P.B.S (pH 7.4) and was then left in a shaking incubator at 37 ± 0.5°C. A known quantity of sample was then withdrawn and replaced with fresh medium in a predetermined time intervals for maintaining the total volume constant. The amount of curcumin released from the hydrogel nanoparticle was then measured using UV spectrophotometer (Perkin Elmer, USA) at 420 nm.

### Cell uptake studies

Cellular uptake of curcumin and folic acid-conjugated PAA (FA-CLAP) nanocurcumin were studied using confocal microscopy. Briefly, $2.0 \times 10^4$ HeLa cells were grown on cover slips placed in 24 well plates. After overnight incubation, when the cells attained their morphology, they were treated with curcumin dissolved in dimethyl sulfoxide (DMSO) (25 μM), folic acid-conjugated PAA nanocurcumin (25 μM) was suspended in aqueous medium and blank polymer. After 2 h of incubation the cells were washed with 1X PBS, fixed with PFA and the nuclei were stained with propidium iodide and were mounted using DPX. Cells were examined for intracellular fluorescence of curcumin using confocal laser scanning microscope in the FITC channel (488 nm).

### MTT assay

Cytotoxicity studies of free curcumin and folic acid-conjugated PAA nanocurcumin were carried out in HeLa cells using MTT assay [44]. HeLa cells were seeded ($3.0 \times 10^3$/well) in a 96-well culture plate and grown for 24 h before the assay. The cells were then treated with different concentrations of curcumin dissolved in DMSO and folic acid-conjugated PAA nanocurcumin (5–50 μM) for 72 h and then 20 μl MTT (5 mg/ml) was added in 80 μl culture medium to each well. After incubating for 2 h at 37°C, cells were lysed using lysis buffer, incubated for 1 h, and the optical densities were measured at 570 nm using a microplate reader (Bio-Rad Laboratories, Hercules, CA). The relative cell viability in percentage was calculated as:

$$\text{Relative Cell Viability } = (\text{A570 of treated samples } / \text{A570 of untreated samples}) \times 100$$

### Acridine orange (AO)/ethidium bromide (EB) staining

Acridine orange/ethidium bromide (AO/EB) double staining was used to detect apoptosis [45]. Briefly, $5 \times 10^3$ cells/well were seeded in a 96-well plate and treated with curcumin in DMSO (25 μM) or folic acid-conjugated PAA (FA-CLAP) nanocurcumin (25 μM) for 24 h. After washing with 1X PBS, the cells were stained with acridine orange (100 μg/ml) and ethidium bromide (100 μg/ml) solutions for 2 min. The cells were then washed with 1X PBS, viewed under an inverted fluorescent microscope (Nikon Eclipse, TE-300) and were photographed.

### Additional file

> **Additional file 1: Supplementary information.**

#### Competing interests
The authors declare that they have no competing interests.

#### Authors' contributions
JPG synthesized, characterized the polymer and nanoparticles. DNC and NA have written the final manuscript. AKTT had done the biological experiments. RJA participated in evaluation of the biological experiments and supplied information for writing the final manuscript. GSVK planned the whole work and corrected the manuscript. All authors read and approved the final manuscript.

#### Acknowledgements
Authors are thankful to Department of Biotechnology, Government of India, for financial support and Arun Kumar T Thulasidasan and Ashwanikumar Narayanan for Council of Scientific and Industrial Research, New Delhi, India for providing Senior Research Fellowship.

#### Author details
[1]Chemical Biology, Rajiv Gandhi Centre for Biotechnology, Thiruvananthapuram-695 014, Poojappura, Kerala, India. [2]Division of Cancer Research, Rajiv Gandhi Centre for Biotechnology, Thiruvananthapuram-695 014, Poojappura, Kerala, India.

#### References
1.  Patel HB, Patel HL, Shah ZH, Modasiya MK: **Review on hydrogel nanoparticles in drug delivery.** *Am J Pharm Res* 2011, 1:19–38.

2.	Kim IS, Jeong YI, Kim DH, Lee YH, Kim SH: Albumin release from biodegradable hydrogels composed of dextran and poly (ethylene glycol) macromer. Arch Pharm Res 2001, 24:69–73.

3.	Hamidi M, Azadi A, Rafiei P: Hydrogel nanoparticles in drug delivery. Adv Drug Deliv Rev 2008, 60:1638–1649.

4.	Ratner BD, Hoffman AS: Synthetic Hydrogels for Biomedical Applications. In Hydrogels for Medical and Related Applications. 31st edition. Edited by Andrade JD. Washington DC: ACS Symposium Series, American Chemical Society; 1976:1–36.

5.	Blanco MD, García O, Trigo RM, Teijón JM, Katime I: 5-Fluorouracil release from copolymeric hydrogels of itaconic acid monoester: I. Acrylamide-co-monomethyl itaconate. Biomaterials 1996, 17:1061–1067.

6.	Chen R, Chen Q, Huo D, Ding Y, Hu Y, Jiang X: In situ formation of chitosan-gold hybrid hydrogel and its application for drug delivery. Colloids Surf B: Biointerfaces 2012, 97:132–137.

7.	Liu Y, Chan-Park MB: Hydrogel based on interpenetrating polymer networks of dextran and gelatin for vascular tissue engineering. Biomaterials 2009, 30:196–207.

8.	Deepa G, Thulasidasan A, Anto RJ, Pillai JJ, Kumar GSV: Cross-linked acrylic hydrogel for the controlled delivery of hydrophobic drugs in cancer therapy. Int J Nanomedicine 2012, 7:4077–4088.

9.	Xiao W, Liu W, Sun J, Dan X, Wei D, Fan H: Ultrasonication and Genipin Cross-Linking to Prepare Novel Silk Fibroin–Gelatin Composite Hydrogel. J Bioact Compat Polym 2012, 27:327–341.

10.	Seliktar D: Designing Cell-Compatible Hydrogels for Biomedical Applications. Science 2012, 336:1124–1128.

11.	Zhang L, Jeong Y, Zheng S, Jang S, Suh H, Kang DH, Kim: Biocompatible and pH-sensitive PEG hydrogels with degradable phosphoester and phosphoamide linkers end-capped with amine for controlled drug delivery. Polym Chem 2013, 4:1084–1094.

12.	Khare AR, Peppas NA: Swelling/deswelling of anionic copolymer gels. Biomaterials 1995, 16:559–567.

13.	Patenaude M, Hoare T: Injectable, mixed natural-synthetic polymer hydrogels with modular properties. Biomacromolecules 2012, 13:369–378.

14.	Burugapalli K, Bhatia D, Koul V, Choudhary V: Interpenetrating polymer networks based on poly (acrylic acid) and gelatin I: swelling and thermal behavior. J Appl Polym Sci 2001, 82:217–227.

15.	Soppimath K, Aminabhavi T, Dave A, Kumbar S, Rudzinski W: Stimulus-responsive "Smart" hydrogels as novel drug delivery systems*. Drug Dev Ind Pharm 2002, 28:957–974.

16.	Gao X, He C, Xiao C, Zhuang X, Chen X: Synthesis and characterization of biodegradable pH-sensitive poly (acrylic acid) hydrogels crosslinked by 2-hydroxyethyl methacrylate modified poly (L-glutamic acid). Mater Lett 2012, 77:74–77.

17.	Gupta P, Vermani K, Garg S: Hydrogels: from controlled release to pH-responsive drug delivery. Drug Discov Today 2002, 7:569–579.

18.	Hennink W, Van Nostrum C: Novel crosslinking methods to design hydrogels. Adv Drug Deliv Rev 2002, 54:13–36.

19.	Kuttan R, Bhanumathy P, Nirmala K, George M: Potential anticancer activity of turmeric (Curcuma longa). Cancer Lett 1985, 29:197–202.

20.	Shishodia S, Sethi G, Aggarwal BB: Curcumin: getting back to the roots. Ann N Y Acad Sci 2005, 1056:206–217.

21.	Strimpakos AS, Sharma RA: Curcumin: preventive and therapeutic properties in laboratory studies and clinical trials. Antioxidants Redox Signaling 2008, 10:511–546.

22.	Anand P, Sundaram C, Jhurani S, Kunnumakkara AB, Aggarwal BB: Curcumin and cancer: an "old-age" disease with an "age-old" solution. Cancer Lett 2008, 267:133–164.

23.	Mulik RS, Mönkkönen J, Juvonen RO, Mahadik KR, Paradkar AR: ApoE3 mediated polymeric nanoparticles containing curcumin: Apoptosis induced in vitro anticancer activity against neuroblastoma cells. Int J Pharm 2012, 437:29–41.

24.	Tuttle S, Hertan L, Daurio N, Porter S, Kaushic C, Li D, Myamoto S, Lin A, O' Malley BW, Koumenis C: The chemopreventive and clinically used agent curcumin sensitizes HPV-but not HPV+ HNSCC to ionizing radiation, in vitro and in a mouse orthotopic model. Canc Biol Ther 2012, 13:0–1.

25.	Chuang S, Kuo M, Hsu C, Chen C, Lin J, Lai G, Hsieh C, Cheng A: Curcumin-containing diet inhibits diethylnitrosamine-induced murine hepatocarcinogenesis. Carcinogenesis 2000, 21:331–335.

26.	Kawamori T, Lubet R, Steele VE, Kelloff GJ, Kaskey RB, Rao CV, Reddy BS: Chemopreventive effect of curcumin, a naturally occurring anti-inflammatory agent, during the promotion/progression stages of colon cancer. Cancer Res 1999, 59:597.

27.	Inano H, Onoda M, Inafuku N, Kubota M, Kamada Y, Osawa T, Kobayashi H, Wakabayashi K: Chemoprevention by curcumin during the promotion stage of tumorigenesis of mammary gland in rats irradiated with γ-rays. Carcinogenesis 1999, 20:1011–1018.

28.	Singh SV, Hu X, Srivastava SK, Singh M, Xia H, Orchard JL, Zaren HA: Mechanism of inhibition of benzo [a] pyrene-induced forestomach cancer in mice by dietary curcumin. Carcinogenesis 1998, 19:1357–1360.

29.	Li N, Chen X, Liao J, Yang G, Wang S, Josephson Y, Han C, Chen J, Huang MT, Yang CS: Inhibition of 7, 12-dimethylbenz [a] anthracene (DMBA)-induced oral carcinogenesis in hamsters by tea and curcumin. Carcinogenesis 2002, 23:1307–1313.

30.	Nasongkla N, Bey E, Ren J, Ai H, Khemtong C, Guthi JS, Chin SF, Sherry AD, Boothman DA, Gao J: Multifunctional polymeric micelles as cancer-targeted, MRI-ultrasensitive drug delivery systems. Nano Lett 2006, 6:2427–2430.

31.	Nair KL, Sankar J, Nair AS, Kumar GSV: Evaluation of triblock copolymeric micelles of δ-valerolactone and poly (ethylene glycol) as a competent vector for doxorubicin delivery against cancer. J Nanobiotechnology 2011, 9:42.

32.	Lilach V, Itai B: In vivo characteristics of targeted drug-carrying filamentous bacteriophage nanomedicines. J Nanobiotechnology 2011, 9:58.

33.	Mehmet HU, Seta K, Bernhard S, Uwe BS: Characterization of CurcuEmulsomes: nanoformulation for enhanced solubility and delivery of curcumin. J Nanobiotechnology 2013, 11:37.

34.	Deepa G, Ashwanikumar N, Pillai JJ, Kumar GSV: Polymer nanoparticles-a novel strategy for administration of paclitaxel in cancer chemotherapy. Curr Med Chem 2012, 19:6207–6213.

35.	Blanco MD, Guerrero S, Benito M, Fernández A, Teijón C, Olmo R, Katime I, Teijón JM: In vitro and in vivo evaluation of a folate-targeted copolymeric submicrohydrogel based on n-isopropylacrylamide as 5-fluorouracil delivery system. Polymers 2011, 3:1107–1125.

36.	Roger E, Kalscheuer S, Kirtane A, Guru BR, Grill AE, Whittum-Hudson J, Panyam J: Folic acid-functionalized nanoparticles for enhanced oral drug delivery. Mol Pharm 2012, 9:2103–2110.

37.	Kumar M, Singh G, Arora V, Mewar S, Sharma U, Jagannathan N, Sapra S, Dinda A, Kharbanda S, Singh H: Cellular interaction of folic acid conjugated superparamagnetic iron oxide nanoparticles and its use as contrast agent for targeted magnetic imaging of tumor cells. Int J Nanomedicine 2012, 7:3503–3516.

38.	Choi SK, Thomas TP, Li MH, Desai A, Kotlyar A, Baker JR: Photochemical release of methotrexate from folate receptor-targeting PAMAM dendrimer nanoconjugate. Photochem Photobiol Sci 2012, 11:653–660.

39.	Vanderhoff J, Bradford E, Tarkowski H, Shaffer J, Wiley R: Inverse emulsion polymerization. Adv Chem 1962, 34:32–51.

40.	Ravichandran P, Shantha KL, Rao KP: Preparation, swelling characteristics and evaluation of hydrogels for stomach specific drug delivery. Int J Pharm 1997, 154:89–94.

41.	Huang H, Yuan Q, Shah JS, Misra RDK: A new family of folate-decorated and carbon nanotube-mediated drug delivery system: synthesis and drug delivery response. Adv Drug Deliv Rev 2011, 63:1332–1339.

42.	Glavas-Dodov M, Goracinova K, Mladenovska K, Fredro-Kumbaradzi E: Release profile of lidocaine HCl from topical liposomal gel formulation. Int J Pharm 2002, 242:381–384.

43.	Qiu Y, Park K: Environment-sensitive hydrogels for drug delivery. Adv Drug Deliv Rev 2001, 53:321–339.

44.	Anto RJ, Venkatraman M, Karunagaran D: Inhibition of NF- B sensitizes A431 cells to epidermal growth factor-induced apoptosis, whereas its activation by ectopic expression of RelA confers resistance. J Biol Chem 2003, 278:25490–25498.

45.	Ribble D, Goldstein NB, Norris DA, Shellman YG: A simple technique for quantifying apoptosis in 96-well plates. BMC Biotechnol 2005, 5:12.

# Characterization of nanoparticle mediated laser transfection by femtosecond laser pulses for applications in molecular medicine

Markus Schomaker[1*], Dag Heinemann[1], Stefan Kalies[1], Saskia Willenbrock[2], Siegfried Wagner[2], Ingo Nolte[2], Tammo Ripken[1], Hugo Murua Escobar[2,3], Heiko Meyer[1,4] and Alexander Heisterkamp[1,5]

## Abstract

**Background:** In molecular medicine, the manipulation of cells is prerequisite to evaluate genes as therapeutic targets or to transfect cells to develop cell therapeutic strategies. To achieve these purposes it is essential that given transfection techniques are capable of handling high cell numbers in reasonable time spans. To fulfill this demand, an alternative nanoparticle mediated laser transfection method is presented herein. The fs-laser excitation of cell-adhered gold nanoparticles evokes localized membrane permeabilization and enables an inflow of extracellular molecules into cells.

**Results:** The parameters for an efficient and gentle cell manipulation are evaluated in detail. Efficiencies of 90% with a cell viability of 93% were achieved for siRNA transfection. The proof for a molecular medical approach is demonstrated by highly efficient knock down of the oncogene HMGA2 in a rapidly proliferating prostate carcinoma *in vitro* model using siRNA. Additionally, investigations concerning the initial perforation mechanism are conducted. Next to theoretical simulations, the laser induced effects are experimentally investigated by spectrometric and microscopic analysis. The results indicate that near field effects are the initial mechanism of membrane permeabilization.

**Conclusion:** This methodical approach combined with an automated setup, allows a high throughput targeting of several 100,000 cells within seconds, providing an excellent tool for *in vitro* applications in molecular medicine. NIR fs lasers are characterized by specific advantages when compared to lasers employing longer (ps/ns) pulses in the visible regime. The NIR fs pulses generate low thermal impact while allowing high penetration depths into tissue. Therefore fs lasers could be used for prospective *in vivo* applications.

**Keywords:** Laser transfection, Plasmonics, Nanoparticles, Permeabilization mechanisms, siRNA, Gene delivery

## Background

The direct modulation of gene expression is essential to establish therapeutic approaches in molecular medicine. Additionally to the development of therapies on the molecular level, the evaluation of target genes as therapeutic agents by combining the technology of RNAi and high throughput screenings is of major interest [1-3].

A major challenge in molecular medicine is the efficient, non-toxic and cell type independent transfection of cells in high throughput. In general a very effective manipulation strategy to achieve this is the transduction of cells via viral vectors. However, despite of the high efficiency this method bears high biological risk as integrational mutagenesis [4]. Alternative existing non-viral transfection methods show specific advantages and disadvantages. Transfection with lipid based reagents is often applied in high throughput assays but this method is cell type dependent and occasionally inefficient, especially for primary- and stem cell transfection [5]. Due to the difficulties in transfection of these cells, the commonly employed manipulation methods are either electroporation or nucleofection [6,7]. Unfortunately, these methods affect cell viability which is crucial when handling sensitive cells. Consequently in this manipulation it is essential to achieve a balance between transfection efficiency and methodical toxicity. Electroporation and

* Correspondence: m.schomaker@lzh.de
[1]Department of Biomedical Optics, Laser Zentrum Hannover, Hollerithallee 8, 30419 Hannover, Germany
Full list of author information is available at the end of the article

nucleofection can also be utilized for high throughput assays, but these physical techniques remain usually limited to well plates with low well numbers being additionally cost ineffective [8].

In order to address these challenges methodicaly, a variety of optical transfection techniques have been developed based on pulsed as well as continuously emitting lasers [9-13]. None of these techniques fulfills the requirements of an efficient and low-toxic transfection method combined with high throughput. Accordingly, there is no laser based technique currently established, that allows routinely laboratory or clinical use. A promising tool for molecular medical applications is the nanoparticle mediated laser transfection using a microchip laser emitting ps laser pulses with a resonant wavelength of 532 nm [14,15]. Herein, gold nanoparticle (AuNP) labeled cells are irradiated with a weakly focused laser beam. This method allows targeting many cells simultaneously, ensuring high throughput while maintaining a high spatial selectivity. Additionally, this physical method using resonant laser pulses is very promising for the manipulation of a variety of cell types.

By applying off-resonant fs laser pulses, the transfection of hematopoietic stem cells (CD34+) can be achieved [16]. Here, the excitation of the membrane adhered AuNP with the incident laser light leads to plasmon resonances which increase the absorption and scattering cross section of the AuNP by several orders of magnitude. When the AuNP is irradiated at a resonant wavelength, the laser energy is absorbed leading predominantly to thermal effects and changes in the particles morphology [15,17]. Using near infrared (NIR) femtosecond (fs) laser systems, off-resonant AuNP excitation can be achieved [18]. At this wavelength the absorption and therefore the thermal impact is reduced and the incident light is scattered into the near field of the particle. Due to this "nanolens" effect, an enhancement of the electric field in the near field takes place [19]. If the AuNP is adhered to the cell membrane, the field enhancement can initiate a spatially confined membrane

permeabilization [18]. In proof of principle experiments we could show the possibility to perforate the cell membrane using off resonant 800 nm fs laser pulses to deliver fluorescent labeled small interfering RNA (siRNA) and plasmid DNA (pDNA) into cells [20,21]. In another fs based study, a DNA-transfection rate of 23% using a melanoma cell line was stated and plasma induced nanocavitation is supposed as the membrane permeabilization effect [22]. The advantage of NIR wavelengths located in the "diagnostic window" regime of the electromagnetic spectrum results in higher penetration depths into biological tissue which might allow *in vivo* applications [23]. Furthermore, the low absorption cross section in the NIR reduces the risk of thermal induced AuNP fragmentation.

Within this work, microscopic analyses were performed to visualize the nanoparticle-cell membrane interaction, such that the co-incubation time for membrane permeabilization and the fundamental binding mechanism could be evaluated. To achieve an efficient uptake of extracellular molecules at high cell viabilities, a detailed parameter evaluation for a transient cell membrane permeabilization was performed. Different radiant exposures, scanning velocities of the laser spot, particle concentrations and particle sizes were applied to determine optimized permeabilization parameters. Additionally, the cell viability on a time scale up to 72 h after laser exposure and AuNP incubation was evaluated. The optimized parameters were used to evaluate the siRNA transfection efficiency, cell viability and functional oncogene knockdown in a cancer cell line. Due to the scanning method (Figure 1) and the automated setup, a high throughput is achieved and thus it is possible to handle all kinds of well plates within several minutes. Additionally to the manipulation experiments, the effects involved in the permeabilization process are investigated by temperature and near field simulations and a particle fragmentation study to further analyze the excitation of AuNP and the perforation mechanisms. The results indicate that both, near field and

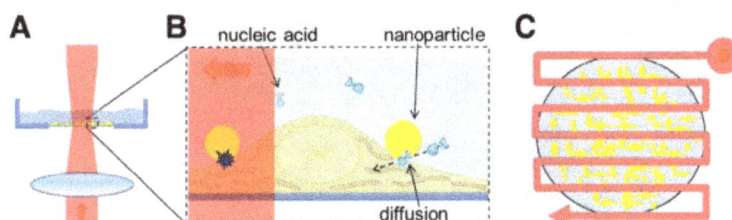

**Figure 1 Principle of AuNP mediated laser cell membrane permeabilization.** Spherical AuNP were incubated with the cells to allow sedimentation of the particles onto the cell membrane. Prepared samples were placed on an automatized stage to move selected wells of a well plate into the laser focus. Selected wells were completely irradiated by a raster shaped pattern with an inter line distance of 55 µm (1/3 of the laser diameter). **A)** Side view: the laser beam is weakly focused on the dish bottom where the AuNP labeled cells are located. **B)** Sketch of manipulation principle: AuNP are in contact with the cell membrane and irradiated by fs-laser pulses (left side). The interaction of the laser pulses with membrane adhered AuNP induces plasmon mediated effects which result in a transient enhanced permeability of the cell membrane. Through this permeabilization, extracellular molecules can cross the cell membrane and diffuse into the cytoplasm (right side). **C)** By applying a meander shaped scanning pattern, a high number of cells can be treated.

heating effects contribute to the mechanism of nanoparticle mediated membrane permeabilization in the fs regime.

## Results

### Interaction of cells with gold nanoparticles

Time lapse multiphoton microscopy was employed to monitor the incubation process. As shown in Figure 2A, bright spots, identified as the luminescence of the AuNP, are visible at the cell membrane after 3 h of incubation. Images which were taken at shorter incubation times show no spots or marginal changes in the background brightness. Increasing the incubation time from 3 to 5 h resulted slightly brighter luminescence. Within 5 to 7 h of co-incubation, the number and brightness of the AuNP signal saturated. The AuNP luminescence was still visible after washing, indicating that the particles remained adhered to the cell membrane.

Scanning electron microscopy (SEM) and environmental scanning electron microscopy (ESEM) provided detailed information about the attachment and distribution of the AuNP at the cell membrane after co-incubation and several washing steps (Figure 2B, C). The results show a loose dispersion of AuNP after 1 h of incubation. The particles were located at the culture dish bottom and on the cell membrane. By increasing the incubation time to more than 3 hours, the particles started to aggregate at the cell membrane. After an incubation time of 5 h, no further increase could be observed. Depending on the location of the particles, some of the particles appeared brighter than others. At higher magnifications, as visible in Figure 2C, some particles were located on the cell membrane (solid ellipse Figure 2C) and some were started to be endocytosed (dashed ellipse Figure 2C), which is demonstrated by the cell membrane covered

particles. Based on this we defined an incubation time of 3 h for our gold nanoparticle mediated laser transfection. Within this time a sufficient number of particles adhere to the cell membrane to induce membrane permeabilization. The number of particles at the cell membrane was counted using ESEM images of ZMTH3 cells taken after 3 h of incubation. An incubation concentration of 11 µg/ml was applied which represents the optimal concentration for cell manipulation. On average $164 \pm 50$ particles at the membrane of a single cell were counted.

### Evaluation of efficient and gentle cell manipulation parameters

To evaluate the optimal process parameters for an efficient and gentle cell manipulation, the cells were treated with different parameters in the presence of 10 kDa FITC labeled dextran and the corresponding fluorescence level was determined. As an indicator for viability, the respective metabolic activities of the manipulated cells were measured after laser treatment using an fluorescence based assay (Qblue). An efficiency ratio of the used parameters was evaluated as the normalized ratio of FITC fluorescent level and viability. The purpose was to optimize the parameters for later transfection experiments and to get an overview of the influence of the different parameters. It was not intended to determine absolute transfection efficiencies.

The influence of the scanning velocity on the molecular uptake targeting ZMTH3 cells is shown in Figure 3A. At a fixed scanning velocity, AuNP size and AuNP concentration of 11 µg/ml, the FITC fluorescence level increased with increasing radiant exposure. The highest efficiency ratio was found at 80 mJ/cm$^2$ for a scanning velocity of 50 mm/s. With higher radiant exposures, the

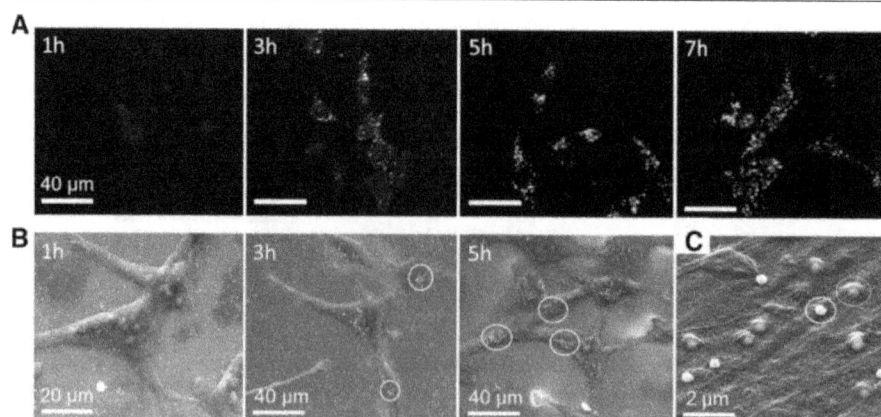

**Figure 2 Nanoparticle - cell interaction. A)** Time lapse multiphoton microscopy of granulosa cells with 150 nm particles after 1 h, 3 h, 5 h and 7 h of co-incubation. **B)** ESEM and **C)** SEM images of ZMTH3 cells after different incubation times with 200 nm gold particles. **B)** ESEM images: After 1 h a loose dispersion of particles is visible. After 3 h the AuNP started to aggregate (ellipse). The formation of particle clusters at the membrane can be observed after 5 h. **C)** SEM image in a higher magnification: After an incubation time of 3 h, particles are either on the cell membrane (solid ellipse) or covered by the membrane (dashed ellipse) [24].

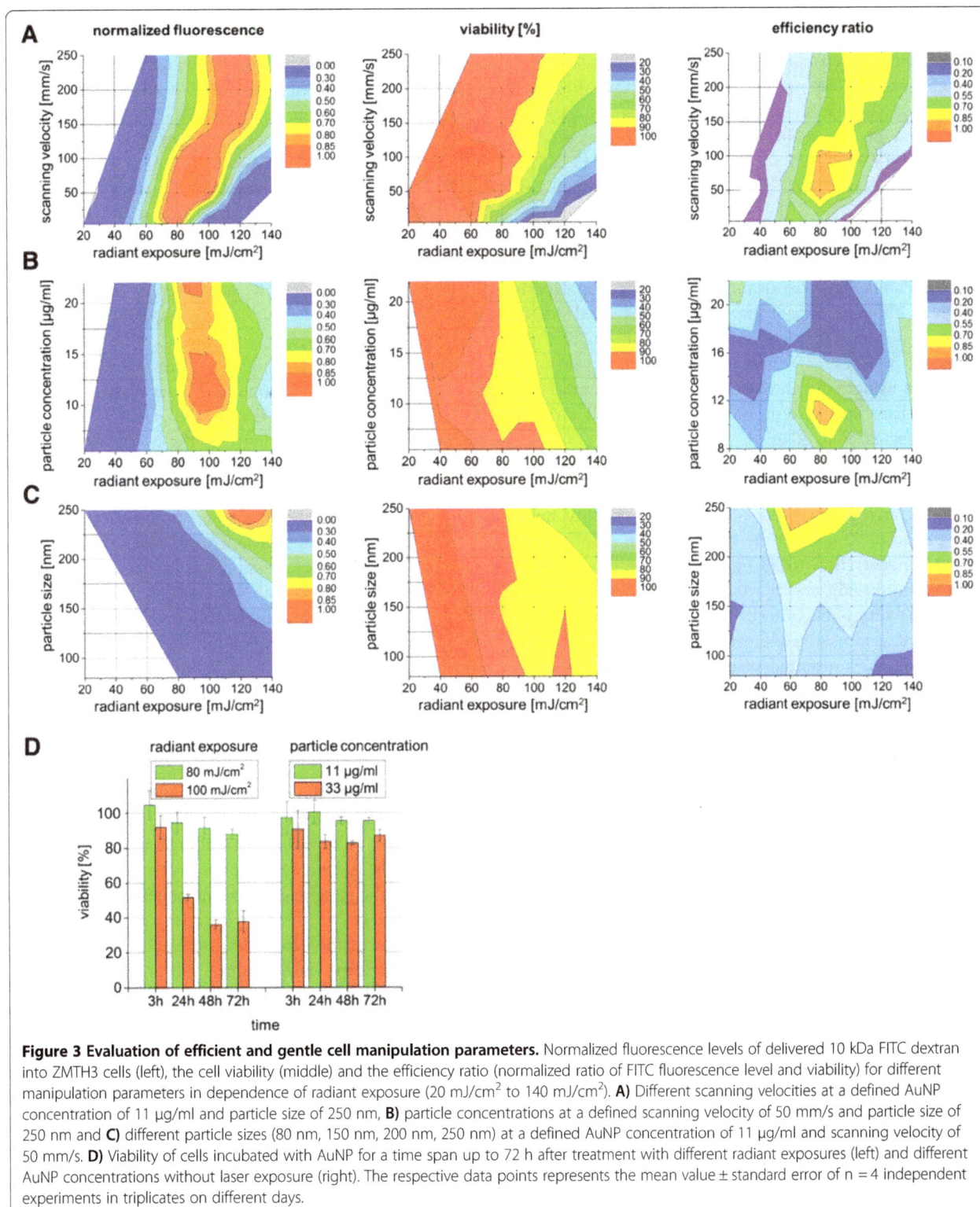

**Figure 3 Evaluation of efficient and gentle cell manipulation parameters.** Normalized fluorescence levels of delivered 10 kDa FITC dextran into ZMTH3 cells (left), the cell viability (middle) and the efficiency ratio (normalized ratio of FITC fluorescence level and viability) for different manipulation parameters in dependence of radiant exposure (20 mJ/cm² to 140 mJ/cm²). **A)** Different scanning velocities at a defined AuNP concentration of 11 µg/ml and particle size of 250 nm, **B)** particle concentrations at a defined scanning velocity of 50 mm/s and particle size of 250 nm and **C)** different particle sizes (80 nm, 150 nm, 200 nm, 250 nm) at a defined AuNP concentration of 11 µg/ml and scanning velocity of 50 mm/s. **D)** Viability of cells incubated with AuNP for a time span up to 72 h after treatment with different radiant exposures (left) and different AuNP concentrations without laser exposure (right). The respective data points represents the mean value ± standard error of n = 4 independent experiments in triplicates on different days.

efficiency ratio decreased due to a loss in cell viability as a consequence of an irreversible damage of the cell membrane and/or the ablation of the cells from the glass bottom. Varying the AuNP concentration (Figure 3B), the highest efficiency ratio was reached at a concentration of 11 µg/ml (6.3 µg/cm²) and a radiant exposure of 80 mJ/cm². When exceeding the threshold of 11 µg/ml the efficiency ratio dropped most likely due to many induced pores which consequently results in irreversible cell damage.

A further parameter impacting the efficiency ratio is the particle size (Figure 3C). A higher efficiency ratio was reached with an increase of particle size. Up to a particle size of 150 nm no efficient permeabilization occurred. Using larger particle sizes, the efficiency ratio peaked at a radiant exposure of 60 mJ/cm$^2$ for 200 nm and 60–80 mJ/cm$^2$ for 250 nm particles before the efficiency ratio dropped due to laser induced cell damage.

### Monitoring of the exposure effects on cell viability

The cell viability after performing permeabilization experiments at different radiant exposures and a fixed AuNP concentration of 11 µg/ml was followed up to 72 h. As presented in Figure 3D (left), the cell viability remained above 80% using radiant exposures up to 80 mJ/cm$^2$. For a higher radiant exposure of 100 mJ/cm$^2$ the cell viability strongly decreased to 40%.

The incubation of cells with AuNP at a concentration of 11 µg/ml for three hours without laser treatment did not show any pronounced effect on the viability for a time period of 72 h. Even the tripling of the AUNP incubation concentration to 33 µg/ml leads only to a slight decrease to 80-85% in cell viability. This negative effect on cell viability is likely to be caused by the residues of chloroauric acid used while particle manufacture.

Based on the presented results in Figure 3, the optimal parameter for an efficient cell permeabilization and tolerable cell loss is to a radiant exposure of 80 mJ/cm$^2$, a particle size of 250 nm and an AuNP concentration of 11 µg/ml.

### Nanoparticle mediated laser transfection

The evaluated parameters allowing an efficient and gentle cell permeabilization were used for cell transfection experiments. In Figure 4A the cell density is visualized by Hoechst 33342 nuclei staining. The successful transfection of CT1258 and ZMTH3 cells with an Alexa Fluor 488 labeled siRNA was performed using the optimized parameter (Figure 4B). Neither in the negative control (with siRNA, no laser treatment (Figure 4C)) nor in the AuNP control (with siRNA and AuNP incubation (Figure 4D)) a fluorescent signal was detected. Within the laser control (with siRNA and laser treatment, no AuNP) a weak fluorescence in individual cells was detected (Figure 4E). For CT1258 cells, a transfection efficiency of 85% ± 9 was evaluated using fluorescence microscopy. Here the fraction of necrotic cells was 3%. Flow cytometry analysis of ZMTH3 cells revealed a transfection efficiency of 90% and a cell viability of 93.5%. A significant difference (* p ≤ 0.05) was found between the siRNA samples and the native cells. The percentage of apoptotic cells was 2.15% and 5% for necrotic cells (Figure 4F).

In order to evaluate a potential gene therapeutic approach, functional siRNAs were used in a proof of principle experiment using high cell numbers. For HMGA2 (high mobility group AT-hook 2) gene knock down experiments the canine HMGA2 overexpressing cell line CT1258 [25] was transfected with four different anti-HMGA2 siRNAs complementary to the 3′-untranslated region of the HMGA2 mRNA and one non-sense scrambled siRNA. Due to the lack of reliable evaluated canine antibodies against the protein and thus potential unspecific cross reactions we opted for quantitative real-time PCR as detection method. This technique allows to measure the canine HMGA2 mRNA expression quantitatively.

The relative *HMGA2* mRNA expression was analyzed 48 h after treatment via one step quantitative real time PCR (qRT-PCR) analysis (Figure 4G). The *HMGA2* expression was quantified relative to the housekeeping gene *Beta-actin (ACTB)*, the non-treated cells were used for calibration (reference value = 1). In all samples treated with *HMGA2* specific siRNAs in combination with the laser manipulation suppression of *HMGA2* could be observed. The highest suppression was induced by using the siRNA 1 and 2. For the siRNA 1 and 3, the gene knock down was significant compared to native cells (p-values < 0.05). In the control samples, no *HMGA2* gene knock down could be observed. A slight increase was found for the scrambled siRNA, potentially resulting from off-target effects. No significant difference between the control samples and native cells was observed.

### Characterization of the nanoparticle mediated membrane permeabilization mechanism

In this section we describe different experiments to address the mechanisms involved in membrane permeabilization focusing on the parameters allowing an efficient and gentle cell manipulation.

Simulations of the near field distribution of the electric field at an incident wavelength of 796 nm for 80 nm and 250 nm particles are shown in Figure 5A and B, mapping the field-enhancement at the particles. For larger particles the dipole emission is distorted due to multipole oscillations within the sphere [17]. The enhancement factors of the different AuNP sizes are presented in Figure 5C (left y axis). For the used particles the highest field enhancement is reached for 150 nm particles. Here the near field is about 10 times higher than the incident field. For the 200 nm and 250 nm particles, the average enhancement is at 6.6 and 4.9, respectively. Furthermore, the near field volume is increasing with an increasing particle size (Table 1) and thereby the interaction zone of the near field with the membrane. This could be a reason for the increasing permeabilization efficiency at larger particle sizes shown in Figure 3C.

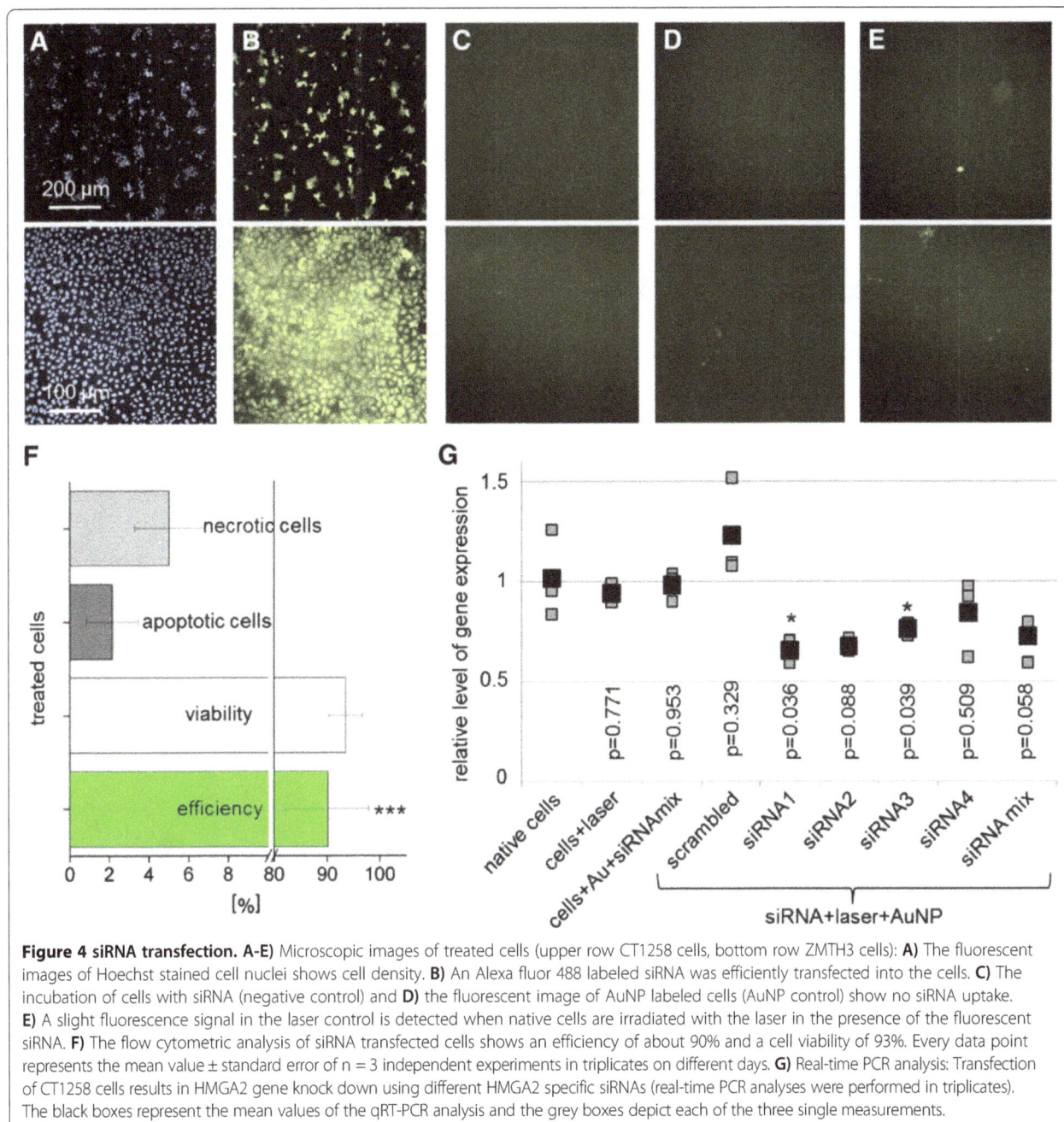

**Figure 4 siRNA transfection. A-E)** Microscopic images of treated cells (upper row CT1258 cells, bottom row ZMTH3 cells): **A)** The fluorescent images of Hoechst stained cell nuclei shows cell density. **B)** An Alexa fluor 488 labeled siRNA was efficiently transfected into the cells. **C)** The incubation of cells with siRNA (negative control) and **D)** the fluorescent image of AuNP labeled cells (AuNP control) show no siRNA uptake. **E)** A slight fluorescence signal in the laser control is detected when native cells are irradiated with the laser in the presence of the fluorescent siRNA. **F)** The flow cytometric analysis of siRNA transfected cells shows an efficiency of about 90% and a cell viability of 93%. Every data point represents the mean value ± standard error of n = 3 independent experiments in triplicates on different days. **G)** Real-time PCR analysis: Transfection of CT1258 cells results in HMGA2 gene knock down using different HMGA2 specific siRNAs (real-time PCR analyses were performed in triplicates). The black boxes represent the mean values of the qRT-PCR analysis and the grey boxes depict each of the three single measurements.

The evaluated enhancement factors and the applied intensity were used to calculate the near field intensity (Figure 5C (right y axis)). The values of the near field intensities of all particle sizes are below the threshold of an optical breakdown (LIOB) in water, which is $6\times10^{12}$ W/cm$^2$ for the used wavelength and pulse duration [26]. The highest near field intensity is reached for 150 nm particles which is close to the LIOB threshold. Intensities below the LIOB threshold in the low density plasma regime can lead to nonlinear effects like multiphoton ionization and avalanche-ionization. This might lead to the permeabilization of the cell membrane [14,22,27].

The accumulation of single pulses can induce the dissociation of biological molecules by forming reactive oxygen species (ROS) which results in membrane permeabilization [27]. Here, the threshold pulse energy $E_N$ depends on the number of pulses (Equation (1)) [14,27].

$$E_N = E_1 \cdot N^{-1/k}. \tag{1}$$

Where $E_1$ describes the threshold energy of a single pulse, N is the number of pulses and k the accumulation strength [28].

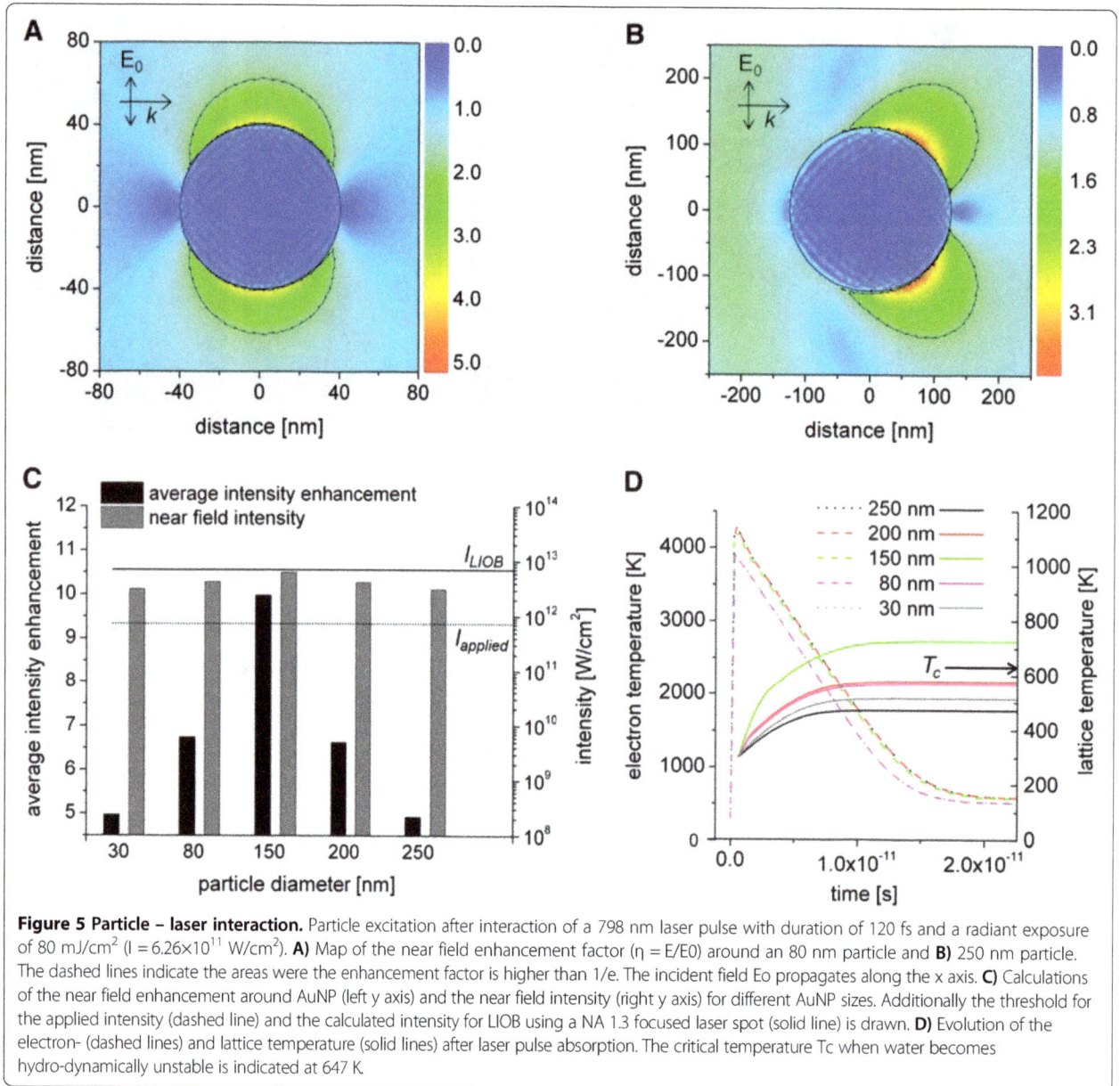

**Figure 5 Particle – laser interaction.** Particle excitation after interaction of a 798 nm laser pulse with duration of 120 fs and a radiant exposure of 80 mJ/cm² (I = 6.26×10¹¹ W/cm²). **A)** Map of the near field enhancement factor (η = E/E0) around an 80 nm particle and **B)** 250 nm particle. The dashed lines indicate the areas were the enhancement factor is higher than 1/e. The incident field Eo propagates along the x axis. **C)** Calculations of the near field enhancement around AuNP (left y axis) and the near field intensity (right y axis) for different AuNP sizes. Additionally the threshold for the applied intensity (dashed line) and the calculated intensity for LIOB using a NA 1.3 focused laser spot (solid line) is drawn. **D)** Evolution of the electron- (dashed lines) and lattice temperature (solid lines) after laser pulse absorption. The critical temperature Tc when water becomes hydro-dynamically unstable is indicated at 647 K.

The dependence of the pulse energy on the number of pulses for standardized fluorescence levels ("fluorescence brightness") is shown in Figure 6. A given fluorescence level corresponds to a specific amount of fluorescence molecules in the cells per well. We analyzed the number of laser pulses and pulse energy to yield four different fluorescence levels.

With an increasing number of pulses, less pulse energy is needed for an efficient permeabilization. An average accumulation strength of k = 5.57 ± 0.02 was evaluated

**Table 1 Near field and temperature related values for AuNP irradiated with 796 nm and 6.26 W/cm²**

| | 30 nm | 80 nm | 150 nm | 200 nm | 250 nm |
|---|---|---|---|---|---|
| Near field volume [nm³] ($I_{max}/e^2$) | $7\times10^3$ | $1.2\times10^5$ | $7.1\times10^5$ | $1.6\times10^6$ | $2.8\times10^6$ |
| Average near field intensity [W/cm²] | $3.8\times10^{12}$ | $2.5\times10^{12}$ | $1.7\times10^{12}$ | $2.5\times10^{12}$ | $3.3\times10^{12}$ |
| Absorption efficiency $Q_{abs}$ | 0.025 | 0.05 | 0.145 | 0.125 | 0.08 |
| Particle temperature [K] | 541 | 561 | 726 | 578 | 471 |

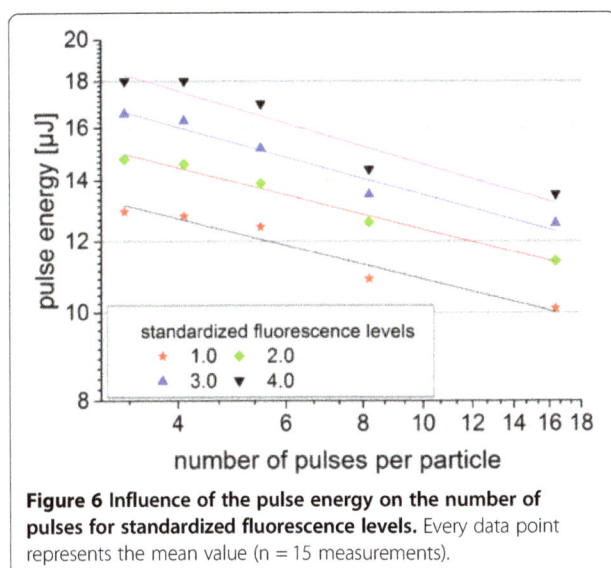

**Figure 6 Influence of the pulse energy on the number of pulses for standardized fluorescence levels.** Every data point represents the mean value (n = 15 measurements).

by a power-law fit (Table 2). This indicates that 5 photons with a photon energy of 1.55 eV at the applied wavelength of 796 nm are absorbed simultaneously to reach the ionization threshold of 6.6 eV for water [26].

When laser radiation is absorbed by the electrons of the AuNP the energy is transferred from the electrons to the particle lattice due to electron phonon coupling within a time span of a few ps and the particle temperature increases [29,30]. The temperature of the electrons and the lattice can be calculated with a two-temperature model (Figure 5D) [31]. The lattice temperature reaches the highest temperature of 726 K for 150 nm particles. This temperature is above the critical temperature ($T_c$) for phase transformation in water. For all other particles sizes this critical temperature is not reached. This reflects the different values for absorption efficiencies $Q_{abs}$ listed in Table 1.

The influence of the laser irradiation and possible changes in the particle morphology due to melting or fragmentation were analyzed by absorbance spectra of irradiated and non-irradiated particles (Figure 7A). After irradiation of 250 nm particles with radiant exposures of 60 mJ/cm$^2$ and 100 mJ/cm$^2$ a blue shift of the peak of 0.5 nm and 1.75 nm, occurred respectively (Table 3)). These shifts were in the SEM range of the untreated control. A reason for small changes can be polishing

effects due to surface melting of the particle, which occurs below the melting point of bulk gold [17]. At radiant exposures of 140 mJ/cm$^2$ and higher values the spectrum were broadly blue shifted (Table 3) and a narrowing of the spectrum occurred (Figure 7A). The spectrum of a 250 nm particle exposed to a radiant exposure of 300 mJ/cm$^2$ is broadly similar to the spectrum of 80 nm particles [32]. This clearly indicates a change in particle size due to laser exposure which can be induced by particle evaporation or near field ablation [17].

The value of the peak shift for different particle sizes after laser radiation in dependence of the radiant exposure is shown in Figure 7B. The highest peak shift of 80 nm was measured for 150 nm particles and barley changes with increasing radiant exposures. Relating to the AuNP size of 250 nm used for transfection a peak shift occurred at radiant exposures ≥ 140 mJ/cm$^2$. Furthermore, the amount of the peak shift for all radiant exposures is lower than for 150 nm particles which correlate with the calculated temperatures and near field enhancement in Figure 5.

## Discussion

In our study, we characterized the underlying mechanism and the potential of nanoparticle mediated cell membrane perforation in combination with fs-laser pulses as an alternative optical transfection method. Therefore the influencing parameters on the achieved perforation rate and cell viability were systematically determined and the successful transfection of cells with a fluorescent siRNA as well as the knock down of the oncogene *HMGA2* in tumor cells with specific siRNAs was demonstrated. Furthermore, the passive binding of AuNP to the cell membrane was studied.

Multiphoton and scanning electron microscopy images show the localization of AuNP near the cell membrane. Depending on the incubation time of the AuNP, single particles or clusters are located near, or associated with, the membrane. After an incubation time of 3 h the AuNP are clearly visible near the cell membrane. Within this time the particles form clusters with enhanced scattering of the laser light proved by multiphoton microscopy [33]. The agglomeration of particles after 3 hours is also visible in the ESEM images. This is in agreement with findings from Chithrani et al. who determined the uptake half-life at 2.24 h for 74 nm AuNP [33]. Furthermore, they evaluated the uptake of the number of particles per cell and also showed that the number of particles per cell saturated after 5 h. In the present study a particle number of approx. 160 was estimated at the membrane of a single cell for an incubation concentration of 11 μg/ml. Baumgart et al. [22] counted per cell 90 ± 23 AuNP with a diameter of 100 nm at an incubation concentration of 8 μg/ml after an incubation time

## Table 2 Power-law fit

|  | Threshold energy E$_1$ [μJ] | k | R$^2$ |
|---|---|---|---|
| 1.0 | 16.06 ± 0.7 | 5.88 ± 0.02 | 0.93 |
| 2.0 | 18.36 ± 0.7 | 5.88 ± 0.01 | 0.98 |
| 3.0 | 20.79 ± 0.7 | 5.55 ± 0.02 | 0.94 |
| 4.0 | 23.27 ± 0.7 | 5.00 ± 0.03 | 0.90 |

Dependence of the pulse energy on the number of pulses for standardized permeabilization efficiencies.

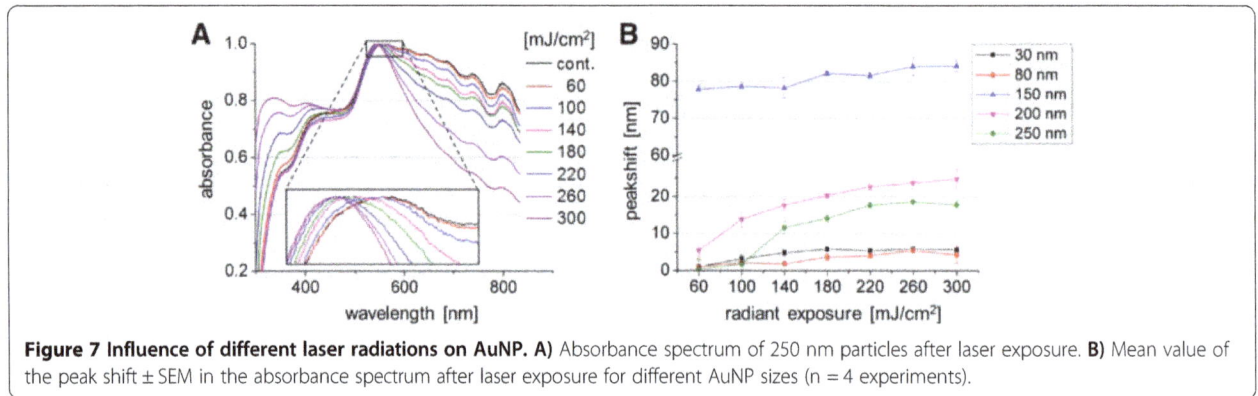

**Figure 7 Influence of different laser radiations on AuNP. A)** Absorbance spectrum of 250 nm particles after laser exposure. **B)** Mean value of the peak shift ± SEM in the absorbance spectrum after laser exposure for different AuNP sizes (n = 4 experiments).

of 6 h using SEM images. Taking into account that in this work a higher particle concentration and a larger diameter was used (and therefore a faster sedimentation of the particles takes place) the results are in a very good agreement.

In addition, Chithrani et al. evaluated the number of AuNP per vesicle and found an average number of 3 AuNP per vesicle for 100 nm particles. In comparison to our SEM images (see Figure 2B) we assume that one 200 nm particle per vesicle get endocytosed by the cell. As bare AuNP are used, a serum protein corona is formed at the particles surface and no specific binding at the cell membrane is likely to occur. Therefore, we suggested the receptor-mediated endocytosis (RME) to be the acting uptake mechanism [34].

The initial mechanism of plasmon mediated cell membrane permeabilization is still a current matter in research. Depending on the parameters, different mechanisms and effects are assumed. These are thermal ("nanoheater effect") [19,35], or near field enhancement effects ("nanolens effect") [18,35]. In addition, the generation of a low density plasma induced by multiphoton ionization combined with thermal effects can possibly lead to membrane permeabilization [14,15]. For short laser pulses in the nanosecond-picosecond regime, where the energy is mainly absorbed by the particle, thermal effects could be the main mechanism for membrane permeabilization [36-38]. After AuNP heating, the water evaporates followed by a shockwave and forming a cavitation bubble around the exposed particles as reported by Pitsillides et al. and Zharov et al. and enabling membrane perforation [39,40]. Using fs laser pulses, nanocavitation bubbles can be formed by the induced field enhancement. This enhancement can lead to an optical breakdown near the

particle and to the generation of a shockwave [18,36]. In this work, the evaluated intensities at the surface of single AuNP are near the threshold for an optical breakdown in the low density plasma regime. In existing studies, different concentrations of AuNP were required to achieve cell membrane perforation [15]. Higher numbers of particles are necessary to manipulate the cells with fs laser pulses [22,41]. Due to the formation of AuNP clusters the near field is further enhanced in comparison to single particles. The neighboring particles interact via the scattered waves and due to plasmon coupling "hot spots" are formed [42,43]. Taking into account that the field enhancement is higher for AuNP clusters compared to single particles, the intensities could be above the optical breakdown threshold [42].

Our assumption herein, that clusters of AuNP at the cell membrane are necessary to induce a field enhancement by fs laser pulses which is high enough to perforate the cell membrane. This is supported by the presented microscopic images and the number of AuNP utilized in this and other studies using fs laser pulses for membrane perforation [22,41]. Within the performed experiments we showed the efficient and transient permeabilization of the cell membrane due to an expected enhancement of the near field at the AuNP clusters. Based on this and the evaluated simultaneous absorption of 5 photons in the pulse number dependent experiments (Figure 6) we understand the near field enhancement followed by the multiphoton ionization of the surrounding medium as the initial perforation mechanism.

The fs laser pulses are enhanced in the near-field of the particle for membrane permeabilization by surface plasmon resonances. NIR fs laser pulses benefit from a

**Table 3 Mean values ± SEM for the peak shift in the absorbance spectrum**

| Radiant exposure [mJ/cm²] | 0 | 60 | 100 | 140 | 180 | 220 | 260 | 300 |
|---|---|---|---|---|---|---|---|---|
| Shift [nm] | 0 | 0.5 | 1.75 | 11.68 | 14.18 | 17.68 | 18.62 | 17.81 |
| SEM [nm] | ±2.98 | ±2.68 | ±2.21 | ±1.71 | ±1.01 | ±0.66 | ±0.13 | ±1.06 |

Irradiation of 250 nm particles with different radiant exposures (n = 4 experiments).

low thermal impact and a high penetration depth into tissue which is important for *in vivo* experiments. Furthermore, laser irradiation mediated fragmentation of nanoparticles is especially for *in vivo* settings an important issue. Fragmentation in small nanoparticles under 5 nm can lead to toxicity by intercalation into the DNA [44]. The comparison of fs pulses and ns pulses reveal a more pronounced change in particle morphology for longer (850 ps, 532 nm) pulses. In absorbance measurements, no pronounced peak shift (as indicator for particle morphology and size change) was detected for a fluence of 100 mJ/cm2, which exceeds the optimal fluence for cell manipulation (80 mJ/cm2) using NIR fs pulses (Table 3). In comparison to this, for 850 ps ($\approx$1 ns) pulses a peak shift of 15.4 nm was determined using the optimal manipulation fluence of 20 mJ/cm2. The change in particle morphology was caused due to thermal effects and the strong linear absorption at 532 nm. Nevertheless, the cell viability stayed above 80% in all the performed experiments suggesting the use of visible ns pulses for *in vitro* experiments [15]. For fs pulses, the cell viability was determined to be above 90%. The presented results and the advantages of NIR fs laser pulses (e.g. a high penetration depth and the avoidance of photo thermal effects) indicate the great potential of fs laser for *in vivo* manipulation. Furthermore the development of endoscopic systems for ultrafast laser microsurgery [45] or fiber based approaches [46] makes the application of ultrashort laser pulses potentially suitable for fs laser *in vivo* cell manipulation. Additionally, first *in vivo* experiments showed the generation of nanobubbles around AuNP clusters for selective cancer cell killing using short, 780 nm laser pulses [47]. Next to the properties of the fs laser pulses, an advantage of the presented method is the double selectivity by the spatial confined radiation (Figure 8A) and the possibility of specific cell targeting by antibody conjugated AuNPs. The latter can be used to induce selective cell manipulation or ablation in both, *in vitro* and *in vivo* models. For example, the treatment of squamous carcinoma cells in the buccal mucosa or at the tongue. Further in tumor scenarios where minimal invasive tissue ablation is essential as malignant glioblastoma, it is crucial to sustain non-target (healthy) tissue. Here the presented method can be a powerful tool. Exemplarily for primary cell manipulation a membrane impermeable fluorescent dye was delivered into a human embryonic stem cell (ES) cell line hES3 and a human induced pluripotent stem cell (iPSC) line hCBiPS2 (Figure 8B)." The results of the siRNA experiments show that fs nanoparticle mediated laser transfection is suitable for high throughput functional gene assays due to the short processing time of approximately 10 min per 96 well plate. As the applied AuNP were shown to be non-toxic, this method is excellent

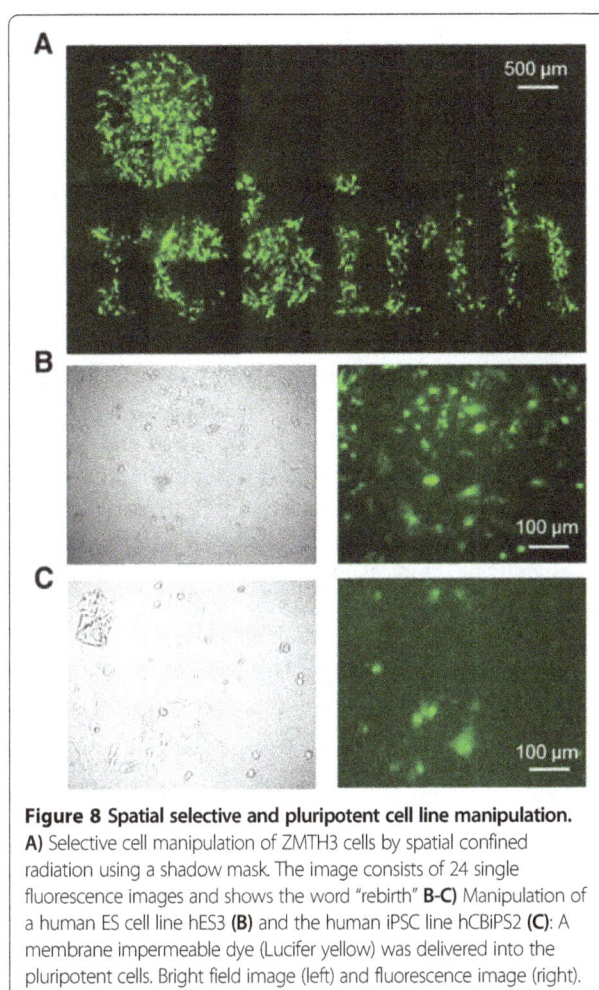

**Figure 8 Spatial selective and pluripotent cell line manipulation.**
**A)** Selective cell manipulation of ZMTH3 cells by spatial confined radiation using a shadow mask. The image consists of 24 single fluorescence images and shows the word "rebirth" **B-C)** Manipulation of a human ES cell line hES3 **(B)** and the human iPSC line hCBiPS2 **(C)**: A membrane impermeable dye (Lucifer yellow) was delivered into the pluripotent cells. Bright field image (left) and fluorescence image (right).

suited for *in vitro* application but also for other applications in molecular medicine. Furthermore, it can be applied for the manipulation of various cell types as shown in our previous work and by Baumgart et al. [16,22]. Additional applications as gene or cell therapeutic approaches can be served by this technique. As an example, it is possible to manipulate high cell numbers required for e.g. tumor vaccination strategies in an appropriate time. The knock down of the oncogene HMGA2 in canine prostate carcinoma cells was carried out successfully as shown by real time PCR expression analyses (Figure 4G). Due to the extraordinary high HMGA2 expression in the CT1258 cell line a incomplete siRNA mediated HMGA2 knock down within the treated cells was to be expected. Conventional HMBA2 knock down in less aggressive human pancreatic cell lines by Watanabe et al. [48] resulted in higher efficiencies. However, we opted to target the canine prostate cancer derived cell line CT1258 as canine prostate cancer represents the only spontaneously arising model for human prostate cancer with considerable incidence. This includes several tumor relevant aspects as biological behavior, marker gene expression and histological presentation [49]. Thus, a successful establishment of a therapeutic approach in dogs will offers high transfer potential to a human clinical setting. Consequently, prior to human clinical trials, a valid clinical trial in dogs as naturally occurring model is of major interest allowing to monitor the therapeutic intervention in an genetic outbreed model with unmanipulated immune system.

## Conclusion

Our studies on nanoparticle mediated fs laser cell perforation show, that this method is suitable for high throughput siRNA transfection with high efficiency and low cell toxicity. To establish this method as an alternative transfection technique, the manipulation of different cell types will be continued in further studies. However, due to the underlying physical mechanism the permeabilization should be cell type independent. Based on the mechanistic investigations, we assume that an enhancement of the near field occurs at AuNP clusters. This leads to the generation of a low density plasma with multiphoton ionization of the surrounding liquid, which in turn perforates the cell membrane. The uptake mechanism of extracellular molecules remains to be investigated in further experiments [50]. The presented method is an alternative transfection method to deliver molecules into living cells being particularly well suited for standardized processes like high throughput or high content screening assays for fundamental and pharmaceutical research.

## Methods
### Cell culture

The canine pleomorphic mammary adenoma cell line ZMTH3 [51] was cultured routinely in RPMI 1640 supplemented with 10% fetal calf serum (FCS) and 1% penicillin/streptomycin (Biochrom AG, Berlin, Germany). Rat granulosa cells (GFSHR-17) were cultivated in DMEM (Dulbecco's Modified Eagle Medium) supplemented with 5% FCS, 1% penicillin/streptomycin (Biochrom AG, Berlin, Germany). The canine prostate adenocarcinoma cell line CT1258 was derived from an extremely aggressive canine prostate carcinoma [52] and cultured in Medium 199 (Life Technologies GmbH, Darmstadt, Germany) supplemented with 10% FCS and 2% penicillin/streptomycin (Biochrom AG, Berlin, Germany). The human ES cell line hES3 and the human iPSC line hCBiPS2 [53] were cultured and expanded on irradiated mouse embryonic fibroblasts (MEF) in knockout DMEM supplemented with 20% knockout serum replacement, 1mM L-glutamine, 0.1mM β-mercaptoethanol, 1% nonessential amino acid stock (all from Life Technologies) and 10ng/ml bFGF (supplied by the Institute for Technical Chemistry, Leibniz University Hannover). One day before laser transfection cells were

detached from the feeder layer by 0.2% collagenase IV (Life Technologies) followed by an incubation step with TrypLE (Life Technologies) for single-cell dissociation and plated onto Matrigel™ (BD Biosciences) coated dishes in MEF-conditioned medium.

### Laser setup

The used automated setup for cell manipulation is operating with a fs amplifier laser system (Spitfire Pro, Newport Corporation, Irvine, USA). The generated laser pulses have a pulse duration of 120 fs at a fixed wavelength of 796 nm. The output power of the system is 2.1 W at a repetition rate of 5 kHz. To irradiate the biological tissue, the laser pulses were guided through an automatized attenuator consisting of a $\lambda/2$-plate and a polarizing beam splitter and reflected by two scanning mirrors (Litrack, JMLaser, Müller Elektronik, Spaiching, Germany). A convex lens with a focal length of 800 mm was used to focus the laser pulses onto the sample, located on the automatized stage (OptiScan, Prior, Jena, Germany), resulting in a spot diameter of 164 μm.

### Nanoparticle incubation

Prior to the laser cell manipulation experiments and to investigate the interaction of AuNP with the cell membrane, the cells were co-incubated with the AuNP at 37°C in a 5% $CO_2$ atmosphere. The AuNP were chemically manufactured in presence of chloroauric acid (PGO, Kisker Biotech, Steinfurt, Germany). Uncoated AuNP of 80 nm, 150 nm, 200 nm, 250 nm were used.

### Multiphoton microscopy

Images were obtained to evaluate the incubation time for AuNP mediated cell permeabilization and the possibility of a passive binding of the particles. Briefly, granulosa cells were incubated with 150 nm gold particles and imaged after different incubation times. After a PBS wash, the cells were observed with a custom built multiphoton microscope which is based on a fs-laser system tunable from $\lambda = 690$ nm to 1040 nm (Chameleon ultra II, Coherent, Göttingen, Germany) [27]. The images were recorded through a 100× oil immersion objective (Carl Zeiss AG, "Plan-Neofluar", NA = 1.3) at an excitation wavelength of $\lambda_{exc} = 700$ nm.

### Scanning electron microscopy (SEM) and environmental scanning electron microscopy (ESEM)

To investigate the interaction of cells and AuNP images of ZMTH3 cells were generated after different times of co-incubation with 200 nm particles. The cells were washed after co-incubation with AuNP and fixed by adding a 4% paraformaldehyde (PFA) solution with 0.2% glutaraldehyde at 4°C. For ESEM imaging the cells were washed after 20 min with distilled water. For SEM, the cells were further treated at room temperature for 20 min with a 2% osmium tetroxide solution. Subsequently, the cells were washed 3 times with water for 5 min before incubation with different ethanol concentrations for 10 min each (30%, 50%, 70%, 90%, 95%, 95% and 3 × 100%). Before sputtering the cells with a 5 nm gold layer, the cells were dried for 30 min under laminar air flow conditions. For counting AuNP at the cell membrane after incubation, ImageJ was used [54]. Values represent the mean of n = 6 images ± SEM.

## Plate reader measurements

To evaluate the optimal parameters of an efficient and gentle transfection, $2.5 \times 10^4$ canine ZMTH3 cells per well were seeded in a black wall/clear bottom 96 well plate (BD Bioscience, Heidelberg, Germany) 24 h before laser treatment. As an indicator of membrane permeabilization, fresh medium with 2 mg/ml of 10 kDa FITC-dextran (Sigma-Aldrich, Steinheim, Germany) was added to the cells. After laser treatment, the cells were incubated for 30 min followed by several washing steps until the background fluorescence from the permeabilization indicator (10 kDa FITC dextran) was eliminated. To measure the metabolic activity of the cells, 10% (v/v) of the resazurin based, fluorometric QBlue viability assay kit (BioCat GmbH, Heidelberg, Germany) was added to the medium. During an incubation time of 1 h, viable cells converted resazurin into the fluorescent form resuorufin. The fluorescence levels of the delivered FITC dextran (EX488/EM520 nm) for molecular delivery and the resorufin (EX570/EM600 nm) as an indicator for viability were measured by the Infinite 200 Pro plate reader (Tecan, Männedorf, Switzerland). The value for FITC dextran delivery was calculated by subtracting the fluorescent background from each sample and afterwards the highest FITC fluorescence level was normalized to 1. The cell viability (V) was determined by the QBlue fluorescence level of the sample ($F_s$), the fluorescence of the untreated control ($F_C$) and the background ($F_B$) (Equation(2)).

$$V = \frac{F_S - F_B}{F_C - F_B} \cdot 100 \qquad (2)$$

The efficiency ratio (E) was calculated by correlating the fluorescence level for molecular delivery ($F_{FITC}$) and viability (V) using equation (3). Afterwards the values were normalized to 1.

$$E = F_{FITC} \cdot V \qquad (3)$$

## Simulation of the particle temperature and near field

For a deeper insight into the mechanisms involved in membrane permeabilization using fs laser pulses, the particle temperature and the near field were analyzed. The temperature of the AuNP during fs irradiation was

calculated based on a two temperature model, employing data for the specific heat capacity of the electrons and the electron phonon coupling constant from Lin et al. [55]. Temperature loss due to interaction with the surrounding medium was not considered due to the short timescales used. The field strength and intensity as well as the near field volume were simulated by the discrete dipole approximation, using the software DDSCAT [56,57]. A dipole separation of less than 3.5 nm was used for the largest sphere with a diameter of 250 nm. Modeling of the optical breakdown intensities in the near field was performed according to the Keldysh theory following the approach used by Vogel et al. [26,58]. The maximum intensity divided by the square of e was considered as near field volume and the enhancement in the modeling of the optical breakdown as well as the near field volume were averaged in the according area.

## UV–Vis spectroscopy

Particle spectra were monitored to evaluate a possible peakshift (as an indicator for a change in particle size/shape) of laser irradiated particles compare to untreated particles. Therefore an UV/Vis spectroscope (UV 1650-PC, Shimadzu, Duisburg, Germany) was used. The particles were diluted in culture media (RPMI as described before) without phenol red at a concentration of 50 µg/ml. Using a 96 well plate, the samples with a total volume of 200 µl per well were irradiated in a meander pattern.

## Fluorescence microscopy

In order to evaluate the transfection efficiency of the CT1258 cells, fluorescence microscopy was applied. 24 h before laser treatment, $1 \times 10^4$ cells were seeded in each well of a 24 well plate (PAA Laboratories, Cölbe, Germany). For siRNA transfection, 10 µM of a fluorescently labeled (AlexaFluor488) siRNA (Qiagen, Hilden, Germany) was added to the extracellular medium before laser treatment. The samples were treated with the optimized parameters as evaluated within the plate reader measurements. After laser treatment, the cells were incubated for 30 min followed by several washing steps until the background fluorescence from the fluorescent siRNA was eliminated. Three independent experiments in duplicates were performed on different days. Three images of each well were analyzed using Image J. By counting the cell nuclei (ca. 546 per image, stained with HOECHST33342) and transfected cells (Alexafluor488 siRNA positive cells) the transfection efficiency was determined. Propidium Iodide was used as an indicator for necrotic cells.

## Flow cytometry analysis

Flow cytometric analysis was performed to evaluate the transfection efficiencies and the necrotic- and apoptotic rate. 24 h before laser treatment, $1.5 \times 10^5$ cells were seeded in each well of a 24 well plate. For siRNA transfection, 10 μM of a fluorescently labeled (AlexaFluor488) siRNA was added to the extracellular medium before laser treatment. The samples were treated with optimized parameters as evaluated within the plate reader measurements. Three hours after laser treatment the samples were prepared for flow cytometric analysis. Therefore, the cells were washed and trypsinized (TrypLE™, Life Technologies (LT), Darmstadt, Germany). A viability staining with Annexin V (V-PE-Cy5 Apoptosis Detection Kit, BioCat, Heidelberg, Germany) to detect the apoptotic cells, and with 1.5 μM Propidium Iodide (Invitrogen, Darmstadt, Germany) to identify necrotic cells, was performed. The positivity of siRNA transfected cells was determined by comparing the AlexaFluor488 fluorescence intensity to native cells, both measured in the FL1-H channel using a FACSCalibur flow cytometer (BD Bioscience, Heidelberg, Germany). Within the native cell population, a gate was set determining 98% of the native cells as non-transfected using the software Cell Quest (BD Bioscience, Heidelberg, Germany). This gate was subsequently applied on the siRNA transfected cell population resulting in the percentage of positive and non-transfected cells. To determine the ratio of apoptotic and necrotic cells within the siRNA transfected samples, the Annexin V and PI labelled cells were analyzed for PE-Cy5 fluorescence in the FL4-H channel and for PI in the FL2-H channel. Within the native cells a gate was set at which a cell population of 2% was identified as Annexin and PI positive and transferred to the sample with siRNA transfected cells to discriminate living from apoptotic and necrotic cells. For statistical analyses, the student's t-test was used. The significance is given as * for $p < 0.05$, ** for $p < 0.01$ and *** for $p < 0.001$.

## HMGA2 suppression analysis

As a proof of principle, that the presented method is suitable for molecular medicine approaches a functional gene knock down experiment was performed. We used the tumor cell line CT1258 which is characterized by overexpression of endogenous HMGA2 [25]. 24 h prior to transfection $3 \times 10^5$ cells were seeded per well into a 6 well plate (Greiner Bio-One GmbH, Frickenhausen, Germany). Cells were laser-transfected with 10 nM of different anti-HMGA2 siRNAs, a scrambled siRNA and a siRNA mix consisting of 10 nM of each of the four anti-HMGA2 siRNAs (Riboxx, Radebeul, Germany). The corresponding siRNA sequences are listed in Table 4. After a time span of 48 h the growth medium was removed from the CT1258 cells and 1 ml Tryp LE Express (Life Technologies GmbH, Darmstedt, Germany) was applied on cells. Once the cells were detached 1 ml cultivation medium was added to stop the reaction. Cell suspension was pelleted at 300 × g for 5 min. The supernatant was discarded and the pellet stored at −80°C until further processing.

**Table 4 Name and sequence of the used siRNAs for HMGA2 knock down**

| siRNA name | sequence |
| --- | --- |
| A2-3UTR 1 | 5′-UUAAUUCUCUCCGUAGCUCCCCC-3′ |
| A2-3UTR 2 | 5′-UCUUACUGUUCCAUUGGCCCCC-3′ |
| A2-3UTR 3 | 5′-AUUAUCCUUAAGAACCUAGCCCCC-3′ |
| A2-3UTR 4 | 5′-UUCUUACUGUUCCAUUGGCCCCC-3′ |
| scrambled siRNA | 5′-UAAGCACGAAGCUCAGAGUCCCCC-3′ |

## RNA extraction

For PCR analysis total RNA was isolated according to the "NucleoSpin miRNA" protocol (Macherey & Nagel, Düren, Germany). Small and large RNAs were finally eluted in 30 μl nuclease free water. Total RNA concentration was measured with the Synergy 2 reader (BioTek Instruments GmbH, Bad Friedrichshall, Germany).

## Quantitative one step real-time PCR analysis

For the relative *HMGA2* / *ACTB* quantification 25 ng total RNA were mixed with SYBR Green, *HMGA2* or *ACTB* specific primers, nuclease free water (Qiagen, Hilden, Germany) and reverse transcriptase according to the "QuantiTect SYBR Green RT-PCR" protocol (Qiagen, Hilden, Germany). The fluorescence of each sample was analyzed in triplicates. As negative controls a non-template and a no-reverse transcriptase control were included. The experiments were performed using the Mastercycler ep realplex (Eppendorf AG, Hamburg, Germany). qRT-PCR conditions were as follows: 30 min at 50°C and 15 s at 95°C, followed by 40 cycles with 15 s at 94°C, 30s at 60°C and 30 s at 72°C. Finally a melting curve analysis was performed to verify specificity and identity of the qRT-PCR products according to the Eppendorf Mastercycler ep realplex instrument instructions. For the comparison of the relative gene expression levels based on the ΔΔCT method the gene expression level of the untreated CT1258 cells was used as calibrator (calibrator expression level was set as 1). Statistical analysis of the qRT-PCR results was done by using the software tool REST 2009, version 2.0.13. A p-value of ≤ 0.05 was considered as statistically significant.

### Competing interests

The authors declare that they have no competing interests.

### Authors' contributions

MS: Conceived and designed the experiments, performed the laser perforation and transfection experiments. Performed multi photon imaging and laser-particle interaction experiments, manuscript drafting and wrote the paper. DH: Conceived and designed the experiments, performance of the SEM imaging experiments, participated in the perforation experiments. SK: Carried out the simulation for the particle temperature and near field enhancement. Wrote parts of the paper. SWi: Performed flow cytometry analysis and analyzed the data, Participated in drafting the transfection experiments, wrote parts of the paper. SWa: Performance of PCR analysis and data processing IN: Contributed reagents/materials/analysis tools and participation at biological study design. TR: Manuscript drafting, Contributed reagents/materials/analysis tools. HME: Donated cell line, partial study design. HM:

Drafting and wrote parts of the manuscript. AH: Conceptional design of the study, reagents/materials/analysis tools, manuscript drafting and finalization. All authors read and approved the final manuscript.

## Acknowledgments
The authors thank Regina Carlson for technical support in flow cytometry and the German Research Foundation DFG (within the Transregio 37 and the excellence cluster REBIRTH) for the financial support. We thank Ulrich Martin (Leibnitz Research Laboratories for Biotechnology and Artificial Organs (LEBAO), Hannover Medical School) for providing the hES3 and hCBiPS2 cells.

## Author details
[1]Department of Biomedical Optics, Laser Zentrum Hannover, Hollerithallee 8, 30419 Hannover, Germany. [2]Small Animal Clinic, University of Veterinary Medicine Hannover, Bünteweg 9, 30559 Hannover, Germany. [3]Department of Hematology, Oncology, and Palliative Medicine, University of Rostock, Ernst- Heydemann-Str. 6, 18057 Rostock, Germany. [4]Department of Cardiothoracic Transplantation and Vascular Surgery, Hannover Medical School, Carl-Neuberg-Str. 1, 30625 Hannover, Germany. [5]Institut für Quantenoptik Leibniz Universität Hannover Welfengarten 1, 30167 Hannover, Germany.

## References
1. Roth JA, Cristiano RJ: **Gene therapy for cancer: what have we done and where are we going?** *J Natl Cancer Inst* 1997, **89:**21–39.
2. Selkirk S: **Gene therapy in clinical medicine.** *Postgrad Med J* 2004, **80:**560–570.
3. Dorsett Y, Tuschl T: **siRNAs: applications in functional genomics and potential as therapeutics.** *Nat Rev Drug Discov* 2004, **3:**318–329.
4. Hacein-Bey-Abina S, Von Kalle C, Schmidt M, McCormack MP, Wulffraat N, Leboulch P, Lim A, Osborne CS, Pawliuk R, Morillon E, Sorensen R, Forster A, Fraser P, Cohen JI, de Saint Basile G, Alexander I, Wintergerst U, Frebourg T, Aurias A, Stoppa-Lyonnet D, Romana S, Radford-Weiss I, Gross F, Valensi F, Delabesse E, Macintyre E, Sigaux F, Soulier J, Leiva LE, Wissler M, *et al*: **LMO2-associated clonal T cell proliferation in two patients after gene therapy for SCID-X1.** *Science* 2003, **302:**415–419.
5. Uchida E, Mizuguchi H, Ishii-Watabe A, Hayakawa T: **Comparison of the efficiency and safety of non-viral vector-mediated gene transfer into a wide range of human cells.** *Biol Pharm Bull* 2002, **25:**891–897.
6. Karra D, Dahm R: **Transfection techniques for neuronal cells.** *J Neurosci* 2010, **30:**6171–6177.
7. Papapetrou EP, Zoumbos NC, Athanassiadou A: **Genetic modification of hematopoietic stem cells with nonviral systems: past progress and future prospects.** *Gene Ther* 2005, **12**(Suppl 1):118–130.
8. Krausz E: **High-content siRNA screening.** *Mol BioSyst* 2007, **3:**232–240.
9. Tsukakoshi M, Kurata S, Nomiya Y, Ikawa Y, Kasuya T: **A novel method of DNA transfection by laser microbeam cell surgery.** *App Phys B* 1984, **35:**135–140.
10. Terakawa M, Ogura M, Sato S, Wakisaka H, Ashida H, Uenoyama M, Masaki Y, Obara M: **Gene transfer into mammalian cells by use of a nanosecond pulsed laser-induced stress wave.** *Opt Lett* 2004, **29:**1227–1229.
11. Tirlapur UK, König K: **Targeted transfection by femtosecond laser.** *Nature* 2002, **418:**290–291.
12. Soughayer JS, Krasieva T, Jacobson SC, Ramsey JM, Tromberg BJ, Allbritton NL: **Characterization of cellular optoporation with distance.** *Anal Chem* 2000, **72:**1342–1347.
13. Stevenson DJ, Gunn-Moore FJ, Campbell P, Dholakia K: **Transfection by Optical Injection.** In *Handbook of Photonics for Biomedical science.* Edited by Tuchin VV. Boca Raton: CRC Press, Taylor and Francis Group; 2010:87–118.
14. Kalies S, Heinemann D, Schomaker M, Escobar HM, Heisterkamp A, Ripken T, Meyer H: **Plasmonic laser treatment for Morpholino oligomer delivery in antisense applications.** *J Biophotonics* 2013, doi:10.1002/jbio.201300056
15. Heinemann D, Schomaker M, Kalies S, Schieck M, Carlson R, Murua Escobar H, Ripken T, Meyer H, Heisterkamp A: **Gold nanoparticle mediated laser transfection for efficient siRNA mediated gene knock down.** *PLoS One* 2013, **8:** doi:10.1371.
16. Schomaker M, Killian D, Willenbrock S, Heinemann D, Kalies S, Ngezahayo A, Nolte I, Ripken T, Junghanss C, Meyer H, Murua Escobar H, Hesterkamp A: **Biophysical effects in off-resonant gold nanoparticle mediated (GNOME) laser transfection of cell lines, primary- and stem cells using fs laser pulses.** *J Biophotonics* 2014, doi:10.1002/jbio.201400065.

17. Hashimoto S, Werner D, Uwada T: **Studies on the interaction of pulsed lasers with plasmonic gold nanoparticles toward light manipulation, heat management, and nanofabrication.** *J Photoch Photobiol C* 2012, **13:**28–54.
18. Boulais E, Lachaine R, Meunier M: **Plasma mediated off-resonance plasmonic enhanced ultrafast laser-induced nanocavitation.** *Nano Lett* 2012, **12:**4763–4769.
19. Nedyalkov NN, Imamova S, Atanasov PA, Tanaka Y, Obara M: **Interaction between ultrashort laser pulses and gold nanoparticles: nanoheater and nanolens effect.** *J Nanopart Res* 2011, **13:**2181–2193.
20. Schomaker M, Fehlauer H, Bintig W, Ngezahayo A, Nolte I, Murua Escobar H, Lubatschowski H, Heisterkamp A: **Fs-laser cell perforation using gold nanoparticles of different shapes.** *Proc SPIE* 2010, **7589:**75890C.
21. Schomaker M, Killian D, Willenbrock S, Diebbold E, Mazur E, Bintig W, Ngezahayo A, Nolte I, Murua Escobar H, Junghanß C, Lubatschowski H, Heisterkamp A: **Ultrashort laser pulse cell manipulation using nano- and micro- materials.** *Proc SPIE* 2010, **7762:**77623G.
22. Baumgart J, Humbert L, Boulais É, Lachaine R, Lebrun JJ, Meunier M: **Off-resonance plasmonic enhanced femtosecond laser optoporation and transfection of cancer cells.** *Biomaterials* 2012, **33:**2345–2350.
23. König K: **Multiphoton microscopy in life sciences.** *J Microsc* 2000, **200:**83–104.
24. Schomaker M: *Plasmonenbasierte Zelltransfektion im Hochdurchsatz mittels ultrakurzer Laserpulse.* Garbsen, Germany: Degree Thesis, University Hannover, PZH Verlag; 2013.
25. Winkler S, Murua Escobar H, Meyer B, Simon D, Eberle N, Baumgartner W, Loeschke S, Nolte I, Bullerdiek J: **HMGA2 expression in a canine model of prostate cancer.** *Cancer Genet Cytogenet* 2007, **177:**98–102.
26. Vogel A, Noack J, Hüttman G, Paltauf G: **Mechanisms of femtosecond laser nanosurgery of cells and tissues.** *Appl Phys B* 2005, **81:**1015–1047.
27. Kuetemeyer K, Rezgui R, Lubatschowski H, Heisterkamp A: **Influence of laser parameters and staining on femtosecond laser-based intracellular nanosurgery.** *Biomed Opt Express* 2010, **1:**587597.
28. Jee Y, Becker MF, Walser RM: **Laser-induced damage on single-crystal metal surfaces.** *J Opt Soc Am B* 1988, **5:**648–659.
29. Ekici O, Harrison RK, Durr NJ, Eversole DS, Lee M, Ben-Yakar A: **Thermal analysis of gold nanorods heated with femtosecond laser pulses.** *J App Phys D* 2008, **41:**1–11.
30. Pelton M, Aizpurua J, Bryant G: **Metal-nanoparticle plasmonics.** *Laser Photon Rev* 2008, **2:**136–159.
31. Anisimov SI, Kapeliovich BL, Perel'man TL: **Electron emission from metal surfaces exposed to ultrashort laser pulses.** *Soviet Physics JETP* 1974, **39:**375–377.
32. Jain PK, Lee KS, El-Sayed IH, El-Sayed MA: **Calculated absorption and scattering properties of gold nanoparticles of different size, shape, and composition: applications in biological imaging and biomedicine.** *J Phys Chem B* 2006, **110:**7238–7248.
33. Chithrani BD, Ghazani AA, Chan WC: **Determining the size and shape dependence of gold nanoparticle uptake into mammalian cells.** *Nano Lett* 2006, **6:**662–668.
34. Nel AE, Mädler L, Velegol D, Xia T, Hoek EM, Somasundaran P, Klaessig F, Castranova V, Thompson M: **Understanding biophysicochemical interactions at the nano-bio interface.** *Nat Mater* 2009, **8:**543–557.
35. Pustovalov VK, Smetannikov AS, Zharov VP: **Photothermal and accompanied phenomena of selective nanophotothermolysis with gold nanoparticles and laser pulses.** *Laser Phys Lett* 2008, **5:**775–792.
36. Bisker G, Yelin D: **Noble-metal nanoparticles and short pulses for nanomanipulations: theoretical analysis.** *JOSA B* 2012, **29:**1383–1393.
37. Lukianova-Hleb E, Hu Y, Latterini L, Tarpani L, Lee S, Drezek RA, Hafner JH, Lapotko DO: **Plasmonic nanobubbles as transient vapor nanobubbles generated around plasmonic nanoparticles.** *ACS Nano* 2010, **4:**2109–2123.
38. Lukianova-Hleb EY, Ren X, Constantinou PE, Danysh BP, Shenefelt DL, Carson DD, Farach-Carson MC, Kulchitsky VA, Wu X, Wagner DS, Lapotko DO: **Improved cellular specificity of plasmonic nanobubbles versus nanoparticles in heterogeneous cell systems.** *Plos one* 2012, **7:**e34537.
39. Pitsillides CM, Joe EK, Wei X, Anderson RR, Lin CP: **Selective cell targeting with light-absorbing microparticles and nanoparticles.** *Biophys J* 2003, **84:**4023–4032.
40. Zharov VP, Galitovsky V, Viegas M: **Photothermal detection of local thermal effects during selective nanophotothermolysis.** *Appl Phys Lett* 2003, **83:**4897–4899.
41. Minai L, Yeheskely-Hayon D, Golan L, Bisker G, Dann EJ, Yelin D: **Optical nanomanipulations of malignant cells: controlled cell damage and fusion.** *Small* 2012, **8:**1732–1739.

42. Quinten M: **Local fields close to the surface of nanoparticles and aggregates of nanoparticles.** *Appl Phys B* 2001, **73**:245–255.

43. Nedyalkov NN, Atanasov PA, Obara M: **Near-field properties of a gold nanoparticle array on different substrates excited by a femtosecond laser.** *Nanotechnology* 2007, **18**:305703.

44. Skuridin SG, Dubinskaya VA, Rudoy VM, Dement'eva OV, Zakhidov ST, Marshak TL, Kuz'min VA, Popenko VI, Evdokimov YM: **Effect of gold nanoparticles on DNA package in model systems.** *Dokl Biochem Biophys* 2010, **432**:141–143.

45. Ferhanoglu O, Yildirim M, Subramanian K, Ben-Yakar A: **A 5-mm piezo-scanning fiber device for high speed ultrafast laser microsurgery.** *Biomed Opt Express* 2014, **5**:2023–2036.

46. Ma N, Gunn-Moore F, Dholakia K: **Optical transfection using an endoscope-like system.** *J Biomed Opt* 2011, **16**:028002.

47. Lukianova-Hleb EY, Ren X, Sawant RR, Wu X, Torchilin VP, Lapotko DO: **On-demand intracellular amplification of chemoradiation with cancer-specific plasmonic nanobubbles.** *Nat Med* 2014, **20**:778–784.

48. Watanabe S, Ueda Y, Akaboshi S, Hino Y, Sekita Y, Nakao M: **HMGA2 maintains oncogenic RAS-induced epithelial-mesenchymal transition in human pancreatic cancer cells.** *Am J Pathol* 2009, **174**:854–868.

49. Withrow JS, Vail DM: Withrow and MacEwen's Small Animal Clinical Oncology. 5th ed. St Louis Missouri: Saunders Company; 2012.

50. Davis AA, Farrar MJ, Nishimura N, Jin MM, Schaffer CB: **Optoporation and genetic manipulation of cells using femtosecond laser pulses.** *Biophys J* 2013, **105**:862–871.

51. Murua Escobar H, Meyer B, Richter A, Becker K, Flohr AM, Bullerdiek J, Nolte I: **Molecular characterization of the canine HMGB1.** *Cytogenet Genome Res* 2003, **101**:33–38.

52. Winkler S, Murua Escobar H, Eberle N, Reimann-Berg N, Nolte I, Bullerdiek J: **Establishment of a cell line derived from a canine prostate carcinoma with a highly rearranged karyotype.** *J Hered* 2005, **96**:782–785.

53. Haase A, Olmer R, Schwanke K, Wunderlich S, Merkert S, Hess C, Zweigerdt R, Gruh I, Meyer J, Wagner S, Maier LS, Han DW, Glage S, Miller K, Fischer P, Schöler HR, Martin U: **Generation of induced pluripotent stem cells from human cord blood.** *Cell stem cell* 2009, **5**:434–441.

54. Schneider CA, Rasband WS, Eliceiri KW: **NIH Image to ImageJ: 25 years of image analysis.** *Nat Methods* 2012, **9**:671–675.

55. Lin Z, Zhigilei LV, Celli V: **Electron–phonon coupling and electron heat capacity of metals under conditions of strong electron–phonon nonequilibrium.** *Phys Rev B* 2008, **77**:075133.

56. Draine BT, Flatau PJ: **Discrete-dipole approximation for scattering calculations.** *J Opt Soc Am A* 1994, **11**:1491–1499.

57. Draine, BT, Flatau PJ: *User Guide to the Discrete Dipole Approximation Code DDSCAT 7.2.* 2012.

58. Keldysh LV: **Ionization in the field of a strong electromagnetic wave.** *J Exptl Theoret Phys (USSR)* 1964, **47**:1945–1957. translation: *Soviet Physics JETP* 1965, **20**: 1307–1314.

# Development of antibody functionalized magnetic nanoparticles for the immunoassay of carcinoembryonic antigen: a feasibility study for clinical use

Che-Chuan Yang[1], Shieh-Yueh Yang[1*], Chia-Shin Ho[1], Jui-Feng Chang[1], Bing-Hsien Liu[1] and Kai-Wen Huang[2,3]

## Abstract

**Background:** Magnetic nanoparticles functionalized antibodies are used for *in-vitro* assays on bio-markers. This work demonstrates the synthesis of high-quality magnetic nanoparticles coated with antibodies against carcinoembryonic antigen (CEA). Various characterizations, such as particle size, particle suspension, bio-activity and the stability of bio-magnetic nanoparticles suspended in liquid, are studied. The properties for the assay of CEA molecules in serum are also studied. The assay method used is so-called immunomagnetic reduction.

**Results:** The results show that the effects of common materials in serum that interfere with detected signals are not significant. The low-detection limit is 0.21 ng/ml, which is well below the clinical threshold of 2.5 ng/ml.

**Conclusions:** The dynamic range for the assay of CEA molecules in serum is 500 ng/ml. By assaying serum CEA molecules from 24 normal controls and 30 colorectal-cancer patients, the threshold for the serum-CEA concentration to diagnose colorectal cancer is 4.05 ng/ml, which results in a clinical sensitivity of 0.90 and specificity of 0.87.

**Keywords:** Bio-magnetic nanoparticles, Carcinoembryonic antigen, Assay, Colorectal cancer

## Background

Bio-functionalized magnetic particles are used in biomedicines. Different bio-applications require different sizes of magnetic particles. For example, because each particle is strongly magnetized, magnetic particles with micrometer diameters are useful for *in-vitro* extraction or purification of bio-molecules such as antibodies, proteins and nucleic acids [1-3]. Magnetic nanoparticles with sub-micrometer diameters are used to sort specific cells *in vitro*, [4-6]. The main reason for the use of sub-micro-particles instead of micro-particles for cell sorting is to suppress the immunological responses from cells that are bound with magnetic particles. Nano-scaled magnetic particles are mostly used for *in-vivo* targeting or delivery, e.g. as a contrast medium for magnetic resonance imaging, vectors for drug delivery and for hyperthermia [7-10]. In the late 1990's, the *in-vitro* quantitative detection of bio-molecules using antibody functionalized magnetic nanoparticles was proposed [11-13]. This is referred to as a magnetically labeled immunoassay (MLI).

There are several types of MLI: sandwiched MLI [12,14,15], wash-free MLI [11,13] and single-probe MLI [11,13,16]. Different types of magnetic signals are detected for various types of MLI, including, ac magnetic susceptibility [15], magnetic relaxation [11], magnetic remanence [12], phase lag for ac magnetization [17], nuclear magnetic resonance [18] and magnetic reduction [13] and these are related to the concentrations of bio-molecules that are to be detected. In addition to this academic innovation, the literature shows that MLI is a promising method for *in-vitro* diagnosis in clinics. Since the early part of this century, some MLI technology has been commercialized in the US [19], France [20], Germany, Sweden [21], Japan, China [22] and Taiwan [23]. There has been continuing investment in the development, the commercialization and the marketing of MLI, worldwide.

* Correspondence: syyang@magqu.com
[1]MagQu Co., Ltd., Sindian Dist, New Taipei City 231, Taiwan
Full list of author information is available at the end of the article

In a MLI, bio-functionalized magnetic nanoparticles are used as labeling markers to target molecules. If a test sample has more target molecules, more magnetic nanoparticles associate with target molecules. Ideally, each magnetic nanoparticle is identical. Every nanoparticle has the same size and magnetization. Each associated magnetic nanoparticle contributes equally to the magnetic signals. If more magnetic nanoparticles associate with target molecules, the magnetic signal is greater. The magnetic signals are exactly correlated to the number of target molecules. The precession of assay target molecules is high. However, if the magnetic nanoparticles obviously differ from each other and there is a broad variation in particle size, magnetic nanoparticles of different sizes contribute differently to the magnetic signals. This results in a significant variation in the magnetic signals for a fixed number of associated magnetic nanoparticles, so the precision the assay of target molecules is poor. For a MLI, it is important that the bio-functionalized magnetic nanoparticles are uniform. For a MLI, magnetic nanoparticles are suspended in solution as a reagent. When these nanoparticles agglomerate, the binding area between the nanoparticles and the target molecules is significantly reduced, which results in a reduced sensitivity and stability for detection, so the agglomeration of nanoparticles in a reagent must be inhibited.

Other required properties for the use of suspended bio-functionalized magnetic nanoparticles as a reagent for *in-vitro* diagnosis in clinics are the life time, the interference, the low-detection limit, the sensitivity and the specificity. Most previous studies have focused on the development of either magnetic nanoparticles or detection methodologies, so there has been no complete study of the feasibility of the clinical use of bio-functionalized magnetic nanoparticles for *in-vitro* diagnosis. This study characterizes both the particle properties and the assay features of antibody functionalized magnetic nanoparticles. The target molecule is the carcinoembryonic antigen (CEA), which is the clinical bio-marker for the *in-vitro* diagnosis of colorectal cancer. The antibodies against CEA (anti-CEA) are immobilized on magnetic nanoparticles. Various characteristics, such as particle size, particle suspension, bio-activity and the stability of the anti-CEA functionalized magnetic nanoparticles suspended in liquid are studied. The assay method used is the so-called immunomagnetic reduction. Assaying CEA in serum allows features such as the interference, the low-detection limit, the dynamic range, the clinic sensitivity and the specificity to be determined.

## Results and discussion
### Stability of magnetic nanoparticle suspension
The schematic composition of anti-CEA functionalized magnetic nanoparticles is shown in Figure 1(a). The distribution of anti-CEA functionalized magnetic nanoparticles suspended in PBS solution in hydrodynamic diameter is

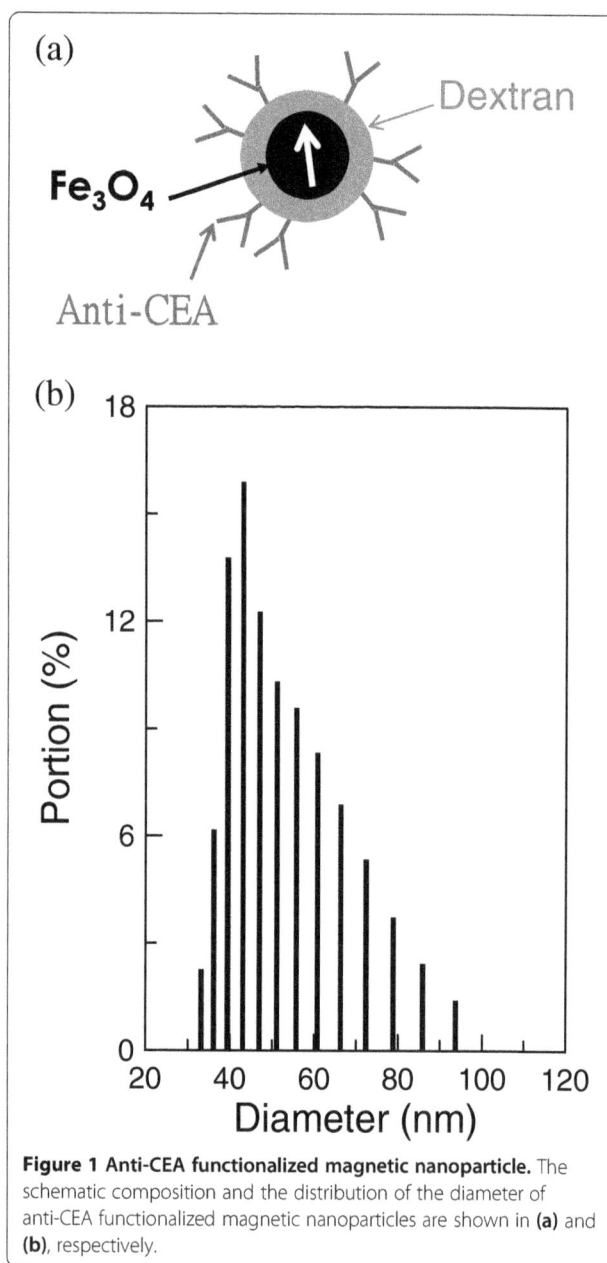

Figure 1 Anti-CEA functionalized magnetic nanoparticle. The schematic composition and the distribution of the diameter of anti-CEA functionalized magnetic nanoparticles are shown in (a) and (b), respectively.

shown in Figure 1(b). The mean value and the standard deviation of the hydrodynamic diameter are found to be 51.3 nm and 13.51 nm, respectively, as measured using dynamic laser scattering. Hereafter, the anti-CEA functionalized magnetic nanoparticles suspended in PBS solution are referred to as CEA reagent. The CEA reagent was stored at 2–8°C. During the storage, the mean value and standard deviation for the hydrodynamic diameter of anti-CEA functionalized magnetic nanoparticles were monitored. The results are shown in Figure 2, as dots with error bars. The error bars correspond to the standard deviation of the hydrodynamic diameter of anti-CEA functionalized magnetic nanoparticles. It is obvious that the particle

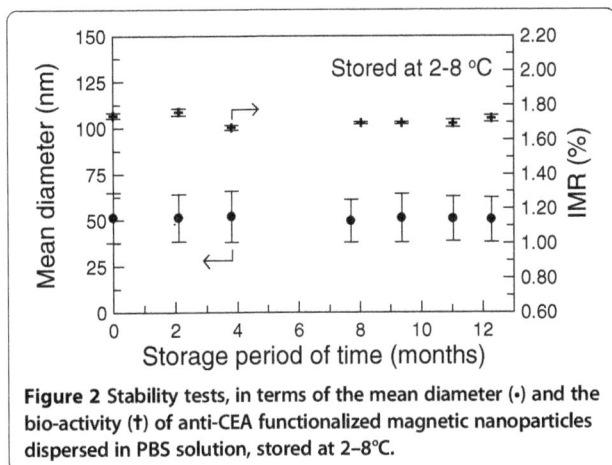

**Figure 2** Stability tests, in terms of the mean diameter (•) and the bio-activity (†) of anti-CEA functionalized magnetic nanoparticles dispersed in PBS solution, stored at 2–8°C.

diameter remains almost unchanged, when it is stored at 2–8°C for 12 months. This shows that there is no significant agglomeration of the anti-CEA functionalized magnetic nanoparticles in CEA reagent that is stored at 2–8°C for 12 months. Namely, the suspension of anti-CEA functionalized magnetic nanoparticles remains stable for 12 months. The stability of the suspension of the nanoparticles in the reagent is important for clinic use. When nanoparticles agglomerate, the association area between antibodies and target molecules varies. The output signal decays as the association area is reduced. The assay result is unreliable, if there is any agglomeration of nanoparticles. Fortunately, the results shown as dots in Figure 2 demonstrate the high stability of the suspension of anti-CEA functionalized magnetic nanoparticles in PBS solution, stored at 2–8°C.

The factors that mainly affect the stability of a nanoparticle suspension in solution are the nano-size and the uniformity of the nanoparticles. If the nano-size is sufficient, the buoyancy of the nanoparticle is strong enough to cancel the gravitational force, so the nanoparticle is suspended in solution. However, for a certain magnetic nanoparticle in the reagent, there can be attractive or repulsive magnetic interactions between the magnetic nanoparticle and neighboring magnetic nanoparticles. If the magnetic nanoparticles are highly uniform, these magnetic interactions are isotropic. The resultant magnetic force that acts on this magnetic nanoparticle is zero and the magnetic interactions with these magnetic nanoparticles can be ignored. This nanoparticle is not attracted by other particles because there are no anisotropic magnetic forces. Magnetic nanoparticles do not agglomerate because of the isotropic magnetic interaction between particles, so highly uniform magnetic nanoparticles exhibit high stability in suspension in solution. The results shown in Figure 1(b) show the nano-size and the high degree of uniformity of the anti-CEA functionalized magnetic nanoparticles synthesized in this

work. As a result, the CEA reagent is highly stable in a suspension in PBS solution.

## Stability of magnetic nanoparticle bio-activity

In addition to the suspension stability, the other important measurement for the CEA reagent is the bio-activity during storage at 2–8°C. To measure this, the IMR signals for 5-ng/ml CEA solution were detected using the CEA reagent, during the storage period. The measurements for the storage period for the IMR signals for the 5-ng/ml CEA solution are plotted in Figure 2, using crosses. The IMR signals range from 1.67% to 1.76%, during storage at 2–8°C for nine months. There is no significant change in the IMR signal for the 5-ng/ml CEA solution during nine months of storage at 2–8°C. Therefore, the bio-activity of the CEA reagent is stable for at least nine months, if the CEA reagent is stored at 2–8°C.

## Room-temperature stability of reagent

For the experimental results shown in Figure 2, the CEA reagent was originally at 2–8°C and was then stored at a room temperature of 25°C. The temperature of the CEA reagent was gradually increased from 2–8°C to 25°C over 5 minutes. 40-μl CEA reagent was used for each IMR measurement. The remainder of the CEA reagent was replace in storage at 2–8°C. When all of the samples were ready, the stored CEA reagent was warmed to 25°C, from 2–8°C, for IMR measurements. This thermal circle could easily damage the bio-activity of CEA reagent, so the CEA reagent was maintained at 25°C, to allow continuous IMR measurements for several samples. In order to determine the bio-activity of CEA reagent stored at 25°C, the CEA reagent was moved from a storage temperature of 2–8°C to 25°C. After 5 minutes, the temperature of the CEA reagent reached 25°C and the CEA reagent was maintained at 25°C for 24 hours. The time period in the x axis in Figure 3 begins at the 5th minute after the reagent was

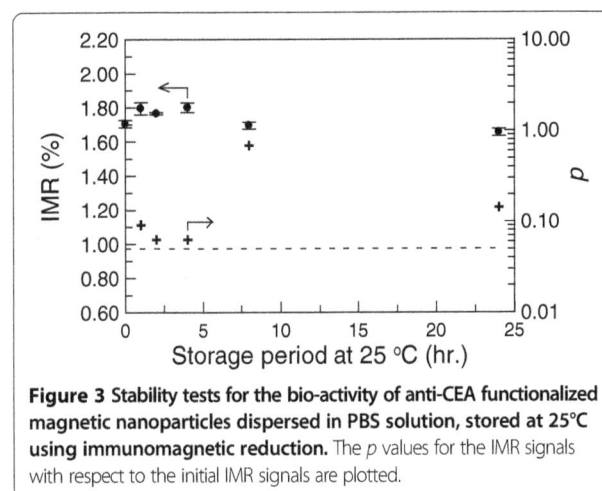

**Figure 3** Stability tests for the bio-activity of anti-CEA functionalized magnetic nanoparticles dispersed in PBS solution, stored at 25°C using immunomagnetic reduction. The *p* values for the IMR signals with respect to the initial IMR signals are plotted.

moved from a storage temperature of 2–8°C to 25°C. The signals for 5-ng/ml CEA solutions for the 25-°C CEA reagent were detected for 24 hours. The results are plotted as dots in Figure 3. The IMR signals at the beginning, i.e. time period =0, are used as a reference. The $p$ values of the IMR signals at other time points with respect to the referenced IMR signal are plotted as crosses in Figure 3. All of the $p$ values are greater than 0.05, which means that there is no significant difference in the IMR signals shown in Figure 3. The results in Figure 3 show that the bioactivity is stable for 24 hours, even if the CEA reagent is stored at 25°C.

### Interference tests

In clinics, serum is the sample that is used to assay CEA. There are many other materials in serum, besides CEA. These materials are referred as to interfering materials. Interfering materials can cause false IMR signals, because of the colors of bio-molecules or the non-specific associations between the interfering materials and antibodies on the magnetic nanoparticles. The accuracy of an assay is adversely affected if false IMR signals occur frequently, so the contributions of the interfering materials to IMR signals for the assay of CEA in serum must be determined.

Serum can contain interfering materials such as hemoglobin, bilirubin, or triglyceride because of common diseases, such as hemolysis, jaundice or hypertriglyceridemia. Other bio-materials that exist naturally in serum, such as uric acid, rheumatoid factor, intra lipid or albumin, are also interfering materials. Other interfering materials include drugs or chemicals in medicine that is used to treat inflammatory diseases, viral and bacteria infections, cancers and cardiovascular disease. All of the natural biomaterials and drugs or chemicals tabulated in Table 1 were spiked into serum that had 5 ng/ml CEA. A 5-ng/ml CEA solution was used because this CEA concentration is approximately the clinical threshold of CEA concentration for the diagnosis of colorectal cancer (~2.5 to 5 ng/ml). The concentrations of these interfering materials are also listed in Table 1. It is worthy of note that the concentrations of the interfering materials are much greater than ordinary levels. For example, the level of hemoglobin in the blood of a patient with hemolysis is around 500 μg/ml. The concentration of hemoglobin used in Sample No. 2 is 1000 μg/ml. The IMR signals for these 5-ng/ml CEA serum solutions are listed in Table 1. The IMR signal for the serum (Sample No. 1) with only 5-ng/ml CEA is used as a reference. All of the other IMR signals for the serum samples (Sample Nos. 2–32) with both 5-ng/ml CEA and the interfering materials are compared with the reference IMR signal. The corresponding $p$ values calculated T-Test and are shown in Table 1. The $p$ values IMR signals for the serum samples with interfering materials are greater than 0.05, as shown in Table 1. This demonstrates that,

with the exception of acetyl cysteine and furosemide, the bio-molecules, drugs and chemicals listed in Table 1 do not interfere with the assay for CEA in serum.

The false IMR signal that is caused by interfering materials is mainly attributable to two factors: the color of the interfering materials and the non-specific associations between the interfering materials and antibodies on the magnetic nanoparticles. The detection signal used for IMR measurement is magnetic ac susceptibility, which is not affected by the colors of the samples, the reagents, or the interfering materials, so the color of the interfering materials does not cause false IMR signals to be generated.

The non-specific associations between the interfering materials and antibodies on the magnetic nanoparticles are inhibited if highly specific antibodies are used. An additional suppression mechanism is activated during IMR measurement. During the IMR measurement, the magnetic nanoparticles oscillate with the external ac magnetic fields. Both the target and other bio-molecules that are bound with antibodies on the oscillating magnetic nanoparticles experience centrifugal forces. At high oscillation frequencies, the centrifugal force is increased. If the centrifugal force is stronger than the binding force between the antibodies and non-target bio-molecules, the non-specific binding is broken, so the centrifugal force must be weaker than the specific binding force between the antibodies and the bio-molecules that are to be detected. As a result, the cross reactions are inhibited during IMR measurement. In principle, this suppression mechanism for non-specific binding between antibodies and non-target bio-molecules is independent of the concentration of the target molecules, such as CEA. A detailed discussion of this suppression mechanism is given in Ref. [24].

### CEA-concentration dependent IMR signals

In addition to the detection of IMR signal for the 5-ng/ml CEA serum sample, the IMR signals for serum samples with CEA at various concentrations, from 0.1 ng/ml to 1000 ng/ml, were measured. The experimental results for the relationship between the CEA-concentration and the IMR signal (IMR(%)-$\phi_{CEA}$) are plotted as dots in Figure 4(a). The detailed results are tabulated in Table 2. The error bar for each data point in Figure 4(a) corresponds to the standard deviation for multiple detections of IMR signals for a given test sample. The IMR signal gradually increases, as the CEA concentration increases from 0.1 ng/ml, and then almost becomes saturated at a CEA concentration of 500 ng/ml. The IMR(%)-$\phi_{CEA}$ relationship is described by the logistic function:

$$IMR(\%) = \frac{A-B}{1+\left(\frac{\varphi_{CEA}}{\varphi_o}\right)^{\gamma}} + B \qquad (1)$$

**Table 1 Materials and concentrations used for interference tests for a CEA assay, using the IMR method**

| Sample no. | Interfering material | Concentration | Mean IMR value (%) | Standard deviation of IMR (%) | p value |
|---|---|---|---|---|---|
| 1 | None | - | 1.70 | 0.021 | - |
| 2 | Hemoglobin | 10000 µg/ml | 1.71 | 0.014 | 0.246 |
| 3 | Bilirubin | 600 µg/ml | 1.66 | 0.021 | 0.100 |
| 4 | Triglyceride | 30000 µg/ml | 1.72 | 0.007 | 0.167 |
| 5 | Uric acid | 200 µg/ml | 1.69 | 0.021 | 0.150 |
| 6 | Rheumatoid factor | 500 IU/ml | 1.68 | 0.014 | 0.246 |
| 7 | Intra lipid | 30000 µg/ml | 1.67 | 0.007 | 0.099 |
| 8 | Albumin | 60000 µg/ml | 1.67 | 0.014 | 0.150 |
| 9 | Acetaminophen | 300 µg/ml | 1.72 | 0.007 | 0.167 |
| 10 | Acetyl cysteine | 150 µg/ml | 1.68 | 0.021 | 0.223 |
| 11 | Acetylsalicylic acid | 500 µg/ml | 1.74 | 0.021 | 0.100 |
| 12 | Ascorbic acid | 300 µg/ml | 1.71 | 0.014 | 0.246 |
| 13 | Atrovastatin | 3 µg/ml | 1.71 | 0.014 | 0.246 |
| 14 | Furosemide | 4000 µg/ml | 1.70 | 0.014 | 0.404 |
| 15 | Ibuprofen | 1000 µg/ml | 1.72 | 0.049 | 0.326 |
| 16 | Levodopa | 20 µg/ml | 1.71 | 0.014 | 0.246 |
| 17 | Methyldopa | 200 µg/ml | 1.72 | 0.014 | 0.150 |
| 18 | Naprosyn sodium | 500 µg/ml | 1.66 | 0.021 | 0.100 |
| 19 | Phenylbutazone | 400 µg/ml | 1.65 | 0.007 | 0.052 |
| 20 | Prednisone | 5 µg/ml | 1.69 | 0.014 | 0.404 |
| 21 | Tegafur with uracil | 50 µg/ml | 1.70 | 0.021 | 0.500 |
| 22 | Theophylline | 50 µg/ml | 1.69 | 0.014 | 0.404 |
| 23 | Warfarin | 50 µg/ml | 1.66 | 0.014 | 0.096 |
| 24 | Ampicillin sodium | 1000 µg/ml | 1.67 | 0.021 | 0.146 |
| 25 | Cefoxitin | 2500 µg/ml | 1.73 | 0.014 | 0.096 |
| 26 | Cyclosporeine A | 10 µg/ml | 1.71 | 0.007 | 0.296 |
| 27 | Doxycycline hyclate | 50 µg/ml | 1.68 | 0.021 | 0.223 |
| 28 | Irinotecan | 100 µg/ml | 1.69 | 0.014 | 0.404 |
| 29 | Lovastatin | 2.5 µg/ml | 1.72 | 0.014 | 0.150 |
| 30 | Metronidazole | 200 µg/ml | 1.70 | 0.021 | 0.500 |
| 31 | Oxaliplatin | 100 µg/ml | 1.72 | 0.014 | 0.150 |
| 32 | Rifampicin | 60 µg/ml | 1.74 | 0.007 | 0.051 |

The concentration of the CEA in each sample is 5 ng/ml. The matrix is serum. The detected mean value and the standard deviation of each sample are listed. The p values of IMR signals for other samples are calculated using the IMR signals for the pure CEA-serum sample as a reference and the results are listed in the right-most column.

where A, B, $\phi_o$ and $\gamma$ are fitting parameters. Fitting the data in Figure 4(a) to Eq. (1) gives values for these parameters of as A =1.05, B =3.22, $\phi_o$ =14.05, and $\gamma$ =0.94. The fitting curve is plotted as a solid line in Figure 4(a). The coefficient of determination, $R^2$, is 0.999.

The stability of the resulting logistic function Eq. (1) depends on the stability of the reagent. Several factors, such as the biodegradability of the antibodies on the magnetic nanoparticles, the agglomeration of the magnetic nanoparticles and the de-magnetization of the magnetic nanoparticles significantly affect the lifetime of the reagent. If these factors do not change, the characteristics of the logistic function Eq. (1) are retained.

In Figure 2, the high stability of the particles' suspension and isolation in the reagent is demonstrated. The particle size is plotted as a function of the storage time at 2–8°C. The IMR signal for 5-ng/ml CEA solution is dependent on storage time, which demonstrates the bio-active stability of the antibodies on the magnetic nanoparticles. The magnetization of the magnetic nanoparticles does not change if the storage temperature remains lower than the Curie temperature of $Fe_3O_4$ (~585°C). The results in

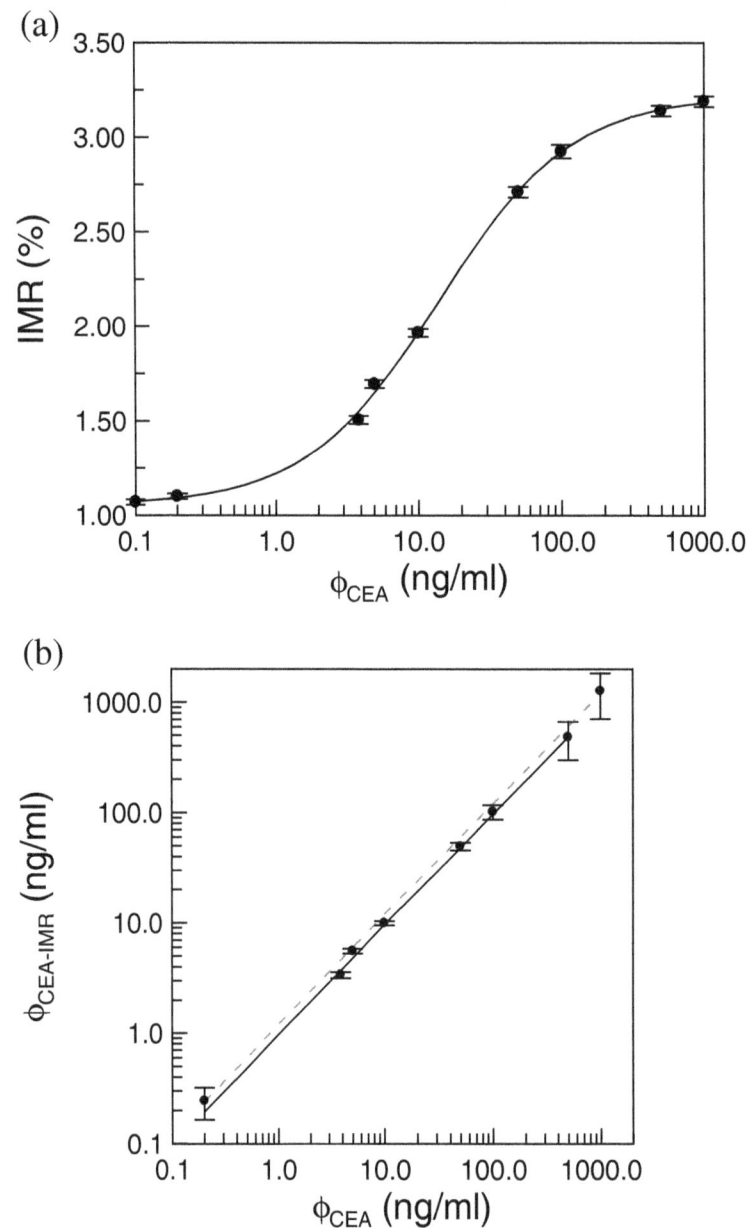

**Figure 4** Spiked-CEA-concentration-in-serum, $\varphi_{CEA}$, and (a) IMR signal and (b) the CEA concentration, $\varphi_{CEA\text{-}IMR}$, derived using the immunomagnetic reduction method.

Figure 2 show that the factors that most greatly affect the lifetime of the reagent are unchanged, if the reagent is stored at 2–8°C for 12 months, so it is expected that the resultant logistic function Eq. (2) is stable over 12 months.

### Low-detection limit of assaying serum CEA

In Eq. (1), A denotes the IMR signal as the CEA concentration approaches zero, so parameter A in Eq. (1) represents the background level for the detection of IMR signals. This non-zero background level is mainly due to the electronic noise of the IMR analyzer and the dynamic equilibrium for

the association between the CEA molecules and anti-CEA on the magnetic nanoparticles. Using the 3-$\sigma$ criterion, the low-detection limit for the assay of CEA in terms of the IMR signal is $(1.05 + 3 \times 0.014)\% = 1.09\%$, where 0.014% is the standard deviation of the IMR signals at low CEA concentrations, such as 0.1 ng/ml. Using Eq. (1), the CEA concentration that corresponds to the IMR signal of 1.09% is 0.21 ng/ml. Therefore, the low-detection limit for the assay of CEA in serum using IMR is 0.21 ng/ml. It is significant that the threshold of CEA concentration in serum for the diagnosis of colorectal cancer is 2.5 ng/ml. The IMR

**Table 2 CEA concentrations, $\varphi_{CEA}$, spiked in serum, for the detections of IMR signals**

| $\varphi_{CEA}$ (ng/ml) | Mean IMR value (%) | Standard deviation of IMR (%) | Converted CEA concentration $\varphi_{CEA\text{-}IMR}$ (ng/ml) |
|---|---|---|---|
| 0.10 | 1.07 | 0.014 | 0.08 ± 0.07 |
| 0.20 | 1.10 | 0.014 | 0.24 ± 0.08 |
| 3.85 | 1.51 | 0.021 | 3.38 ± 0.21 |
| 5.00 | 1.70 | 0.021 | 5.58 ± 0.28 |
| 10.0 | 1.97 | 0.021 | 9.99 ± 0.43 |
| 50.0 | 2.71 | 0.028 | 49.49 ± 3.83 |
| 100 | 2.93 | 0.035 | 101.7 ± 15.0 |
| 500 | 3.14 | 0.028 | 482.6 ± 184.7 |
| 1000 | 3.19 | 0.028 | 1269.6 ± 560 |

The mean values and the standard deviations of the detected IMR signals are shown. Using the detected IMR signals, the CEA concentrations, $\varphi_{CEA\text{-}IMR}$, derived using Eq. (1), are listed in the right-most column.

method allows sufficiently sensitive blood tests for the *in-vitro* diagnosis of colorectal cancer.

### Linearity of assaying serum CEA

A careful inspection for Figure 4(a) shows that not every data point lies on the solid line. If the experimental IMR signals are used to derive the CEA concentration, using Eq. (1), the derived CEA concentrations, $\phi_{CEA\text{-}IMR}$, are not exactly the same as those $\phi_{CEA}$ values that are shown in Table 2. It is noted that $\phi_{CEA}$ denotes the spiked CEA concentration in serum, but $\phi_{CEA\text{-}IMR}$ denotes the CEA concentration in serum, detected using the IMR method. The correlation between $\phi_{CEA\text{-}IMR}$ and $\phi_{CEA}$ is shown in Figure 4(b). Since the low-detection limit for the assay of CEA using IMR method is 0.21 ng/ml, a $\phi_{CEA\text{-}IMR}$ of 0.1-ng/ml CEA solution is not used in Figure 4(b). Figure 4(b) shows the linear relationship between $\phi_{CEA\text{-}IMR}$ and $\phi_{CEA}$. If the $\phi_{CEA\text{-}IMR}$ values for CEA concentration $\phi_{CEA}$ values from 0.2 ng/ml to 1000 ng/ml are used in Figure 4(b), the slope of the $\phi_{CEA\text{-}IMR}$-$\phi_{CEA}$ curve is 1.21 and the coefficient of determination, $R^2$, is 0.989, as plotted with the dashed line in Figure 4(b). The US Food and Drug Administration (FDA) regulations state that the slope of the line in Figure 4(b) must be between 0.90 and 1.10. The slope of the dashed line in Figure 4(b) does not meet the requirement of the US FDA. However, if the $\phi_{CEA\text{-}IMR}$ for a CEA concentration $\phi_{CEA}$ of 1000 ng/ml is ignored, the curve for $\phi_{CEA\text{-}IMR}$ against $\phi_{CEA}$ is linear and is plotted with a solid line in Figure 4(b). The slope of this solid line is 0.97 and the coefficient of determination, $R^2$, is 0.999. It is worthy of note that the slope of the solid line meets the requirement of the US FDA. The range of CEA concentrations used for the solid line in Figure 4(b) is from 0.2 ng/ml to 500 ng/ml, so the dynamic range of the CEA concentration for IMR assay is 500 ng/ml.

A comparison of the low-detection limit and the dynamic range of a CEA assay for commercially available kits (e.g. Siemens, Abbott, and Roche) used in the work is listed in Table 3. It is clear that the IMR assay for CEA is highly sensitive and has a broad dynamic range, which renders it suitable for clinical use.

### Clinical tests for assaying serum CEA

Using the relationship shown in Figure 4(a), the CEA concentrations in human serum samples can be determined using the IMR signals. 24 serum samples from healthy subjects (Normal control) and 30 serum samples from patients with colorectal cancer (CRC) were used for the CEA assay, using the IMR method. CRC patients were identified using either pathological evidence or an immunoassay. The detected CEA concentrations $\phi_{CEA\text{-}IMR}$ of these serum samples are plotted in Figure 5(a). The $\phi_{CEA\text{-}IMR}$ values for the normal control group are distributed over a relatively lower range than those for CRC patients. Most of $\phi_{CEA\text{-}IMR}$ values for the normal control group are within the range, 0.6 ng/ml to 1.5 ng/ml, but the $\phi_{CEA\text{-}IMR}$ values for CRC patients range from 6.0 ng/ml to 20 ng/ml. An analysis of the receiver operating characteristic (ROC) curve shown in Figure 5(b) shows that the threshold for the diagnosis of CRC by an assay of CEA in serum, using the IMR method, is 4.05 ng/ml, which results in the clinic sensitivity of 0.90 and a specificity of 0.87.

### Conclusions

Antibodies against carcinoembryonic antigen (CEA) are conjugated onto magnetic nanoparticles, to synthesize a magnetic reagent for the assay of CEA in serum. The reagent gives a highly stable particle suspension in pH-7.4 phosphate buffered saline (PBS) solution and CEA molecules with a highly stable bio-activity, when the reagent is stored at 2–8°C. The immunomagnetic reduction method gives a low-detection threshold for the assay of CEA is 0.21 ng/ml and the dynamic range is 500 ng/ml. There is no significant interference with the assay of CEA in serum by bio-molecules that commonly occur in serum, or by

**Table 3 Comparison of the low-detection limit and the dynamic range of a CEA assay using commercially available kits (e.g. Siemens, Abbott, and Roche) and those for this work (denoted as this work)**

| Company/Model | Low-detection limit | Dynamic range | Approval |
|---|---|---|---|
| Siemens/ADVIA Centuar CEA assay | 0.5 ng/ml | 0.5 - 100 ng/ml | USFDA |
| Abbott/AXSYM system CEA assay | 0.5 ng/ml | 0.5 - 500 ng/ml | USFDA |
| Roche/Elecsys CEA assay | 0.2 ng/ml | 0.2 - 1,000 ng/ml | USFDA, CE |
| This work | 0.21 ng/ml | 0.21 - 500 ng/ml | None |

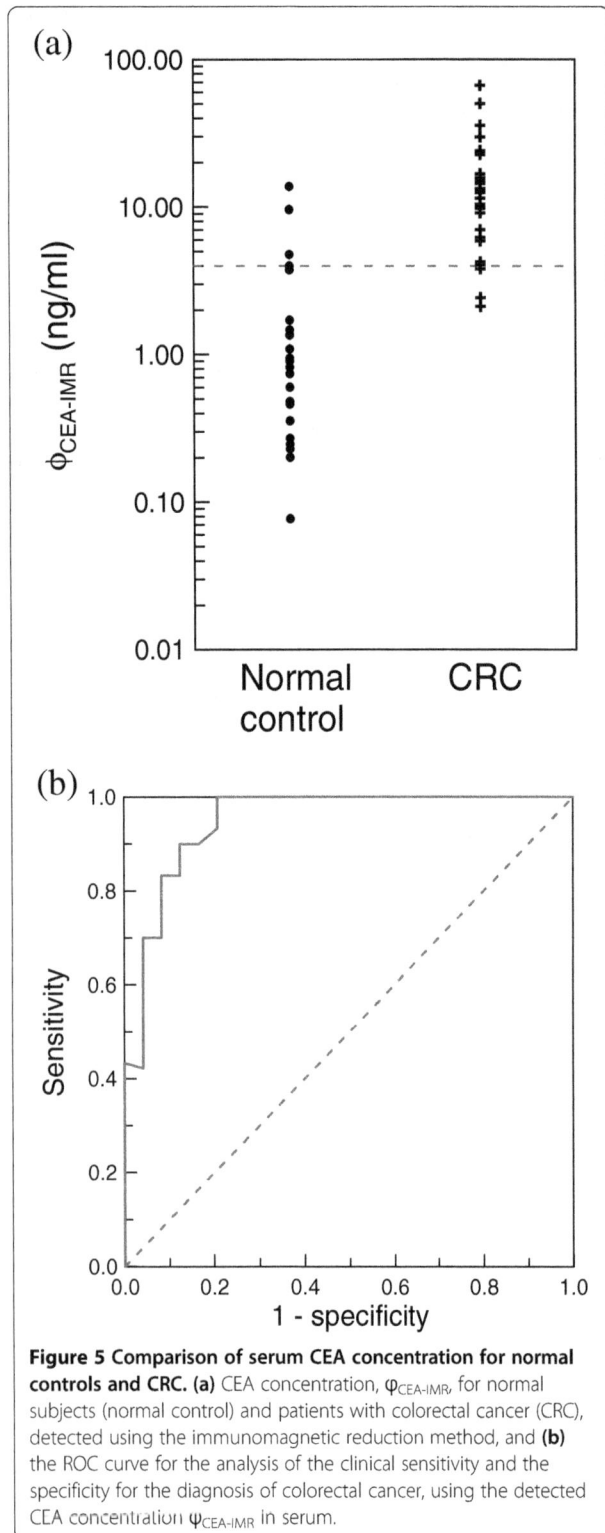

**Figure 5 Comparison of serum CEA concentration for normal controls and CRC.** (a) CEA concentration, $\varphi_{CEA-IMR}$, for normal subjects (normal control) and patients with colorectal cancer (CRC), detected using the immunomagnetic reduction method, and **(b)** the ROC curve for the analysis of the clinical sensitivity and the specificity for the diagnosis of colorectal cancer, using the detected CEA concentration $\psi_{CEA-IMR}$ in serum.

## Methods

### Synthesis of bio-magnetic nanoparticles

The protocol for the synthesis of magnetic $Fe_3O_4$ nanoparticles is proposed by MagQu Co., Ltd [25]. A ferrite solution containing ferrous sulphate hepta-hydrate ($FeSO_4 \cdot 7H_2O$) and ferric chloride hexa-hydrate ($FeCl_3 \cdot 6H_2O$) in a stoichiometric ratio of 1:2 was mixed with an equal volume of aqueous dextran, which acts as a surfactant for $Fe_3O_4$ particles dispersed in water. The mixture was heated to 70–90°C and titrated with a strong base solution, to form black $Fe_3O_4$ particles. Aggregates and excess unbound dextran were removed by centrifugation and gel filtration chromatography, to produce a highly concentrated homogeneous magnetic fluid. The reagent (MF-DEX-0060, MagQu) with the desired magnetic concentration was obtained by diluting the highly concentrated magnetic fluid with pH-7.4 phosphate buffered saline (PBS) solution. To ensure that the antibodies against carcinoembryonic antigen (CEA) for colorectal cancer, i.e. anti-CEA (AT-CEA, MagQu), bound to the dextran on the outmost shell of magnetic nanoparticles, $NaIO_4$ solution was added into the magnetic solution to oxidize the dextran, which then creates aldehyde groups (–CHO). The dextran then reacts with anti-CEA via the linking of –CH = N-, so anti-CEA is bound covalently to dextran, as schematically shown in Figure 1(a). Unbound anti-CEA was separated from the solution by magnetic separation.

### Characterizations of bio-magnetic nanoparticles

The distribution of the size of $Fe_3O_4$ magnetic nanoparticles bio-functionalized with anti-CEA was determined by dynamic laser scattering (Nanotrac 150, Microtrac). To determine the immuno reactivity of anti-CEA functionalized $Fe_3O_4$ magnetic nanoparticles, so-called immunomagnetic reduction was used [13,26,27]. In immunomagnetic reduction, antibody functionalized magnetic nanoparticles were mixed with a solution of target bio-molecules. Before the nanoparticles and CEA molecules associated, the ac magnetic susceptibility $\chi_{ac,o}$ of the mixture was detected, using an ac magnetosusceptometer (XacPro-E, MagQu). Nanoparticles associate with target bio-molecules, via the antibodies on the magnetic nanoparticles. This association results in a reduction in the ac magnetic susceptibility of the mixture. The ac susceptibility of the mixture after association is denoted by $\chi_{ac,\phi}$. The reduction in ac susceptibility is referred to as the IMR signal and is expressed as:

$$IMR(\%) = \left[\left(\chi_{ac,o} - \chi_{ac,\varphi}\right)/\chi_{ac,o}\right] \times 100\% \qquad (2)$$

For each IMR signal measurement, 40-μl reagent and 60-μl CEA solution or sample were used.

According to Ref. [28], the total number of antibody functionalized magnetic nanoparticles in 1-ml, 8-mg-Fe/ml magnetic bio-reagent is roughly $10^{13}$ particles. There

frequently used drugs or chemicals. The results for CEA concentration in 54 serum samples show that the clinical sensitivity and the specificity for the diagnosis of colorectal cancer are 0.90 and 0.87, respectively, with a threshold of 4.05 ng/ml.

are averagely 6 antibodies immobilized on one magnetic nanoparticle. For IMR measurement, the used volume of reagent is 40 μl. Hence, $2.4 \times 10^{12}$ anti-CEA molecules are used for each IMR test.

## Preparation of standard CEA solutions

Standard CEA (Human CD66e) protein was obtained from AdD Serotec (Cat. No. PHP282). Various concentrations of CEA protein were prepared by serially diluting standard CEA protein with PBS buffer or normal free serum and the resulting solution was stored at −80°C. The concentration of CEA protein was then quantified using a spectrophotometer (NanoDrop2000; Thermo Scientific.).

## Assessment of human serum CEA

24 serum samples from healthy subjects (Normal control) and 30 serum samples from patients with colorectal cancer (CRC) were used for the CEA assay. The CEA concentrations in human serum samples will be determined using the IMR signals. CRC patients were identified using either pathological evidence or an immunoassay. All of the enrolled patients provided informed consent before undergoing the procedure and this study was approved by National Taiwan University Hospital Research Ethics Committee (No.201105996RC).

### Competing interests

The authors declare that they have no competing interests.

### Authors' contributions

CC carried out the IMR measurements. SY participated the characterization of bio-magnetic nanoparticles. CS prepared the bio-magnetic particles. JF participated the characterization of bio-magnetic nanoparticles. BH analyzed the experimental data. KW carried out the assessment of human serum CEA. All authors read and approved the final manuscript.

### Acknowledgements

This work is supported by the Ministry of Economic Affairs of Taiwan, under Grant Numbers 101-EC-17-A-17-I1-0074, 1Z970688 and 1Z0990415 (SBIR), by New Taipei City Government, under Grant Number 103049, and by the Council of Agriculture, under Grant Number 103-a5.2-08.

### Author details

[1]MagQu Co., Ltd., Sindian Dist, New Taipei City 231, Taiwan. [2]Department of Surgery & Hepatitis Research Center, National Taiwan University Hospital, Taipei 100, Taiwan. [3]Graduate Institute of Clinical Medicine, College of Medicine, National Taiwan University, Taipei 100, Taiwan.

### References

1. Hultman T, Ståhl S, Homes E, Uhlén M: Direct solid phase sequencing of genomic and plasmid DNA using magnetic beads as solid support. *Nucleic Acids Res* 1989, 17:4937–4946.
2. Kondo A, Kamura H, Higashitani K: Development and application of thermo-sensitive magnetic immunomicrospheres for antibody purification. *Appl Microbiol Biotechnol* 1994, 41:99–105.
3. Franzreb M, Siemann-Herzberg M, Hobley TJ, Thomas ORT: Protein purification using magnetic adsorbent particles. *Appl Microbiol Biotechnol* 2006, 70:505–516.
4. Gånshirt-Ahlert D, Börjesson-Stoll R, Burschyk M, Garritsen HSP, Helmer E, Miny P, Velasco M, Walde C, Patterson D, Teng N, Bhat NM, Bieber MM, Holzgreve W: Detection of fetal trisomies 21 and 18 from maternal blood using triple gradient and magnetic cell sorting. *Am J Reprod Immunol* 1993, 30:194–201.
5. Pamme N, Wilhelm C: Continuous sorting of magnetic cells via on-chip free-flow magnetophoresis. *Lab Chip* 2006, 6:974–980.
6. Adamsa JD, Kim U, Soh HT: Multitarget magnetic activated cell sorter. *Proc Natl Acad Sci U S A* 2008, 105:18165–18170.
7. Kim DK, Zhang Y, Kehr J, Klason T, Bjelke B, Muhammed M: Characterization and MRI study of surfactant-coated superparamagnetic nanoparticles administered into the rat brain. *J Magn Magn Mater* 2001, 225:256–261.
8. Huang KW, Chieh JJ, Lin IT, Horng HE, Yang HC, Hong CY: Anti-CEA-functionalized superparamagnetic iron oxide nanoparticles for examining colorectal tumors *in vivo*. *Nanoscale Res Lett* 2013, 8:413–416.
9. Dobson J: Magnetic nanoparticles for drug delivery. *Drug Dev Res* 2006, 67:55–60.
10. Hergt R, Dutz S, Müller R, Zeisberger M: Magnetic particle hyperthermia: nanoparticle magnetism and materials development for cancer therapy. *J Phys Condens Matter* 2006, 18:S2919–S2934.
11. Kotitz R, Matz H, Trahms L, Koch H, Weitschies W, Rheinlander T, Semmler W, Bunte T: SQUID based remanence measurements for immunoassays. *IEEE Trans Appl Supercond* 1997, 7:3678–3681.
12. Enpuku K, Minotani T, Gima T, Kuroki Y, Itoh Y, Yamashita M, Katakura Y, Kuhara S: Detection of magnetic nanoparticles with superconducting quantum interference device (SQUID) magnetometer and application to immunoassays. *Jpn J Appl Phys* 1999, 38:L1102–L1105.
13. Hong CY, Wu CC, Chiu YC, Yang SY, Horng HE, Yang HC: Magnetic susceptibility reduction method for magnetically labeled immunoassay. *Appl Phys Lett* 2006, 88:1–3. 212512.
14. Baselt DR, Lee GU, Natesan M, Metzger SW, Sheehan PE, Colton RJ: A biosensor based on magnetoresistance technology. *Biosens Bioelectron* 1998, 13:731–739.
15. Krause HJ, Wolters N, Zhang Y, Offenhäusser A, Miethe P, Meyer MHF: Magnetic particle detection by frequency mixing for immunoassay applications. *J Magn Magn Mater* 2007, 311:436–444.
16. Horng HE, Yang SY, Huang YW, Jiang WQ, Hong CY, Yang HC: Nanomagnetic particles for SQUID-based magnetically labeled immunoassay. *IEEE Trans Appl Supercond* 2005, 15:668–671.
17. Liao SH, Yang HC, Horng HE, Chieh JJ, Chen KL, Chen HH, Chen JY, Liu CI, Liu CW, Wang LM: Time-dependent phase lag of biofunctionalized magnetic nanoparticles conjugated with biotargets studied with alternating current magnetic susceptometor for liquid phase immunoassays. *Appl Phys Lett* 2013, 103:1–3. 243703.
18. Shao H, Yoon TJ, Liong M, Weissleder R, Lee H: Magnetic nanoparticles for biomedical NMR-based diagnostics. *Beilstein J Nanotechnol* 2010, 1:142–154.
19. MagnaBioSciences, LLC. http://www.magnabiosciences.com/
20. Magnisense Co., Ltd. http://www.magnisense.com/
21. Lifeassays. http://www.lifeassays.com/
22. Xi'an Goldmag Nanobiotech Co., Ltd. http://www.goldmag.com.cn/
23. MagQu Co., Ltd. http://www.magqu.com/
24. Yang SY, Wang WC, Lan CB, Chen CH, Chieh JJ, Horng HE, Hong CH, Yang HC, Tsai CP, Yang CY, Cheng IC, Chung WC: Magnetically enhanced high-specificity virus detection using bio-activated magnetic nanoparticles with antibodies as labeling markers. *J Virol Methods* 2010, 164:14–18.
25. Jiang WQ, Yang HC, Yang SY, Horng HE, Hung JC, Chen YC, Hong CY: Preparation and properties of superparamagnetic nanoparticles with narrow size distribution and biocompatible. *J Magn Magn Mater* 2004, 283:210–214.
26. Chieh JJ, Yang SY, Horng HE, Yu CY, Lee CL, Wu HL, Hong CY, Yang HC: Immunomagnetic reduction assay using high-$T_c$ superconducting-quantum-interference-device-based magnetosusceptometry. *J Appl Phys* 2010, 107:1–5. 074903.
27. Yang CC, Yang SY, Chen HH, Weng WL, Horng HE, Chieh JJ, Hong CY, Yang HC: Effect of molecule-particle binding on the reduction in the mixed-frequency ac magnetic susceptibility of magnetic bio-reagents. *J Appl Phys* 2012, 112:1–4. 24704.
28. Yang SY, Chieh JJ, Huang KW, Yang CC, Chen TC, Ho CS, Chang SF, Chen HH, Horng HE, Hong CY, Yang HC: Molecule-assisted nanoparticle clustering effect in immunomagnetic reduction assay. *J Appl Phys Lett* 2013, 113:1–5. 144903.

# Gefitinib loaded folate decorated bovine serum albumin conjugated carboxymethyl-beta-cyclodextrin nanoparticles enhance drug delivery and attenuate autophagy in folate receptor-positive cancer cells

Yijie Shi[1†], Chang Su[2†], Wenyu Cui[3], Hongdan Li[4], Liwei Liu[1], Bo Feng[1], Ming Liu[1], Rongjian Su[4] and Liang Zhao[1*]

## Abstract

**Background:** Active targeting endocytosis mediated by the specific interaction between folic acid and its receptor has been a hotspot in biological therapy of many human cancers. Various studies have demonstrated that folate and its conjugates could facilitate the chemotherapeutic drug delivery into folate receptor (FR)-positive tumor cells *in vitro* and *in vivo*. In order to utilize FA-FR binding specificity to achieve targeted delivery of drugs into tumor cells, we prepared Gefitinib loaded folate decorated bovine serum albumin conjugated carboxymethyl-β-cyclodextrin nanoparticles for enhancing drug delivery in cancer cells. On this context, the aim of our study was to develop a novel nano-delivery system for promoting tumor-targeting drug delivery in folate receptor-positive Hela cells.

**Results:** We prepared folic acid (FA)-decorated bovine serum albumin (BSA) conjugated carboxymethyl-β-cyclodextrin (CM-β-CD) nanoparticles (FA-BSA-CM-β-CD NPs) capable of entrapping a hydrophobic Gefitinib. It was observed that nanoparticles are monodisperse and spherical nanospheres with an average diameter of 90.2 nm and negative surface charge of −18.6 mV. FA-BSA-CM-β-CD NPs could greatly facilitate Gefitinib uptake and enhance the toxicity to folate receptor-positive Hela cells. Under the reaction between FA and FR, Gefitinib loaded FA-BSA-CM-β-CD NPs induced apoptosis of Hela cells through elevating the expression of caspase-3 and inhibited autophagy through decreasing the expressing of LC3. It also confirmed that clathrin-mediated endocytosis and macropinocytosis exerted great influence on the internalization of both NPs.

**Conclusions:** These results demonstrated that FA may be an effective targeting molecule and FA-BSA-CM-β-CD NPs provided a new strategy for the treatment of human cancer cells which over-expressed folate receptors.

**Keywords:** Folate, Folate receptors, Carboxymethyl-β-Cyclodextrin, Bovine serum albumin, Nanoparticles, Gefitinib

## Background

Nanosized drug carriers functionalized with moieties specifically targeting tumor cells are promising tools in cancer therapy, due to their ability to circulate in the bloodstream for longer periods and their selectivity for tumor cells, enabling the sparing of healthy tissues [1-5]. Many synthetic biomimetic nanocrystalline apatites are used as nanocarriers to produce multifunctional nanoparticles, by coupling them with the chemotherapeutic drug, such as Gefitinib, Dox or membrane antibody DO-24 monoclonal antibody (mAb) directed against the c-Met/Hepatocyte Growth Factor Receptor (Met/HGFR), which is over-expressed on different kinds of carcinomas and thus represent a useful tumor target recently [6-8]. Gefitinib, a tyrosine kinase inhibitor of Epithelial Growth Factor Receptor (EGFR) usually expressed in solid tumors of epithelial origin, can prevent tumor growth, metastasis and angiogenesis, and promote apoptosis of tumor cells [9-11]. The main mechanism includes that it

* Correspondence: liangzhao79@163.com
†Equal contributors
[1]College of Pharmacy, Liaoning Medical University, Jinzhou 121000, P R China
Full list of author information is available at the end of the article

can block the signal transmission by competitive binding Mg-ATP situated on catalytic domain of EGFR-TK, then inhibit the activation of mitogen activated protein kinase, inducing the apoptosis of cancer cells [12]. However, Gefitinib is absorbed slowly and widely distributed in bodies following oral administration, resulting in the serious side effects and lower bioavailability. Moreover, the solubility of Gefitinib is decreased with the decline of pH in medium [13].

Cyclodextrins (CD), a family of carbohydrate polymers which are produced from starch by enzymatic conversion and commonly used in food, pharmaceutical, drug delivery, and chemical industries, as well as agriculture and environmental engineering, is cyclic oligosaccharide with cone barrel structure composed of seven glucopyranose units with cylindrical cavity [14-16]. The exterior of this cone is polar and hydrophilic, whereas the interior cavity is relatively nonpolar and hydrophobic. Small hydrophobic molecules as the guest molecules can be completely or partially embedded into CD cavity to form complexes, improving water solubility, stability and biological activity of the guest molecules [17-21]. Bovine serum albumin (BSA), a carrier protein, plays an important role in drug storage and transport, for its superior biocompatibility it has been widely used in biomedical research, such as Nano carrier, nanoparticle surface engineering and temples for preparation of nanoparticles [22-25].

To improve the solubility and stability of Gefitinib, we synthesize the amphiphilic BSA-CM-β-CD conjugates to prepare the assembled nanoparticles capable of entrapping hydrophobic Gefitinib into the cavity of CD through the host-guest interaction. Folate receptor (FR), as a transmembrane glycoprotein, promotes the transportation of folate (FA) or its conjugates into the cells by active targeting endocytosis mediated through FA-FR interaction [26-28]. FA is expressed at basal levels in normal adult organs such as brain, lung and liver, but it is over-expressed in many human cancers including ovarian cancer, breast cancer, endometrial cancer, lung cancer, kidney cancer, colon cancer and nasopharyngeal carcinoma cells [29-31]. Several lines of evidence have demonstrated that FA and its conjugates could significantly enhance the drug delivery efficiency into FR-positive tumor cells both *in vitro* and *in vivo* [32-34]. Herein, FA is adopted as the coupling molecule to improve FR-positive tumor-targeted drug delivery (Figure 1). Properties of NPs such as size, morphology and surface potential were examined. Using Gefitinib as the model drug, we prepared drug-loaded nanoparticles. We found that FA-BSA-CM-β-CD NPs greatly facilitated Gefitinib uptake and enhanced the toxic effect in folate receptor-positive Hela cells. Our results demonstrated that FA-BSA-CM-β-CD NPs might be a higher efficiency drug delivery system than the conventional delivery system for the targeting therapy of FR positive human cancers.

## Results and discussion
### The preparation and characteristics of various kinds of NPs
Conjugation of CM-β-CD to BSA was obtained by carbodiimide coupling. Carboxylic group of CM-β-CD reacted with EDAC to form unstable reactive ester. With addition

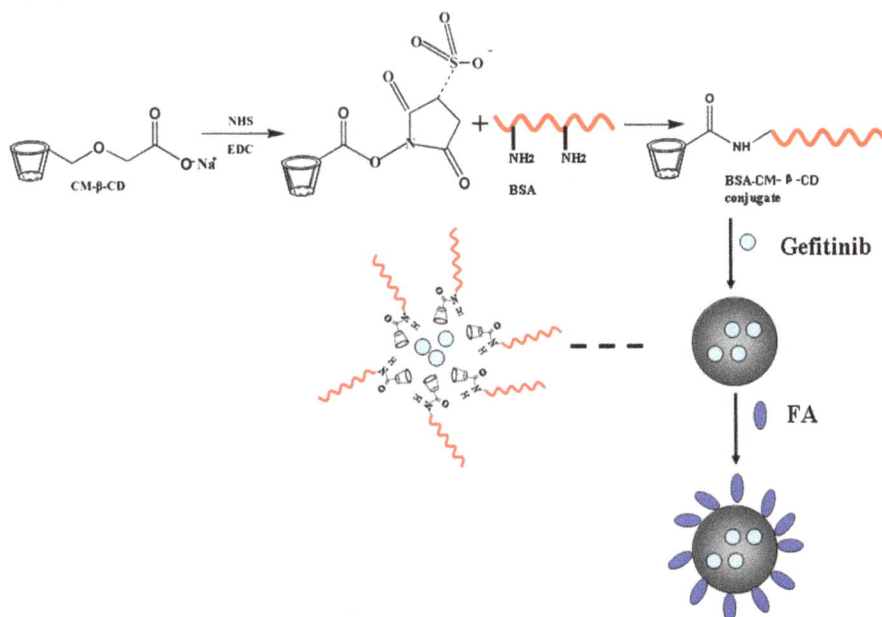

**Figure 1** Schematic formation of Gefitinib loaded folate-decorated bovine serum albumin conjugated carboxymethyl-β-cyclodextrin nanoparticles.

of NHS, semi-stable amine-reactive NHS-ester was synthesized and then mixed with BSA which containing amino group to obtain CM-β-CD conjugated BSA by stable amide bond [35,36].

The characterization of BSA-CM-β-CD conjugates was investigated by infrared spectroscopy (Figure 2). The result showed the FT-IR spectra of BSA, CM-β-CD, and BSA-CM-β-CD conjugates. The characteristic peak of BSA-CM-β-CD conjugates appeared at 1650 $cm^{-1}$ and 1540 $cm^{-1}$ should be ascribed to the newly formed amide bond between CM-β-CD molecules and BSA. These data supported that CM-β-CD has grafted to BSA, and they are correspond to the results of former literatures [37].

Spectrum of infrared absorption of Gefitinib loaded FA-BSA-CM-β-CD NPs was shown in Figure 3. It can be seen that when BSA-CM-β-CD NPs was bonded with FA, its spectrum demonstrated that the aromatic amine groups ($vNH_2$, 3415 $cm^{-1}$ and 3323 $cm^{-1}$) from FA disappeared, suggesting that amine groups from FA reacted with carboxylic group of BSA. Furthermore, the characteristic peak of secondary amine group ($vNH$, 3398 $cm^{-1}$) from Gefitinib disappeared because of the encapsulation of Gefitinib into the core of NPs.

## Development and properties of Gefitinib-loaded FA-BSA-CM-β-CD NPs

Using transmission electronic microscope (TEM), we observed that Gefitinib-loaded FA-BSA-CM-β-CD NPs we prepared were monodisperse spheres, and further analysis revealed that the diameters of NPs ranged from 52.1 to 105.6 nm (Figure 4). Table 1 summarized the average diameters measured by dynamic light scattering (DLS) and surface charge information of these prepared nanoparticles. It was remarkable that Gefitinib-loaded FA-BSA-CM-β-CD NPs showed smaller particle size, negative zeta potential. The average encapsulation efficiency of Gefitinib in FA-BSA-CM-β-CD NPs was 89.2%

and about 70.1% of FA was conjugated on the surface of NPs.

## In vitro drug release study

Gefitinib loaded FA-BSA-CM-β-CD NPs exhibited similar release profiles in the medium with different pH. The release curve in PBS could be divided into two phases: initial fast drug release stage and later stable release stage. Gefitinib was released rapidly in the initial fast release stage, and was released slowly in the later stable stage through diffusion because of the continuous degradation of the polymer (Figure 5). The release speed of Gefitinib decreased with the increase of pH as polymer degraded faster in acid medium. Thus, it possibly suggested that the matrix of NPs tended to be eroded as a result of depolymerization of BSA at pH 5.0 which was closer to the isoelectric points of BSA (pH 4.9), and then drug could be more easily released from NPs. The release ratio during the first 48 h accounted for over 40% of the total drug and the remnants were released over longer time of incubation. It suggested that Gefitinib-loaded FA-BSA-CM-β-CD NPs could be used as a long-lasting and effective drug delivery system.

## Cell viability assays

The cytotoxic effects of Gefitinib loaded FA-BSA-CM-β-CD NPs and BSA-CM-β-CD NPs were evaluated by MTT assay using Hela cell line. MTT analysis showed that in the absence of FA in culturing medium, treatment of Hela cells with Gefitinib loaded FA-BSA-CM-β-CD NPs caused a markedly increase in the cell cytotoxic activities as compared with free Gefitinib and Gefitinib loaded FA unconjugated NPs (Figure 6B). The $IC_{50}$ values of Gefitinib loaded FA-BSA-CM-β-CD NPs treated Hela cells was 4.63 μg/mL, 7.85 μg/mL for free Gefitinib and 13.55 μg/mL for Gefitinib loaded BSA-CM-β-CD NPs. However, no obvious cytotoxic activities were observed when treating the cells with blank FA-BSA-CM-β-CD NPs in Hela cells (Figure 6A). These

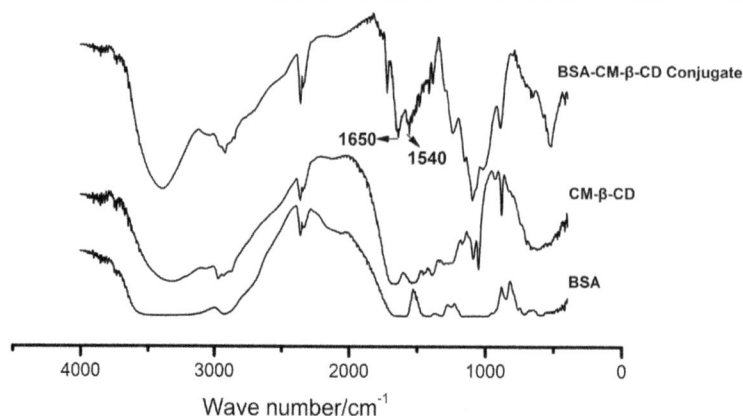

**Figure 2** FT-IR spectra of BSA, CM-β-CD, and BSA-CM-β-CD conjugates.

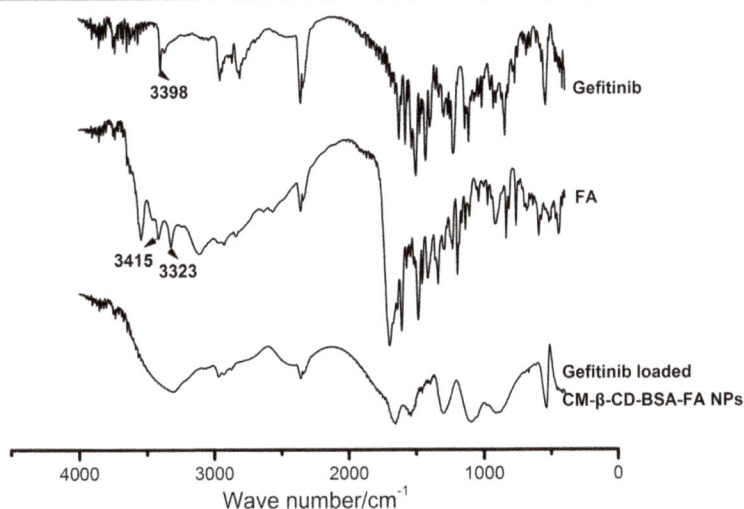

**Figure 3** FT-IR spectra of FA, Gefitinib and Gefitinib loaded FA-BSA-CM-β-CD NPs.

data suggested that more drug loaded FA conjugated NPs could be internalized into Hela cells which expressed FA at higher level by the interaction between FA and FR, further leading to the significant cytotoxicity by the accumulation of drug in cells.

We next examined whether inhibition of FR, which expressed on the cell surface, affected the cytotoxic activities of Gefitinib loaded FA-BSA-CM-β-CD NPs. Hela cells were cultured in the medium containing FA at 5 µg/mL. MTT analysis (Figure 6C) revealed that the presence of FA caused a significant decrease in the cytotoxic effect of Gefitinib loaded FA-BSA-CM-β-CD NPs compared with that without FA in Hela cells. However, pretreatment of FA had little effect on the cytotoxic activity of free Gefitinib and Gefitinib loaded BSA-CM-β-CD NPs. The IC$_{50}$ values of Gefitinib loaded FA-BSA-CM-β-

CD NPs treated Hela cells was 13.02 µg/mL, 8.63 µg/mL for free Gefitinib and 14.76 µg/mL for Gefitinib loaded BSA-CM-β-CD NPs. These data further demonstrated that FA conjugation played critical roles in accumulating NPs inside FR-positive tumor cells and could be used as a targeting molecule in the treatment of human cancers which over-expressed FR on the cell surface.

### *In vitro* uptake ability analysis

To visualize whether FA conjugation could enhance the uptake of BSA-CM-β-CD NPs, The NPs were labeled with Rodamine B and the uptake ability was evaluated in Hela cells. Using confocal laser scanning microscopy analysis, Hela cells showed increased number of red fluorescence patches in the cytoplasm when incubating Rhodamine B-labeled FA-BSA-CM-β-CD NPs in the

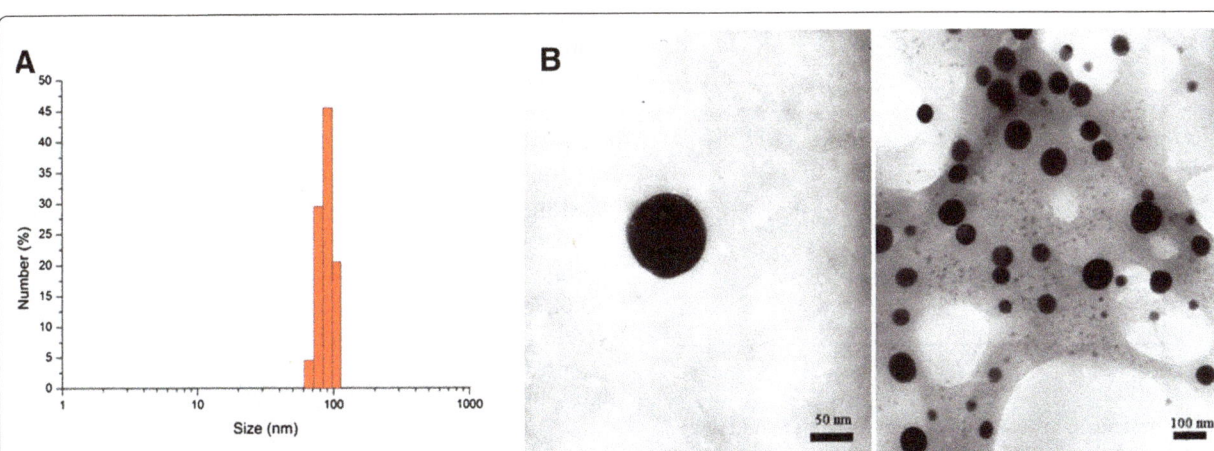

**Figure 4** Particle size distribution (A) and TEM image (B) of the obtained Gefitinib-loaded FA-BSA-CM-β-CD NPs.

**Table 1 Key parameters of Gefitinib-loaded FA-BSA-CM-β-CD NPs**

| Parameters | Data |
| --- | --- |
| Average diameter (nm) | 90.2 ± 10.01 |
| Zeta potential (mv) | −18.6 ± 5.8 |
| Encapsulating efficiency of Gefitinib (%) | 89.2 ± 4.7 |
| Entrapment efficiency of FA (%) | 70.1 ± 4.3 |
| Polydispersity Index (PDI) | 0.093 |

FA-free medium for 6 h compared with that of Rhodamine B-labeled BSA-CM-β-CD NPs. However, the uptake of FA-BSA-CM-β-CD NPs was significantly reduced by addition of FA in the medium (Figure 7). The free FA competition study suggested that free FA in medium competed to bind FR on the surface of Hela cells with FA conjugated NPs, leading to the lower uptake of NPs.

### Intracellular ATP level assay

After cells were treated with free Gefitinib, Gefitinib loaded BSA-CM-β-CD NPs, Gefitinib loaded FA-BSA-CM-β-CD NPs, the changing rates of intracellular ATP level were presented in Figure 8. It can be seen that compared with ATP level of untreated Hela cells as the control group, The changing rates of intracellular ATP level for free Gefitinib, Gefitinib loaded BSA-CM-β-CD NPs and Gefitinib loaded FA-BSA-CM-β-CD NPs were decreased to 70.5%, 75.4% and 50.1%, respectively. The results showed that Gefitinib and Gefitinib loaded NPs were internalized to induce the apoptosis of cells by lowering ATP level rates. It also confirmed that with the interaction between FA conjugated on the surface of

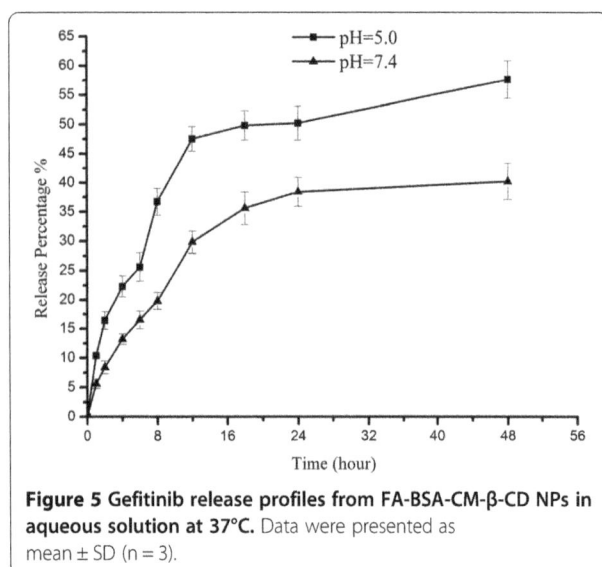

**Figure 5 Gefitinib release profiles from FA-BSA-CM-β-CD NPs in aqueous solution at 37°C.** Data were presented as mean ± SD (n = 3).

NPs and FR situated at Hela cells, more drug loaded FA conjugated NPs were transported into the interior of cells to inhibit energy generation and accelerate the apoptosis of cells by accumulation of drugs in cells.

### Cell apoptosis analysis

To identify the effect of Gefitinib and Gefitinib loaded NPs on cell apoptosis and autophagy, we detected the expression of caspase-3, Bax, and LC3 by western blot (Figure 9). Compared with free Gefitinib and Gefitinib loaded NPs, Gefitinib loaded FA-BSA-CM-β-CD NPs induced the highest caspase-3 protein expression. It also illustrated that with the mediation of FA, a large amount of drug loaded FA conjugated NPs were accumulated in Hela cells and caspase-3 as the main apoptosis relevant protein was increased, corresponding with the results of MTT experiments. However, there was no obvious difference on the Bax protein expression in the treated groups and the control group, confirming that Bax was not involved in Gefitinib induced cell apoptosis (Figure 9A). LC3 (microtubule-associated protein light chain 3) is a specific autophagic marker in mammalian cells during autophagy. So, to identify whether Gefitinib affects autophagy, expression of LC3 was detected in Hela cells, and found that free Gefitinib did not influence the expression of LC3, but with the addition of NPs, the expression of LC3 has been inhibited, also, with the mediation of FA, the inhibition rate increased obviously (Figure 9B). So, the results suggested that through autophagy, Hela cells may be survival and resist free Gefitinib, and FA-NPs mediated accumulation of Gefitinib in cells inhibits LC3 expression. Taken together, through inhibition of autophagy, Gefitinib loaded FA-BSA-CM-β-CD NPs induced cells apoptosis.

### Inhibition of various endocytosis assay

To get more insight to know which uptake mechanisms were implied in NPs uptake, Hela cells were pretreated with various endocytic inhibitors specific for a particular endocytic pathway. Figure 10 showed that when genistein as an inhibitor to block caveolae-mediated endocytosis (CvME) was added into cells, there was no significant difference in both NPs internalization suggesting a minor role of CvME. When cells were treated with cytochalasin D (30 μM, macropinocytosis), the uptake ability of both NPs were significantly decreased to 55.4% and 60.2%. It was also observed that internalization of both NPs in cells with chlorpromazine treatment (clathrin-mediated endocytosis) was significant lower than that in untreated cells. Moreover, 40.1% reduction in FA-BSA-CM-β-CD NPs was observed in comparison with 32.1% reduction of intracellular uptake of BSA-CM-β-CD NPs. Some previous study have

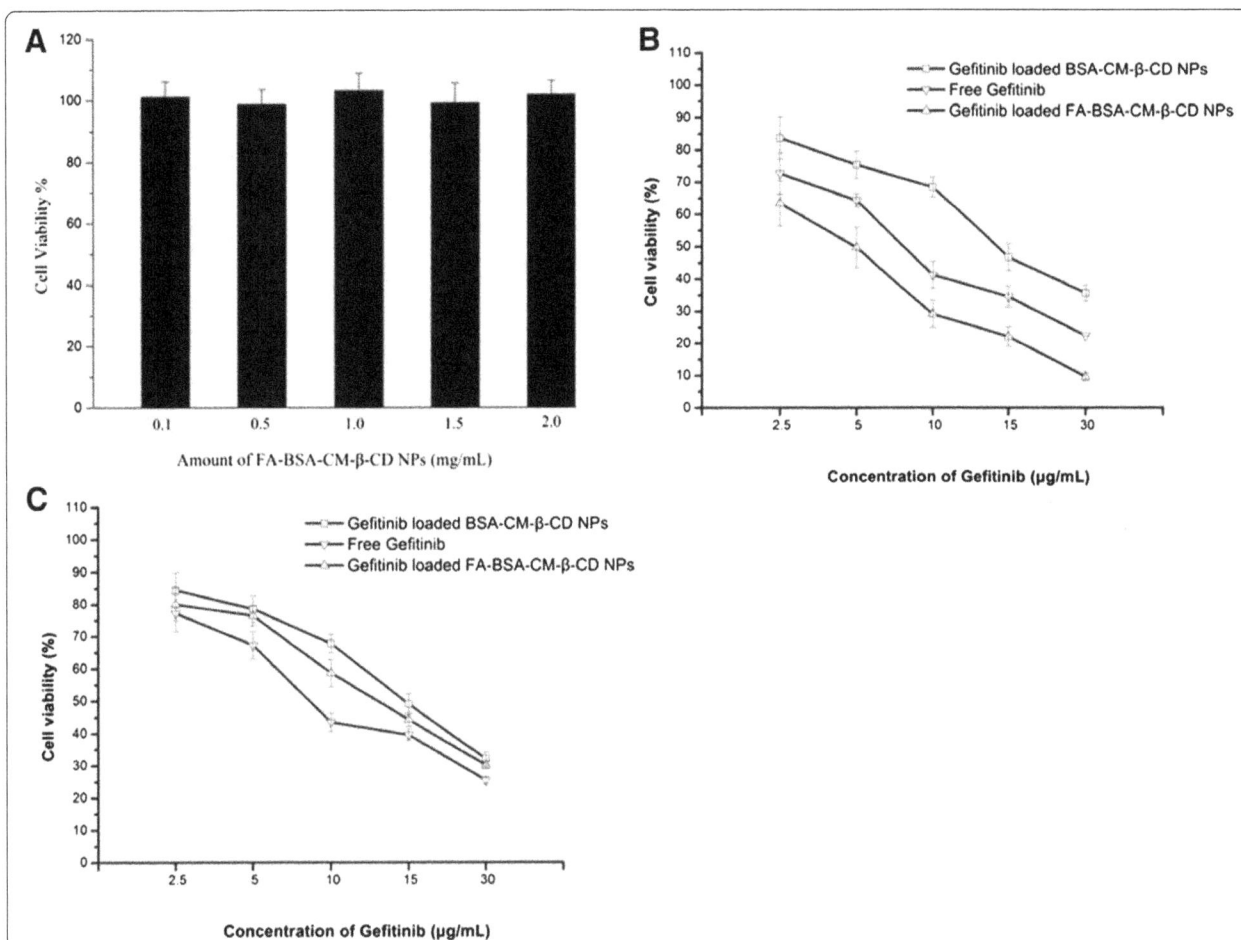

**Figure 6** *In vitro* **viability of NPs in Hela cells.** Data represents mean ± SD (n = 3). **(A)** Viability of Hela cells after incubation with different amounts of naked FA-BSA-CM-β-CD NPs after 48 h. **(B)** Cell viability cultured with NPs loaded at various concentrations of Gefitinib in folate-free medium after 48 h. **(C)** Cell viability cultured with Gefitinib loaded NPs at various concentrations in medium containing FA at 5 μg/mL after 48 h.

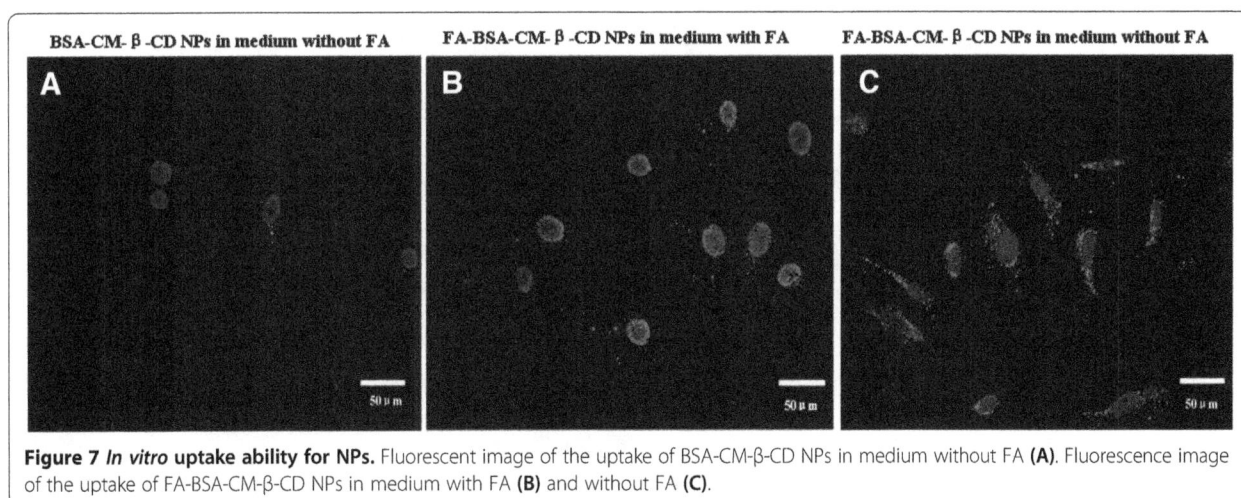

**Figure 7** *In vitro* **uptake ability for NPs.** Fluorescent image of the uptake of BSA-CM-β-CD NPs in medium without FA **(A)**. Fluorescence image of the uptake of FA-BSA-CM-β-CD NPs in medium with FA **(B)** and without FA **(C)**.

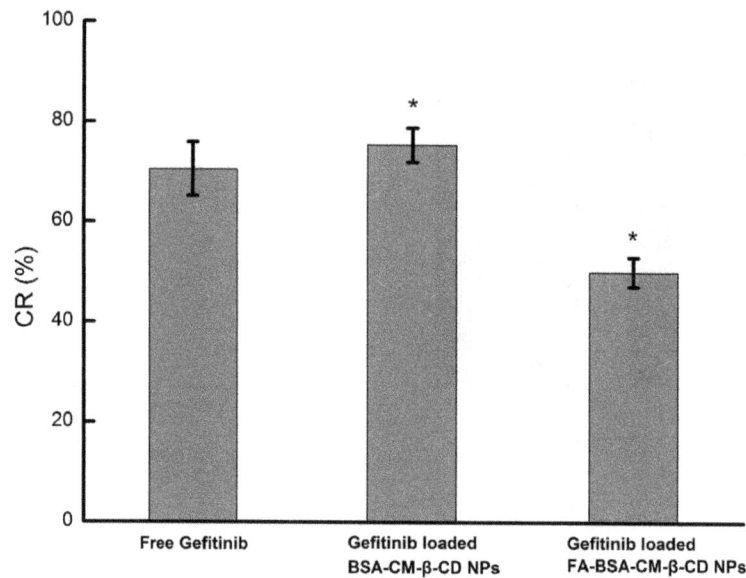

**Figure 8** Results of intracellular ATP level assay after 48 h incubation with different preparations. Data were expressed as mean ± SD (n = 3). *P <0.05, vs the free Gefitinib group.

reported that different conjugation with targeting ligands, such as iRGD, siRNA and disaccharide, could enhance uptake or change the endocytosis pathway of NPs resulting in improving cytotoxicity to cancer cells [38-41]. The results demonstrated that both NPs were internalized into cells mainly depending on clathrin-mediated endocytosis and macropinocytosis being proved by the significant uptake reduction of both NPs in treated cells with chlorpromazine and cytochalasin D. In contrast, the regulation of caveolae-mediated endocytosis on NPs internalization was not significantly different from untreated group.

## Conclusions

In summary, CM-β-CD was conjugated with BSA by carbodiimide coupling. FA as a small targeting molecule, was bond to the surface of NPs. Gefitinib loaded FA-BSA-CM-β-CD NPs showed good monodispersity, negative charge and homogenous particle size. The encapsulating efficiency of Gefitinib and the release pattern were investigated *in vitro*. MTT results showed that no obvious cytotoxicity was observed when incubating naked FA-BSA-CM-β-CD NPs with Hela cells. The free folic acid competition study showed that the cell inhibition of FA conjugated NPs in FR positive cells was significantly enhanced

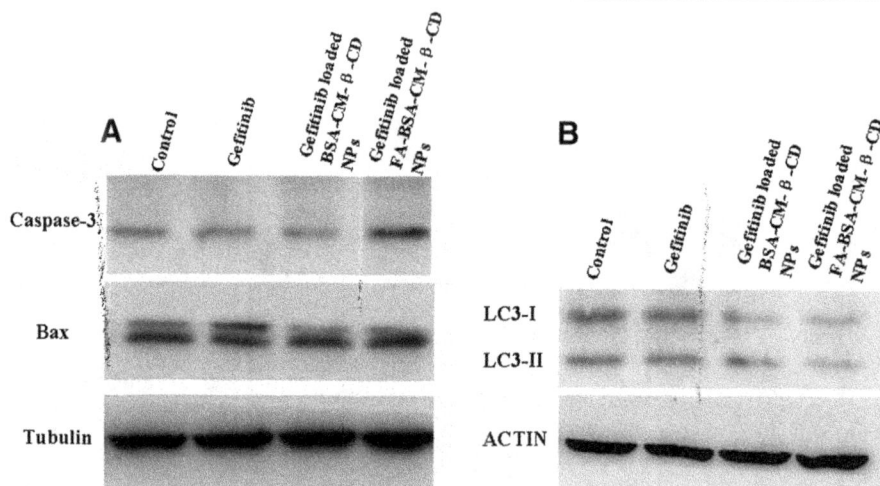

**Figure 9** Apoptotic effects of various Gefitinib formulations on Hela cells. (A) Western blot analysis of the expression levels of Bax and caspase-3 proteins in Hela cells after treatments. (B) Western blot analysis of the expression levels of LC3 proteins in Hela cells after treatments.

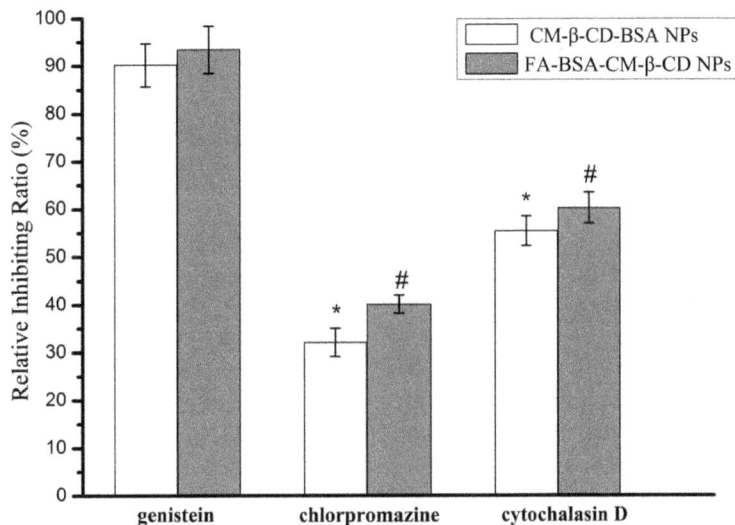

**Figure 10 Effects of endocytic inhibitors on the uptaking ability of the two NPs in Hela cells.** $^{*}$P <0.05, vs the BSA-CM-β-CD NPs group treated with genistein in Hela cells, $^{#}$P <0.05, vs the FA-BSA-CM-β-CD NPs group treated with genistein in Hela cells.

when FA was removed from the medium. Gefitinib loaded FA-BSA-CM-β-CD NPs inhibited cells autophagy by down-regulating LC3, and promoted apoptosis of Hela cells through the prevention of ATP generation and elevating the expression of caspase-3 protein. It also confirmed that clathrin-mediated endocytosis and macropinocytosis played an important role on the internalization of both NPs. Taken together, FA-BSA-CM-β-CD NPs presented the promising candidates as a folate receptor-positive tumor-targeting carrier via folate mediation.

## Methods
### Materials
BSA was purchased from Sigma (USA), Carboxymethyl-β-Cyclodextrin Sodium Salt (CM-β-CD) was purchased from Zhiyuan Bio-Technology Co., Ltd (China), 1-ethyl-3-(3-dimethylaminopropyl) carbodiimide (EDAC) and folic acid were obtained from Sigma Chemicals (St Louis, US). Gefitinib was purchased from Eastbang Pharmaceutical Co., Ltd (China). All other chemicals were of reagent grade and were used as received.

### Synthesis of BSA-CM-β-CD conjugates
8.0 mg of CM-β-CD was dissolved in 8.0 mL PBS buffer solution (pH 5.8). Then, the solution was added into a centrifuge tube in the presence of 40.0 mg EDC and 16.0 mg NHS. After the tube was rotated constantly for 1 h, 8.0 mg BSA were added into the tube. Subsequently, the tube was rotated overnight. Finally, the BSA-CM-β-CD conjugates were collected by dialysis filter with a

dialysis bag with 1000 molecular weight cutoff to remove the uncoupled CM-β-CD.

### Preparation of Gefitinib loaded FA-BSA-CM-β-CD self-assembled nanoparticles
20 mg conjugates were suspended in 20 mL of distilled water to achieve a solution with concentration of 1 mg/mL. Drug solution (0.4 mg/mL) was prepared by 2 mg Gefitinib was dissolved in 5 ml dichloromethane. Gefitinib loaded BSA-CM-β-CD NPs were prepared by quickly dropping 5.0 mL of drug solution into 20 mL distilled water containing 20 mg conjugates at 30°C under continuously stirring for 24 h to remove dichloromethane. FA was conjugated with BSA-CM-β-CD NPs as the following: 5 mg folic acid was dissolved in 10 mL phosphate buffer suspension (pH 7.4), then 15.0 mg EDC and 5.0 mg NHS were added under stirring constantly for 1 h. Entrapment efficiency of FA conjugated with BSA-CM-β-CD NPs was determined as the ratio of actual FA loading amount to the initial added FA amount. The solution was centrifuged at 16,000 rpm for 30 min. NPs collected were washed 3–4 times with deionized water and centrifuged at 16,000 rpm for 20 min, freeze drying to obtain powders.

### Characterization of Gefitinib loaded FA-BSA-CM-β-CD NPs
The characterization of Gefitinib loaded FA-BSA-CM-β-CD NPs was investigated by using AFFINITY-1 IR spectroscopy (Shimadzu, Kyoto, Japan). Its morphology was observed by using transmission electron microscope (TEM) (JEM-1200EX, Tokyo, Japan) and the mean diameter and zeta potential were determined by Zetasizer (Nano ZS90, Malvern, UK). The encapsulation efficiency (EE) of Gefitinib

in FA-BSA-CM-β-CD NPs was calculated using the equation listed below.

$$EE(\%) = \frac{\text{Weight of initially added drug-Weight of free drug in supernatant}}{\text{Weight of initially added drug}} \times 100$$

## Assessment of drug release

The drug releases were carried out in PBS containing 10% serum with different pH at $37.0 \pm 0.5°C$ under gentle agitation. 10 mL PBS (pH 7.4) in which accurate weighed 10 mg dried Gefitinib-loaded FA-BSA-CM-β-CD NPs were suspended was put into a dialysis bag with 1000 molecular weight cutoff and the dialysis bag was immersed into 100 mL phosphate buffer solution containing 10% serum maintained at pH 7.4 or 5.0 at $37.0 \pm 0.5°C$. At predetermined intervals, 5 mL of release medium was withdrawn and the same volume of fresh buffer solution was added. Samples were filtered through 0.45 μm filter and the concentrations of Gefitinib released were analyzed by spectrophotometry at 338 nm.

## Cell viability assays

A 3-(4,5-dimethylthiazol-2-yl)-2,5- diphenyltetrazolium bromide (MTT) assay was used to investigate cell viability. Hela cells were chosen and used as a model folate receptor-positive cell line in angiogenesis targeting delivery and treatment for their high FR expression [42,43]. Hela cells were seeded into the 96-well plate at a density of $5 \times 10^4/mL$ and attached for 24 h at 37°C in both folate-free medium and the medium containing folate at 5 μg/mL under 5% $CO_2$. Then, the cells were treated with free Gefitinib and Gefitinib-loaded NPs for 48 h, followed by addition of 20 μL MTT (5 mg/mL) and incubated for 4 h at 37°C. Then, the supernatant was carefully removed and 150 μL DMSO was added to each well and stirred for 30 min. The absorbance was measured using microplate reader at 490 nm.

## Uptaking ability of different kinds of NPs in Hela cells

Hela cells, (a folate receptor-positive cell line) a model cell line, were applied to investigate cell uptake ability of different kinds of nanoparticles. Rhodamine B as the fluorescent marker was encapsulated in NPs. Cells were cultured in flasks supplemented with both folate-free medium and the medium containing folate 5 μg/mL at 37°C and 5% $CO_2$. When the cell concentrations reached $5 \times 10^4/mL$, 100 μL of medium containing cells was transferred to the 96-well plate and treated with different Rhodamine B-labeled nanoparticles. At specified time, NPs were withdrawn and the wells were washed with PBS. Nucleus was stained with Hoechst for 15 min at 37°C followed by double washing with PBS. The internalization

of RhB-loaded NPs into cells was observed using fluorescent microscopy (DMI400B, Leica, Germany).

## Intracellular ATP level assay

Free Gefitinib, Gefitinib loaded BSA-CM-β-CD NPs, Gefitinib loaded FA- BSA-CM-β-CD NPs at the same drug concentration were added into the 96-well plate filled with Hela cells at a density of $5 \times 10^4/mL$ for 48 h. The luciferin-luciferase-based ATP luminescence assay kit was applied to determine the changing rates of intracellular ATP level (CR%) calculated using equation below.

$$CR(\%) = \frac{\text{ATP level of Hela cells treated with free drug or NPs}}{\text{ATP level of untreated Hela cells}} \times 100$$

## Tracking of uptake pathways using various endocytic inhibitors

In order to analyze the potential mechanism on uptake pathways of nanoparticles, three types of endocytic inhibitors including cytochalasin D (30 μM, macropinocytosis), genistein (1 μg/mL, caveolae mediated endocytosis) and chlorpromazine (10 μg/mL, clathrin mediated endocytosis) were preincubated with Hela cells in 96-well plate for 30 min, respectively. Then both FITC labeled BSA-CM-β-CD NPs and FA- BSA-CM-β-CD NPs were treated with cells to track the uptake pathways. The effects of various inhibitors on the uptake pathway of the NPs were evaluated by comparing the intracellular fluorescent intensity between treatment of adding inhibitors and non-inhibitors.

## Western blot assay

After treated with free Gefitinib, Gefitinib loaded BSA-CM-β-CD NPs, Gefitinib loaded FA-BSA-CM-β-CD NPs, cells were harvested, washed twice with ice cold PBS, then lysed in RIPA buffer (150 mM NaCl, 1% NP-40, 1% SDS, 1 mM PMSF, 10 μg/mL leupeptin, 1 mM aprotinin, 50 mM Tris-Cl, pH 7.4). The cell lysate was cleared by centrifugation at $12,000 \times g$ for 25 min. Cell lysate containing 50 μg protein in 20 μL was separated by 10% SDS-PAGE and the protein was transferred onto polyvinylidene fluoride (PVDF) membrane. After blocking with 1% BSA, the PVDF membrane was incubated with the primary antibodies (caspase-3, Bax, tubulin, LC3) at 4°C overnight. Subsequently, incubated with appropriate secondary antibody for 1 h and stained with ECL. The level of the targeted proteins were photographed and analyzed by UVP gel analysis system.

## Abbreviations

FA: Folic acid; FR: Folate receptor; BSA: Bovine Serum Albumin; CM-β-CD: Carboxymethyl-β-Cyclodextrin; NPs: Nanoparticles.

## Competing interests

The authors declare that they have no competing interests.

## Authors' contributions

YS and CS performed the preparation and characteristics of various kinds of NPs and co- drafted the manuscript. LZ supervised the whole work. WC, LL, BF and ML helped with the biological study. HL and RS helped in the analysis of biological data. All authors read and approved the final manuscript.

## Acknowledgements

This work is supported by Foundation of Liaoning Educational Committee (No. L2014339) and Innovative Program of University Students of Liaoning Province (No. 201410160008).

## Author details

[1]College of Pharmacy, Liaoning Medical University, Jinzhou 121000, P R China. [2]College of Veterinary Medicine, Liaoning Medical University, Jinzhou 121000, P R China. [3]National Vaccine & Serum Institute, Beijing 100024, China. [4]Central Laboratory of Liaoning Medical University, Jinzhou 121000, P R China.

## References

1. Iafisco M, Delgado-Lopez JM, Varoni EM, Tampieri A, Rimondini L, Gomez-Morales J, Prat M: **Cell Surface Receptor Targeted Biomimetic Apatite Nanocrystals for Cancer Therapy.** *Small* 2013, **9**(22):3834–3844.
2. Chen H, Zhao Y, Wang H, Nie G, Nan K: **Co-delivery strategies based on multifunctional nanocarriers for cancer therapy.** *Curr Drug Metab* 2012, **13**(8):1087–1096.
3. Danhier F, Feron O, Préat V: **To exploit the tumor microenvironment: Passive and active tumor targeting of nanocarriers for anti-cancer drug delivery.** *J Control Release* 2010, **148**(2):135–146.
4. Torchilin VP: **Multifunctional nanocarriers.** *Adv Drug Deliv Rev* 2012, **64**:302–315.
5. Gao H, Zhang Q, Yu Z, He Q: **Cell-penetrating peptide-based intelligent liposomal systems for enhanced drug delivery.** *Curr Pharm Biotechnol* 2014, **15**:210–219.
6. Mattheolabakis G, Taoufik E, Haralambous S, Roberts ML, Avgoustakis K: **In vivo investigation of tolerance and antitumor activity of cisplatin-loaded PLGA-mPEG nanoparticles.** *Eur J Pharm Biopharm* 2009, **71**(2):190–195.
7. Hyung Park J, Kwon S, Lee M, Chung H, Kim JH, Kim YS, Park RW, Kim IS, Bong Seo S, Kwon IC, Young Jeong S: **Self-assembled nanoparticles based on glycol chitosan bearing hydrophobic moieties as carriers for Gefitiniborubicin: in vivo biodistribution and anti-tumor activity.** *Biomaterials* 2006, **27**(1):119–126.
8. Yu Z, Schmaltz RM, Bozeman TC, Paul R, Rishel MJ, Tsosie KS, Hecht SM: **Selective Tumor Cell Targeting by the Disaccharide Moiety of Bleomycin.** *J Am Chem Soc* 2013, **135**:2883–2886.
9. William P, Vincent M, Maureen Z, Jennifer D, Katerina P, Inderpal S, Bhuvanesh S, Robert H, Valerie R, Lucinda F, Elaine M, Doris K, Richard W, Mark K, Harold V: **EGF receptor gene mutations are common in lung cancers from "never smokers" and are associated with sensitivity of tumors to gefitinib and erlotinib.** *Proc Natl Acad Sci USA* 2004, **101**(36):13306–13311.
10. Morabito A, Costanzo R, Rachiglio AM, Pasquale R, Sandomenico C, Franco R, Montanino A, De Lutio E, Rocco G, Normanno N: **Activity of Gefitinib in a Non–Small-Cell Lung Cancer Patient with Both Activating and Resistance EGFR Mutations.** *J Thorac Oncol* 2013, **8**(7):e59–e60.
11. Ozao-Choy J, Ma G, Kao J, Wang GX, Meseck M, Sung M, Schwartz M, Divino CM, Pan PY, Chen SH: **The novel role of tyrosine kinase inhibitor in the reversal of immune suppression and modulation of tumor microenvironment for immune-based cancer therapies.** *Cancer Res* 2009, **69**(6):2514–2522.
12. Sordella R, Bell DW, Haber DA, Settleman J: **Gefitinib-sensitizing EGFR mutations in lung cancer activate anti-apoptotic pathways.** *Science* 2004, **305**(5687):1163–1167.
13. Cohen MH, Williams GA, Sridhara R, Chen G, McGuinn WD, Morse D, Abraham S, Rahman A, Liang C, Lostritto R, Baird A, Pazdur R: **United States Food and Drug Administration drug approval summary gefitinib (ZD1839; Iressa) tablets.** *Clin Cancer Res* 2004, **10**(4):1212–1218.
14. Kakuta T, Takashima Y, Nakahata M, Otsubo M, Yamaguchi H, Harada A: **Preorganized Hydrogel: Self-Healing Properties of Supramolecular Hydrogels Formed by Polymerization of Host–Guest-Monomers that Contain Cyclodextrins and Hydrophobic Guest Groups.** *Adv Mater* 2013, **25**(20):2849–2853.
15. Loftsson T, Brewster ME: **Cyclodextrins as functional excipients: methods to enhance complexation efficiency.** *J Pharm Sci* 2012, **101**(9):3019–3032.
16. Loftsson T, Duchêne D: **Cyclodextrins and their pharmaceutical applications.** *Int J Pharm* 2007, **329**:1–11.
17. Kurkov SV, Loftsson T: **Cyclodextrins.** *Int J Pharm* 2013, **453**(1):167–180.
18. Szente L, Szemán J: **Cyclodextrins in Analytical Chemistry: Host–Guest Type Molecular Recognition.** *Anal Chem* 2013, **85**(17):8024–8030.
19. Del Valle EM: **Cyclodextrins and their uses: a review.** *Process Biochem* 2004, **39**(9):1033–1046.
20. Agasti SS, Liong M, Tassa C, Chung HJ, Shaw SY, Lee H, Weissleder R: **Supramolecular host-guest interaction for labeling and detection of cellular biomarkers.** *Angew Chem Int Ed Engl* 2012, **51**(2):450–454.
21. Dorokhin D, Hsu SH, Tomczak N, Reinhoudt DN, Huskens J, Velders AH, Vancso GJ: **Fabrication and luminescence of designer surface patterns with β-cyclodextrin functionalized quantum dots via multivalent supramolecular coupling.** *ACS Nano* 2010, **4**:137–142.
22. Zhang B, Jin H, Li Y, Chen B, Liu S, Shi D: **Bioinspired synthesis of gadolinium-based hybrid nanoparticles as MRI blood pool contrast agents with high relaxivity.** *J Mater Chem* 2012, **22**(29):14494–14501.
23. Sun SK, Dong L, Cao Y, Sun H, Yan X: **Fabrication of multifunctional Gd2O3/Au hybrid nanoprobe via a one-step approach for near-infrared fluorescence and magnetic resonance multimodal imaging in vivo.** *Anal Chem* 2013, **85**(17):8436–8441.
24. Zhang B, Li Q, Yin P, Rui Y, Qiu Y, Wang Y, Shi D: **Ultrasound-triggered BSA/SPION hybrid nanoclusters for liver-specific magnetic resonance imaging.** *ACS Appl Mater Interfaces* 2012, **4**(12):6479–6486.
25. Zhang B, Wang X, Liu F, Cheng Y, Shi D: **Effective reduction of nonspecific binding by surface engineering of quantum dots with bovine serum albumin for cell-targeted imaging.** *Langmuir* 2012, **28**(48):16605–16613.
26. Cagle PT, Zhai QJ, Murphy L, Low PS: **Folate receptor in adenocarcinoma and squamous cell carcinoma of the lung: potential target for folate-linked therapeutic agents.** *Arch Pathol Lab Med* 2013, **137**(2):241–244.
27. Chen C, Ke J, Zhou XE, Yi W, Brunzelle JS, Li J, Yong EL, Xu HE, Melcher K: **Structural basis for molecular recognition of folic acid by folate receptors.** *Nature* 2013, **500**(7463):486–489.
28. Leamon CP: **Folate-targeted drug strategies for the treatment of cancer.** *Curr Opin Investig Drugs* 2008, **9**(12):1277–1286.
29. Coney LR, Tomassetti A, Carayannopoulos L, Frasca V, Kamen BA, Colnaghi MI, Zurawski VR Jr: **Cloning of a tumor-associated antigen: MOv18 and MOv19 antibodies recognize a folate-binding protein.** *Cancer Res* 1991, **51**(22):6125–6132.
30. Weitman SD, Frazier KM, Kamen BA: **The folate receptor in central nervous system malignancies of childhood.** *J Neurooncol* 1994, **21**(2):107–112.
31. Campbell IG, Jones TA, Foulkes WD, Trowsdale J: **Folate-binding protein is a marker for ovarian cancer.** *Cancer Res* 1991, **51**(19):5329–5338.
32. Reddy JA, Low PS: **Folate-mediated targeting of therapeutic and imaging agents to cancers.** *Crit Rev Ther Drug Carrier Syst* 1998, **15**(6):587–627.
33. Chen H, Ahn R, Van den Bossche J, Thompson DH, O'Halloran TV: **Folate-mediated intracellular drug delivery increases the anticancer efficacy of nanoparticulate formulation of arsenic trioxide.** *Mol Cancer Ther* 2009, **8**(7):1955–1963.
34. Chu BC, Kramer FR, Orgel LE: **Synthesis of an amplifiable reporter RNA for bioassays.** *Nucleic Acids Res* 1986, **14**(14):5591–5603.
35. Ghosh SS, Kao PM, McCue AW, Chappelle HL: **Use of maleimide-thiol coupling chemistry for efficient syntheses of oligonucleotide-enzyme conjugate hybridization probes.** *Bioconjug Chem* 1990, **1**(1):71–76.
36. Staros JV, Wright RW, Swingle DM: **Enhancement by N-hydroxysulfosuccinimide of water-soluble carbodiimide-mediated coupling reactions.** *Anal Biochem* 1986, **156**(1):220–222.

37. Khalil SK, El-Feky GS, El-Banna ST, Khalil WA: **Preparation and evaluation of warfarin-β-cyclodextrin loaded chitosan nanoparticles for transdermal delivery.** *Carbohydr Polym* 2012, **90**(3):1244–1253.

38. Joo KI, Xiao L, Liu S, Liu Y, Lee CL, Conti PS, Wong MK, Li Z, Wang P: **Crosslinked multilamellar liposomes for controlled delivery of anticancer drugs.** *Biomaterials* 2013, **34**(12):3098–3109.

39. Schroeder BR, Ghare MI, Bhattacharya C, Paul R, Yu Z, Zaleski PA, Bozeman TC, Rishel MJ, Hecht SM: **The disaccharide moiety of bleomycin facilitates uptake by cancer cells.** *J Am Chem Soc* 2014, **136**(39):13641–13656.

40. Qi R, Liu S, Chen J, Xiao H, Yan L, Huang Y, Jing X: **Biodegradable copolymers with identical cationic segments and their performance in siRNA delivery.** *J Control Release* 2012, **159**(2):251–260.

41. Xiao H, Qi R, Liu S, Hu X, Duan T, Zheng Y, Huang Y, Jing X: **Biodegradable polymer - cisplatin(IV) conjugate as a pro-drug of cisplatin(II).** *Biomaterials* 2011, **32**(30):7732–7739.

42. Song Y, Shi W, Chen W, Li X, Ma H: **Fluorescent carbon nanodots conjugated with folic acid for distinguishing folate-receptor-positive cancer cells from normal cells.** *J Mater Chem* 2012, **22**(25):12568–12573.

43. Feng D, Song Y, Shi W, Li X, Ma H: **Distinguishing Folate-Receptor-Positive Cells from Folate-Receptor-Negative Cells Using a Fluorescence Off–On Nanoprobe.** *Anal Chem* 2013, **85**(13):6530–6535.

# Green silver nanoparticles of *Phyllanthus amarus*: as an antibacterial agent against multi drug resistant clinical isolates of *Pseudomonas aeruginosa*

Khushboo Singh[1], Manju Panghal[1], Sangeeta Kadyan[1], Uma Chaudhary[2] and Jaya Parkash Yadav[1*]

## Abstract

**Background:** *Pseudomonas aeruginosa* infection is a leading cause of morbidity and mortality in burn and immune-compromised patients. In recent studies, researchers have drawn their attention towards ecofriendly synthesis of nanoparticles and their activity against multidrug resistant microbes. In this study, silver nanoparticles were synthesized from aqueous extract of *Phyllanthus amarus*. The synthesized nanoparticles were explored as a potent source of nanomedicine against MDR burn isolates of *P. aeruginosa*.

**Results:** Silver nanoparticles were successfully synthesized using *P. amarus* extract and the nature of synthesized nanoparticles was analyzed by UV-Vis spectroscopy, transmission electron microscopy, energy dispersive X-ray spectroscopy, dynamic light scattering, zeta potential, X- ray diffraction and fourier transform infra-red spectroscopy. The average size of synthesized nanoparticles was 15.7, $24 \pm 8$ and 29.78 nm by XRD, TEM and DLS respectively. The antibacterial activity of AgNPs was investigated against fifteen MDR strains of *P. aeruginosa* tested at different concentration. The zone of inhibition was measured in the range of $10 \pm 0.53$ to $21 \pm 0.11$ mm with silver nanoparticles concentration of 12.5 to 100 μg/ml. The zone of inhibition increased with increase in the concentration of silver nanoparticles. The MIC values of synthesized silver nanoparticles were found in the range of 6.25 to12.5 μg/ml. The MIC values are comparable to the standard antibiotics.

**Conclusion:** The present study suggests that silver nanoparticles from *P. amarus* extract exhibited excellent antibacterial potential against multidrug resistant strains of *P. aeruginosa* from burn patients and gives insight of their potential applicability as an alternative antibacterial in the health care system to reduce the burden of multidrug resistance.

**Keywords:** *Pseudomonas aeruginosa*, Burn isolates, MDR, *Phyllanthus amarus*, Silver nanoparticles, Antibacterial

## Background

*Pseudomonas aeruginosa*, a gram negative bacterium, is the leading cause of morbidity and mortality in burn patients as they are more susceptible to infections because of immune-suppression and loss of cutaneous coverage [1]. Since *P. aeruginosa* has innate potential to develop resistance, virtually to any antibiotics to which it is exposed, due to the presence of multiple resistance mechanisms and it becomes a multidrug resistant (MDR) strain.

Infections caused by MDR *P. aeruginosa* are often severe; life threatening and these strains have frequently been reported as the cause of nosocomial infections. These MDR have been emerged as a major problem in burn units as burn injury disrupts both the normal skin barrier and many of systemic host defence mechanism which make burn patients the ideal hosts for opportunistic infections [2]. The importance to prevent these infections has been recognized since its inception thus it becomes difficult to treat the infection caused by *P. aeruginosa* MDR strains due to their narrow range of susceptibility to antimicrobial agents. Therefore, currently, researchers started to develop

* Correspondence: yadav1964@rediffmail.com
[1]Department of Genetics, M.D. University, Rohtak 124001, Haryana, India
Full list of author information is available at the end of the article

alternative therapies to aid patients to recover from the infections. In future, these alternatives may be useful in treating not only burn infections but other antibiotic resistant infections as well.

Nanotechnology provides a good platform to modify and develop the important properties of silver metal in the form of nanoparticles having promising applications as an antibacterial agent [3,4]. Silver nanoparticles have high surface area to volume ratio and the unique chemical, physical properties [5,6]. Nowadays, they have been widely used as an effective bactericidal agent against broad spectrum of bacteria, including antibiotic resistant strains [7]. Hence, researchers are shifting towards nanoparticles in general and silver nanoparticles (AgNPs) in particular to solve the problem of emergence of MDR bacteria [8]. Also the development of biological approach for the synthesis of nanoparticles is evolving in to an important branch of nanotechnology [9,10]. The biological method has advancement over chemical and physical method as it is cost effective and ecofriendly [11,12]. *Phyllanthus amarus* is an important plant of Indian Ayurvedic system of medicine, belongs to the family Euphorbiaceae. It is a small herb well known for its medicinal properties and has been used worldwide [13].

This study aims to explore the efficacy of synthesized silver nanoparticles from *P. amarus* as a potent source of nanomedicine against MDR burn isolates of *P. aeruginosa* and establish the therapeutic antibacterial potential of plant with nanotechnology; thereby justify the folklore claim of the plant used in the traditional system of Indian medicine.

## Results

### Synthesis of AgNPs

The AgNPs were successfully synthesized using aqueous plant extract of *P. amarus* by mixing with silver nitrate solution (1mM). The colour changes from pale yellow to dark brown (Additional file 1: Figure S1). This was observed due to the reduction of $Ag^+$ and it indicates the formation of AgNPs.

### Characterization of Ag nanoparticles

The synthesis of AgNPs was confirmed by UV-VIS spectrophotometer (Shimadzu). The UV-VIS absorption spectra of the AgNPs were monitored in a range of 300-800 nm. A strong peak specific for the synthesis of silver nanoparticles was obtained at 420-430 nm. Additional file 2: Figure S2 shows the absorption spectra of AgNPs synthesized by *P. amarus*. The TEM results (Figure 1) showed that all synthesized AgNPs were spherical in shape with $24 \pm 8$ nm size and found to be well dispersed in aqueous medium. EDX characterization has shown absorption of strong silver signal along with other elements, which may be originated from the

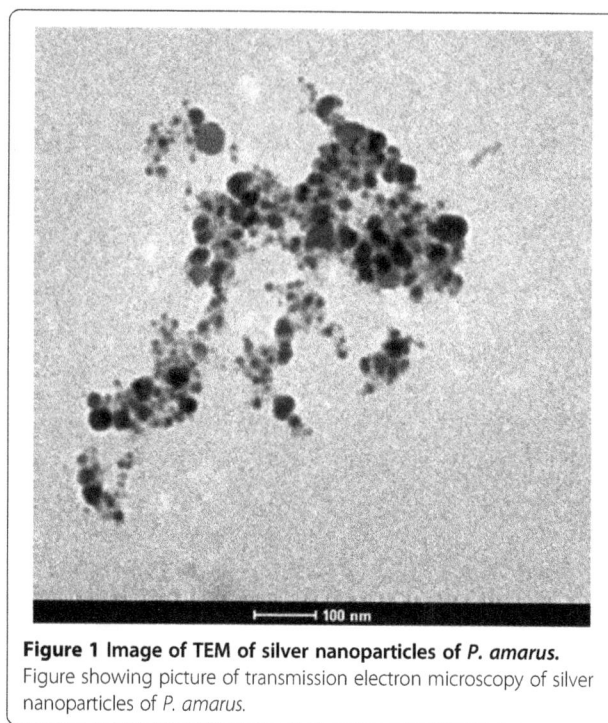

**Figure 1 Image of TEM of silver nanoparticles of *P. amarus*.** Figure showing picture of transmission electron microscopy of silver nanoparticles of *P. amarus*.

biomolecules that are bound to the surface of silver nanoparticles. EDX performed by energy and intensity distributions of X-ray signals generated by focused electron beam on a specimen. From EDX spectra, showed in Figure 2, it is clear that silver nanoparticles reduced by *P. amarus*.

Dynamic light scattering (DLS) technique and zeta potential has been used to determine the size of particles and measure the potential stability of the particles in the colloidal suspension respectively. Figure 3 and Figure 4 have shown the DLS and zeta potential graph of AgNPs of *P. amarus* with an average size of 29.78 nm and the particles carry a charge of -11.9 mV respectively. Silver nanoparticles generally carry a negative charge. All silver nanoparticles synthesized from *P. amarus* showed negative charge and were stable at room temperature. The particle size and nature of AgNPs was determined by XRD. The mean particle diameter of AgNPs was calculated using the Debye-Scherrer's equation. An average size of the silver nanoparticles synthesized by *P. amarus* was 15.7 nm (Figure 5 and Table 1). The FT-IR spectrum of AgNPs from *P. amarus* showed the characteristics absorbance bands (Figure 6) due to aldehydic C–H stretch (2,915 and 2,848 $cm^{-1}$), C-O stretch (1,634 $cm^{-1}$), N-H (1517 $cm^{-1}$, 1462 $cm^{-1}$ N-O stretch (1,377 $cm^{-1}$) and C-O stretch (dialkyl) (1,169 $cm^{-1}$), C-N (1,037 $cm^{-1}$), C-H stretch (718 $cm^{-1}$).

### Antibacterial assay

The 15 multidrug resistant strains of *P. aeruginosa* isolated from burn patients tested at various concentrations

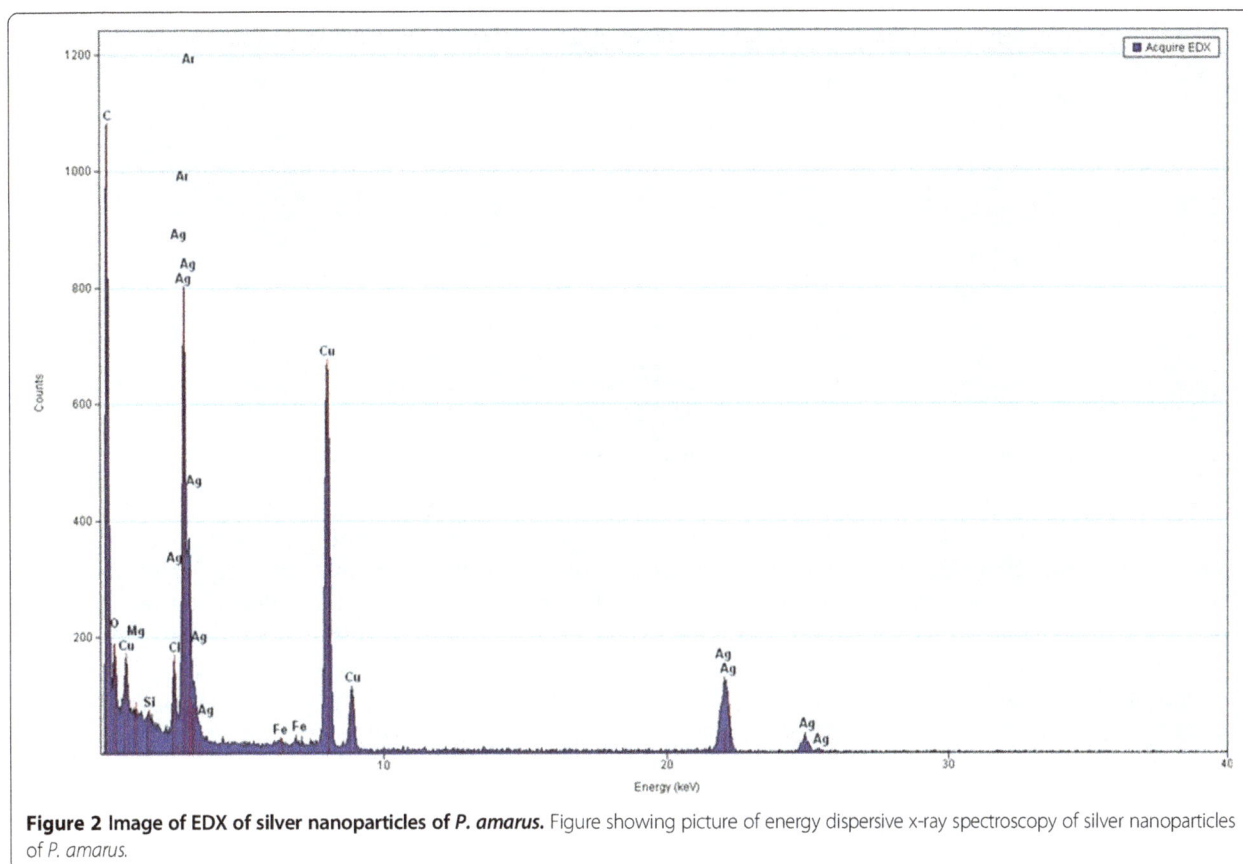

**Figure 2** Image of EDX of silver nanoparticles of *P. amarus.* Figure showing picture of energy dispersive x-ray spectroscopy of silver nanoparticles of *P. amarus.*

of AgNPs i.e. 12.5, 25, 50 and 100 µg/ml to determine the antibacterial effect by agar well diffusion method. The AgNPs showed (Additional file 3: Figure S3) antimicrobial activity against all the tested pathogens. The antibacterial activity is concentration dependent as it increased with the concentration of AgNPs (Figure 7). The zone of inhibition measured in a range of 10 ± 0.53 to 21 ± 0.11 mm. MDR Strain1 was found (Figure 8) to be most susceptible where zone of inhibition ranged from 13 ± 1 to 21 ± 0.11 mm at AgNPs concentration of 12.5 to 100 µg/ml. MDR strain 10 was least susceptible with 10 ± 0.53 to 13 ± 0.41mm zone of inhibition.

**Minimum Inhibitory Concentration (MIC)**

The MIC of AgNPs from *P. amarus* against MDR strains of *P. aeruginosa* was 6.25-12.5 µg/ml. MDR strains 6, 10,12,13,14 and 15 showed the MIC values of 12.5 µg/ml. The remaining nine MDR strains have shown the MIC at 6.25 µg/ml (Table 2) which is lower than standard antibiotic.

**Discussion**

The biosynthesis of nanoparticles has received considerable attention due to the growing need to develop environmentally benign technologies in material synthesis [14]. The phytochemicals derived from plant products

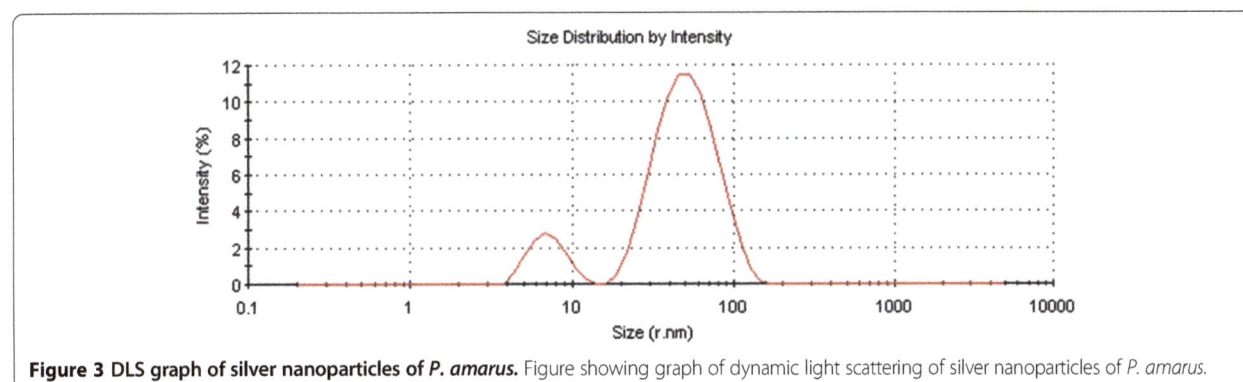

**Figure 3** DLS graph of silver nanoparticles of *P. amarus.* Figure showing graph of dynamic light scattering of silver nanoparticles of *P. amarus.*

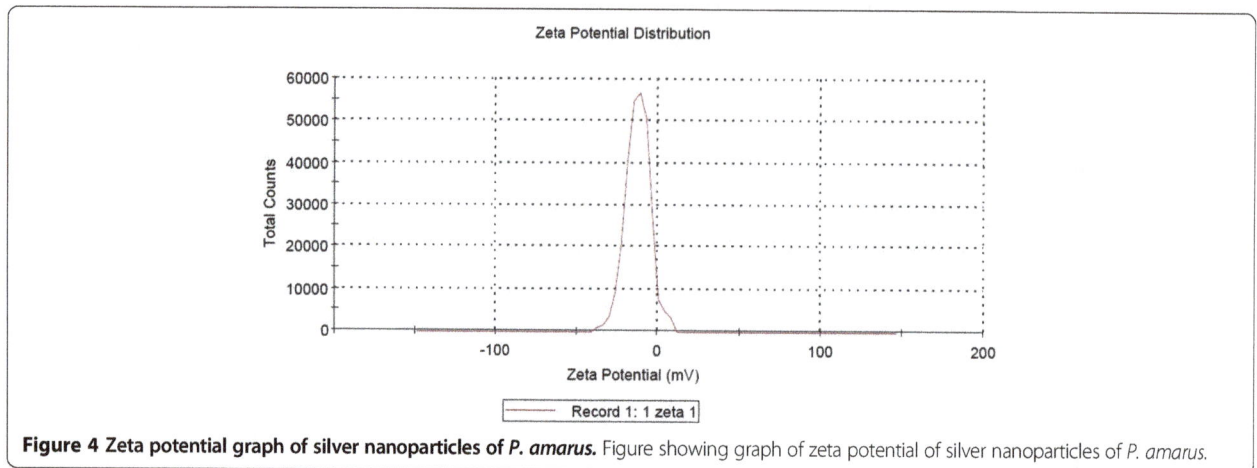

**Figure 4 Zeta potential graph of silver nanoparticles of *P. amarus.*** Figure showing graph of zeta potential of silver nanoparticles of *P. amarus.*

serve as a prototype to develop less toxic and more effective medicines for controlling the growth of microorganisms [15]. These compounds have significant therapeutic application against human pathogens. Numerous studies have been conducted with the extracts of various plants for screening of antimicrobial activity in search of new antimicrobial compounds [16]. *P. amarus* was also reported to have antibacterial efficacy against some drug resistant pathogenic bacterial strains [17]. But there are still limited studies regarding antibacterial activity of AgNPs from this plant. The beauty of the present study is that AgNPs reduced by *P. amarus* were highly effective against MDR burn isolates of *P. aeruginosa* in term of novelty. We synthesized AgNPs from *P. amarus*, which is easily available

in rainy season, safe, non-toxic and have a variety of secondary metabolites that can help in the reduction of silver ions. The main mechanism considered for the process is plant-assisted reduction due to phytochemicals. The main phytochemicals involved are terpenoids, flavones, ketones, aldehydes, amides, and carboxylic acids. Flavones, organic acids, and quinones are water-soluble phytochemicals that are responsible for the immediate reduction of the ions [18]. Studies have revealed that *P. amarus* contain mainly phyllanthin, hypophyllanthin, phyltertralin and many more other phytochemicals [19]. It was also suggested that the phytochemicals are involved directly in the reduction of the ions and formation of silver nanoparticles [20]. Though the exact

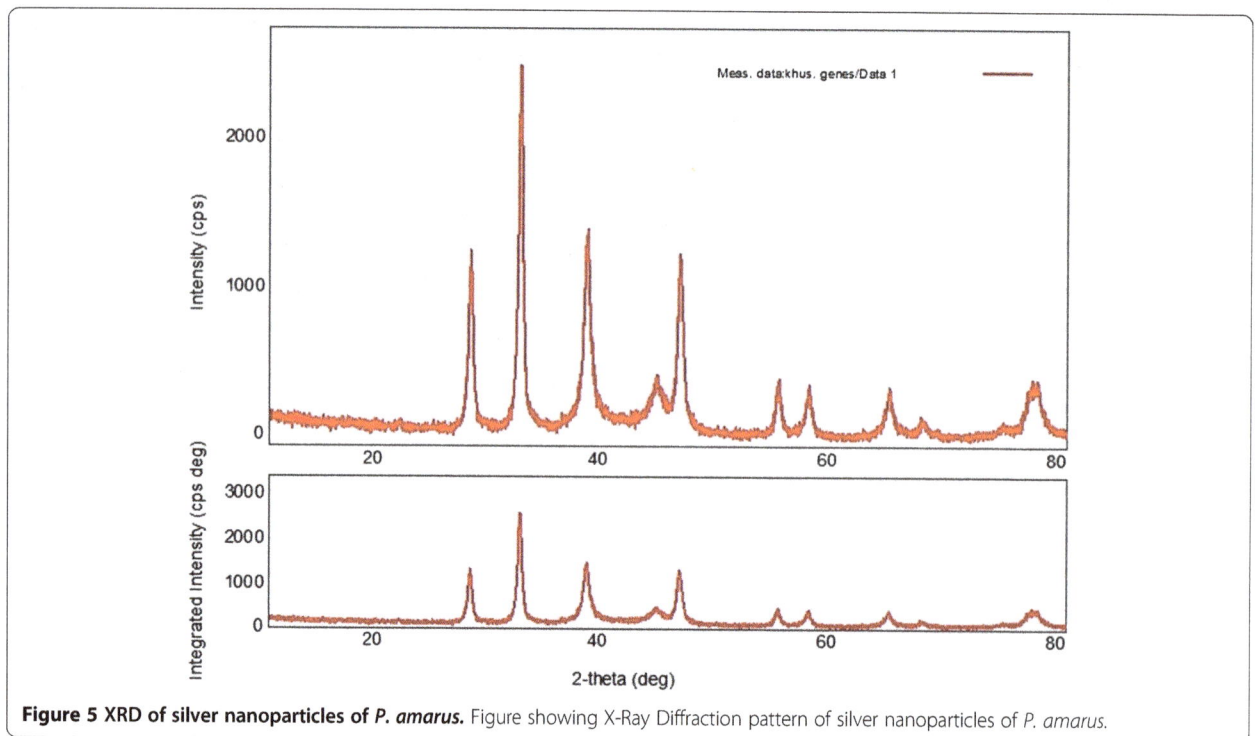

**Figure 5 XRD of silver nanoparticles of *P. amarus.*** Figure showing X-Ray Diffraction pattern of silver nanoparticles of *P. amarus.*

**Table 1 Size of AgNPs of *P. amarus* by using Debye-Scherrer's equation**

| S. No. | 2-theta(deg) | D (ang.) | FWHM(deg) | Int. I(cps deg) | Int. W(deg) | Size(nm) |
|--------|--------------|----------|-----------|-----------------|-------------|----------|
| 1 | 27.797 | 3.206 | 0.464 | 488.7 | 0.651 | 18.4 |
| 2 | 32.210 | 2.776 | 0.450 | 1008.65 | 0.622 | 19.1 |
| 3 | 38.094 | 2.306 | 0.647 | 845.25 | 0.992 | 13.5 |
| 4 | 44.195 | 2.047 | 1.204 | 224.79 | 1.535 | 7.43 |
| 5 | 46.250 | 1.961 | 0.576 | 492.67 | 0.702 | 15.6 |
| 6 | 54.750 | 1.675 | 0.532 | 152.66 | 0.722 | 17.5 |
| 7 | 57.450 | 1.602 | 0.610 | 148.96 | 0.825 | 15.4 |
| 8 | 64.485 | 1.443 | 0.367 | 171.27 | 0.758 | 26.6 |
| 9 | 77.068 | 1.236 | 1.285 | 258.17 | 1.368 | 8.25 |

mechanism involved in each plant varies as due to the presence of different phytochemicals which are involved in the reduction of the ions leads to the synthesis of AgNPs. A strong peak was obtained at 420-430 nm showing the absorption spectra of AgNPs synthesized by *P. amarus*. Further EDX has shown absorption of strong silver signal along with other elements that are bound to the surface of silver nanoparticles. TEM, XRD, DLS revealed the size and zeta potential contributed towards the stability of AgNPs [21]. FTIR confirms the presence of different functional groups absorb characteristic frequencies of IR radiations [22].

The exact mechanism by which silver nanoparticles employ to cause antimicrobial effect is not clearly known. However, there are various theories suggested about the action of AgNPs on microbes to cause the antimicrobial effect. The AgNPs have ability to anchor to the bacterial cell wall and subsequently penetrate it, thereby causing structural changes in the cell membrane like the permeability of cell membrane and death of the cell. There is formation of 'pits' on the cell surface where accumulation of the nanoparticles takes place [23]. The formation of free radicals by AgNPs may be considered to be another mechanism by which the cells die [24,25]. It has also been proposed that there can be release of silver ions by the nanoparticles [26], and these ions can interact with the thiol groups of many vital enzymes and inactivate them [27]. The bacterial cells in contact with silver absorb silver

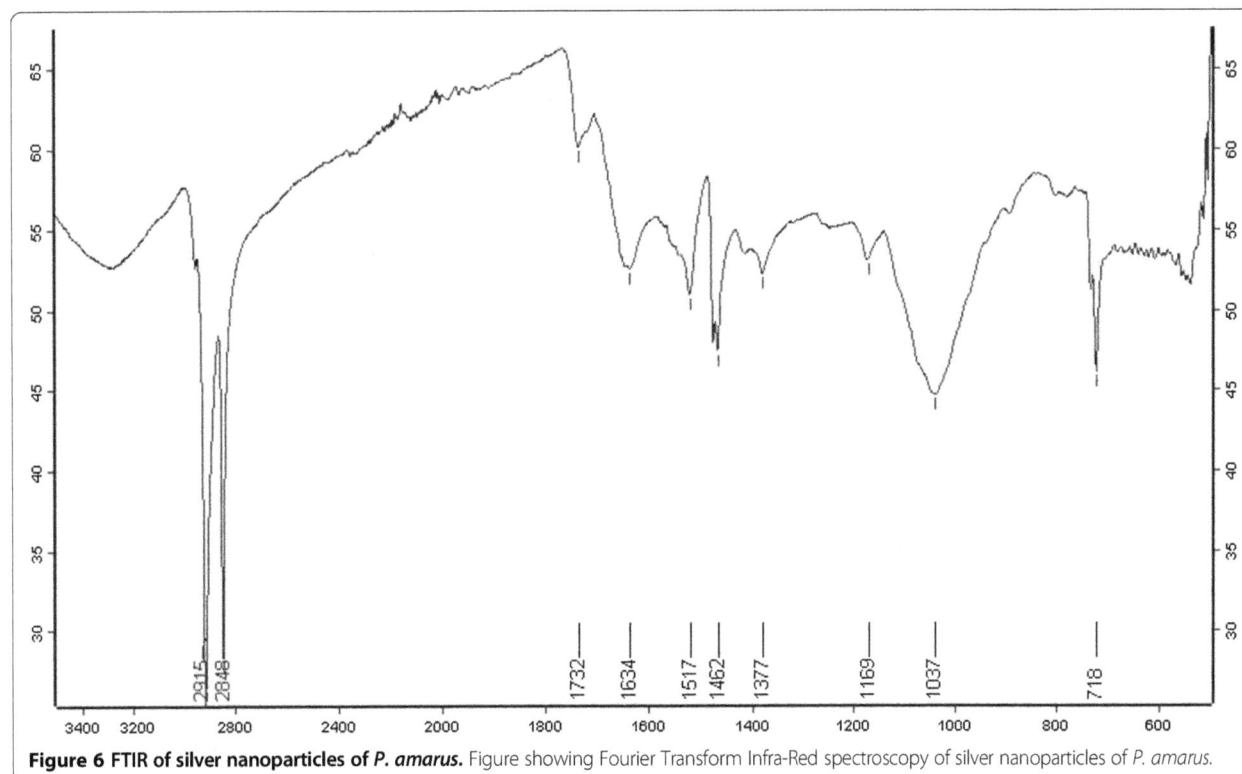

**Figure 6 FTIR of silver nanoparticles of *P. amarus*.** Figure showing Fourier Transform Infra-Red spectroscopy of silver nanoparticles of *P. amarus*.

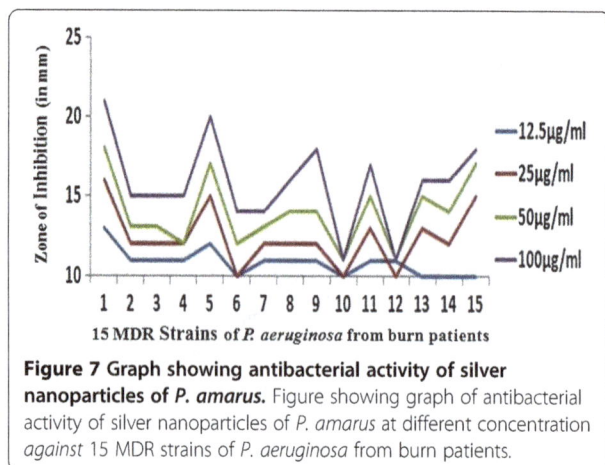

**Figure 7 Graph showing antibacterial activity of silver nanoparticles of *P. amarus.*** Figure showing graph of antibacterial activity of silver nanoparticles of *P. amarus* at different concentration *against* 15 MDR strains of *P. aeruginosa* from burn patients.

ions, which inhibit several functions in the cell and damage the cells.

In recent years, due to the development of resistant strains, antibiotic resistance also has been increased. MDR *P. aeruginosa* strains from burn patients are causing serious infections and exhibit innate resistance to many antibiotics. These can develop new resistance after exposures to antimicrobial agents. Some antimicrobial agents are extremely irritant and toxic. The studies on drug resistant bacteria in this facet are still limited. Also AgNPs have gained insight as an excellent antimicrobial agent due to its non-toxic effect on human cells in its low concentration and weaker ability to develop resistance towards silver ions [28-30].

The various researchers showed that AgNPs of *P. amarus* were found to be good antibacterial agent. Humberto et al. [31] showed the antibacterial activity of AgNPs against multidrug-resistant *P. aeruginosa, E. coli, Streptococcus* sp.

and *S. pyogens.* Kathireshwari et al. [32] showed the antimicrobial activity against multi drug resistant human pathogens from leaf mediated synthesis of AgNPs using *Phyllanthus niruri.* Durairaj et al. [33] studied the antibacterial activity of purchased AgNPs (size 20-30 nm) against 10 isolates of *P. aeruginosa* comprising of 5 MDR strains with an inhibition zone of 11 mm observed with10 µg dose of the nanoparticles. In our results, AgNPs showed excellent antibacterial activity which is better than our previous study [34], which showed the good antibacterial activity of AgNPs prepared using *T. cordifolia* aqueous extract against *P. aeruginosa* MDR strain from burn patient with maximum concentration of 200 µg/ml. However, there is vital need and much interest in finding ways to formulate new types of safe and cost-effective biocidal materials [22]. Therefore, in this study, we used different plant as biomaterial and evaluated its antibacterial effects. The synthesized AgNPs showed significant antibacterial activity at concentration of 12.5-100 µg/ml against MDR strains of *P. aeruginosa* isolates. The MIC of AgNPs was found to be in a range from 6.25-12.5 µg/ml, almost nine MDR strains have shown the MIC at 6.25 µg/ml which was lower than that of the standard antibiotic (10 µg). As infection of *P. aeruginosa* always remains one of the most challenging concerns in burn units and the synthesized AgNPs of *P. amarus* are highly effective antibacterial agent against these MDR burn isolates.

## Conclusion

In conclusion, we have demonstrated that AgNPs from *P. amarus* exhibit excellent antibacterial potential against MDR *P. aeruginosa* strains isolated from burn patients. Therefore these AgNPs may act as ecofriendly antibacterial agent against these nosocomial strains and can

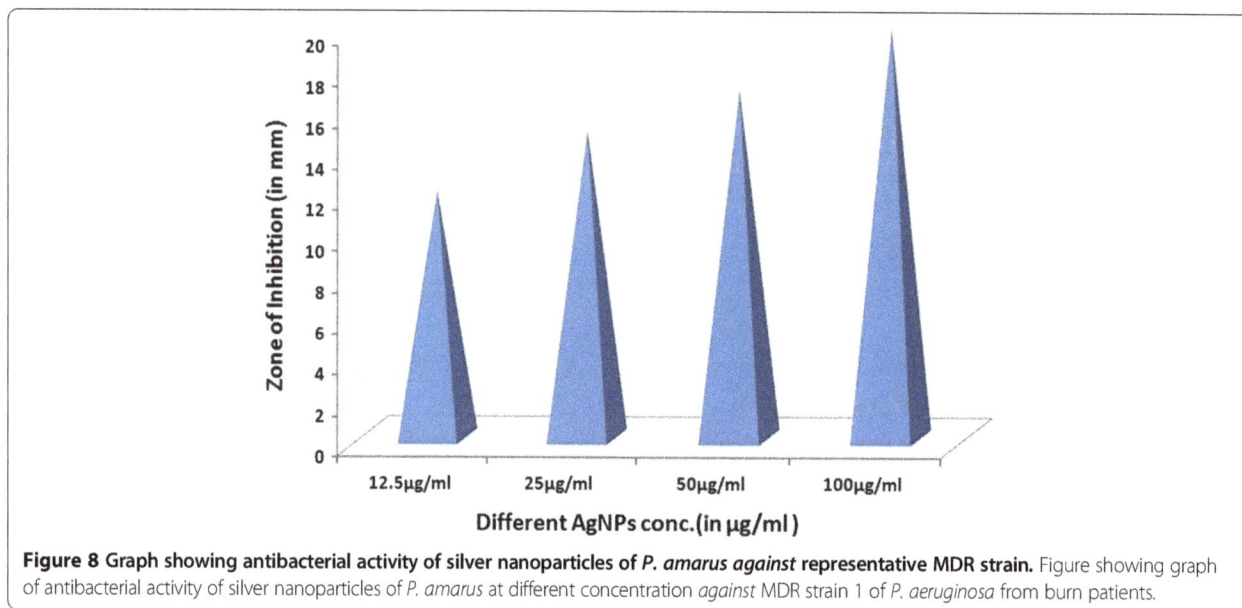

**Figure 8 Graph showing antibacterial activity of silver nanoparticles of *P. amarus against* representative MDR strain.** Figure showing graph of antibacterial activity of silver nanoparticles of *P. amarus* at different concentration *against* MDR strain 1 of *P. aeruginosa* from burn patients.

Green silver nanoparticles of Phyllanthus amarus: as an antibacterial agent against multi drug...

73

**Table 2 MIC of silver nanoparticles of *P. amarus* against MDR strains of *P. aeruginosa* from burn patients**

| S.No | MIC(in µg/ml) |
|------|---------------|
| *P. aeruginosa* MDR Strain 1 | 6.25 |
| *P. aeruginosa* MDR Strain 2 | 6.25 |
| *P. aeruginosa* MDR Strain 3 | 6.25 |
| *P. aeruginosa* MDR Strain 4 | 6.25 |
| *P. aeruginosa* MDR Strain 5 | 6.25 |
| *P. aeruginosa* MDR Strain 6 | 12.5 |
| *P. aeruginosa* MDR Strain 7 | 6.25 |
| *P. aeruginosa* MDR Strain 8 | 6.25 |
| *P. aeruginosa* MDR Strain 9 | 6.25 |
| *P. aeruginosa* MDR Strain 10 | 12.5 |
| *P. aeruginosa* MDR Strain 11 | 6.25 |
| *P. aeruginosa* MDR Strain 12 | 12.5 |
| *P. aeruginosa* MDR Strain 13 | 12.5 |
| *P. aeruginosa* MDR Strain 14 | 12.5 |
| *P. aeruginosa* MDR Strain 15 | 12.5 |

provides a potent alternative nanomedicine in the health care system to reduce the burden of multidrug resistance.

## Material and methods
### Synthesis of silver nanoparticles from plant extract
*Preparation of the extract*
The whole plant of *Phyllanthus amarus* was collected locally from Botanical Garden, M.D. University, Rohtak, Haryana, India. It was thoroughly washed in distilled water, cut into fine pieces. 10g of fresh plant material was boiled into 100 ml sterile distilled water for 10 minutes and filtered through Whatman's No.1 filter paper. The extract was stored at 4°C for further experiments.

### Synthesis of AgNPs from plant extract
For synthesis of AgNPs, the above plant extract of *P. amarus* was used and 15 ml of this extract was added to 200 ml of aqueous silver nitrate solution (1mM). This solution was kept for 20 minutes at 70°C (in water bath). The plant extract act as reducing as well as stabilizing agent in the solution and leads to the formation of AgNPs.

### Characterization of synthesized AgNPs
The seven different characterization techniques were used for AgNPs. At first, AgNPs were characterized by UV-VIS Spectroscopy using Shimadzu UV-VIS Spectrophotometer. The scanning range for the samples was 300-800 nm. The double distilled water used as a blank reference. To remove any free biomass residue or compound that is not the capping ligand of the nanoparticles, after complete reduction, silver nanoparticles were

concentrated by repeated centrifugation (3 times) of the reaction mixture at 15,000rpm for 20 min. The supernatant was replaced by distilled water each time. Thereafter, the purified suspension was freeze dried to obtain dried powder. The shape and size of AgNPs was determined by transmission electron microscopy (TEM). A drop (2 ul) of water dissolved synthesized nanoparticles was placed on a copper grid. The images were obtained with a Tecnai, Twin 200 KV (FEI, Netherlands) at a bias voltage of 200 kV used to analyze samples. The composition of the AgNPs was determined using the Energy Dispersive X-Ray Spectroscopy (EDX) coupled to the TEM. The size distribution or average size of the synthesized AgNPs were determined by dynamic light scattering (DLS) and zeta potential measurements were carried out using DLS (Malvern). For DLS analysis the samples were diluted 10 folds using 0.15M PBS (pH 7.4) and the measurements were taken in the range between 0.1 and 10,000 nm. X- Ray Diffraction (XRD) was done with the help of by X-Pert Pro Diffractometer. The X-ray diffraction data were obtained using step scan technique and with Cu-Ka radiation (1.500 Å, 40 kV, 30 mA) in h–2h configuration. The AgNPs were coated on to the glass substrate and after drying, the sample was analyzed by X-ray diffractometer. The crystallite domain size was calculated using the Debye–Scherrer's formula. Finally, Fourier Transform Infra-red Spectroscopy (FTIR) was used for detection of different functional groups. The dried AgNPs were analyzed by ALPHA FT-IR Spectrometer (from Bruker, Germany) for the detection of different functional groups by showing peaks from the region of 4000 cm$^{-1}$ to 500 cm$^{-1}$.

### Multi drug resistant clinical isolates of *P. aeruginosa* from burn patients
Fifteen clinical isolates were obtained from the various samples of burn patients receiving in Microbiology Department of Pt. B.D.S. Post Graduate Institute of Medical Sciences, Rohtak, Haryana, India. The purity and identity of each isolate was confirmed in laboratory by standard microbiological methods [35-37]. The sources of the clinical isolates were urine, wounds, blood, and body fluids of burn patients. The approval of SRAC (Scientific & Research Advisory Committee) of the institute was taken for the study with reference no. UHS/OSD/2010/1 dated 27/02/2012. The 10 most cost-effective antibiotics routinely used to treat *P. aeruginosa* infections were employed in the susceptibility test. The antibiotics included were amikacin, aztreonam, ceftizoxime, cefepime, gentamicin, imipenem, netilmicin, ofloxacin, piperacillin and tazobactum. For isolation of MDR strains, these antibiotics were used and susceptibility was checked by Kirby-Bauer disc method [38]. The strain which were resistant to 6 or 7 antibiotics was taken as MDR strain.

## Antibacterial assay of AgNPs

4 Test samples of the AgNPs were prepared in DMSO (Dimethyl Sulfoxide). The concentrations of AgNPs were ranges from 12.5-100 μg/ml i.e. 12.5, 25, 50 and 100 μg/ml. The antimicrobial activities were determined by agar well diffusion assay [39]. Under aseptic conditions, in to the Bio safety chamber, 20 ml of MHA medium was dispensed in to pre-sterilized petridishes. Once the media solidifies it was then inoculated with micro-organism suspended in peptone water. The media was then punched with 6mm diameter hole and filled with different dilutions (varying from 12.5 to 100 μg/ml) of AgNPs extract from stock of 20 mg/ml. Streptomycin (10 μg/ml) was used as positive control and DMSO was used as a negative control. Finally, the petridishes were incubated for 24 hours at 37°C. The diameter of zone of inhibition was measured as indicated by clear area devoid of growth of microbes. Each experiment was done in triplicate.

Minimum inhibitory concentration method (MIC) was calculated by micro broth dilution method in 96 multi-well microtitre plates with slight modifications [40]. Qualitative experimentation was done by resazurin indicator solution prepared by dissolving a 270 mg tablet in 40 ml of sterile distilled water. Purple colour of indicator (resazurin) reduced in the presence of living bacteria. Colour change from purple to pink or to colourless. In the absence of living bacteria the colour of the indicator were remain purple. The lowest conc. at which colour change occurred was taken as MIC.

## Consent

Written informed consent was obtained from the patient for the publication of this report.

## Additional files

**Additional file 1: Figure S1.** Formation of silver nanoparticles of *P. amarus.* Figure showing colour change from pale yellow to dark brown.

**Additional file 2: Figure S2.** Uv-Vis Spectra of silver nanoparticles of *P. amarus.* Figure showing Uv-Vis absorption spectra of silver nanoparticles at range of 300-800.

**Additional file 3: Figure S3.** Picture of antibacterial activity of AgNPs against 15 MDR strains of *P aeruginosa.* Figure showing antibacterial activity of AgNPs against 15 MDR strains of *P aeruginosa* at concentration of 12.5-100 μg/ml.

## Competing interests

The authors declare that they have no competing interests.

## Authors' contributions

KS contributed to the design of the study, performed the experiment, analyzed the data and prepared the manuscript. MP maintained the bacterial sample culture. SK contributed in the analysis of data. UC provided the bacterial samples. JPY was responsible for the research and the manuscript. All authors read and approved the final manuscript.

## Acknowledgements

The authors are thankful to National Medicinal Plant Board (Grant no & Date- Z.18017/187/CSS/R&D/HR-01/2011-12-NMPB/24/11/2011), New Delhi for the award of Major Research Project grant and Department of Science & Technology (DST) for providing fund for project (Grant no - SR/WOS- A/LS-259/2011(G) & Date- 19/12/2011).

## Author details

[1]Department of Genetics, M.D. University, Rohtak 124001, Haryana, India. [2]Department of Microbiology, Pt. B.D.S Post Graduate Institute of Medical Sciences Rohtak, Rohtak 124001, Haryana, India.

## References

1. Santucci SG, Gobara S, Santos CR, Fontana C, Levin AS: **Infections in a burn intensive care unit: experience of seven years.** *J Hosp Infect* 2003, **53**:6–13.
2. Cochran A, Morris SE, Edelman LS, Saffle JR: **Systemic** *Candida* **infection in burn patients.** *Surg Infect Larch* 2002, **3**:367–374.
3. Marcato PD, Duran N: **New aspects of nanopharmaceutical delivery systems.** *J Nanosci Nanotechnol* 2008, **8**:2216–2229.
4. Singh R, Singh NH: **Medical applications of nanoparticles in biological imaging, cell labeling, antimicrobial agents, and anticancer nanodrugs.** *J Biomed Nanotechnol* 2008, **7**:489–503.
5. Morones JR, Elechiguerra JL, Camacho A, Ramirez JT: **The bactericidal effect of silver nanoparticles.** *Nanotechnology* 2005, **16**:2346–2353.
6. Kurek A, Grudniak AM, Kraczkiewicz-Dowjat A, Wolska KI: **New antibacterial therapeutics and strategies.** *Pol J Microbiol* 2011, **60**:3–12.
7. Percival Steven L, Bowler PG, Dolman J: **Antimicrobial activity of silver-containing dressings on wound microorganisms using an in vitro biofilm model.** *Int Wound J* 2007, **4**:186–191.
8. Gemmell CG, Edwards DI, Frainse AP: **Guidelines for the prophylaxis and treatment of methicillin-resistant** *Staphylococcus aureus* **(MRSA) infections in the UK.** *J Antimicrob Chemother* 2006, **57**:589–608.
9. Shankar SS, Rai A, Ahmad A, Sastry MJ: **Rapid synthesis of Au, Ag and bimetallic Au-shell nanoparticles using Neem.** *J Colloid Interf Sci* 2004, **275**:496–502.
10. Raut RW, Lakkakula JR, Kolekar NS, Mendhulkar VD, Kashid SB: **Phytosynthesis of silver nanoparticle using** *Gliricidia sepium* **(Jacq.).** *Curr Nanosci* 2009, **5**:117–122.
11. David SG: *Bionanotechnology: Lessons from Nature.* New York: Wiley; 2004.
12. Talebi S, Ramezani F, Ramezani M: **Biosynthesis of metal nanoparticles by micro-organisms.** *Nanocon Olomouc, Czech Republic, EU* 2010, **10**:12–18.
13. Patel JR, Tripathi P, Sharma V, Chauhan NS, Dixit VK: *Phyllanthus amarus*: **ethnomedicinal uses, phytochemistry and pharmacology: a review.** *J Ethnopharmacol* 2011, **138**:286–313.
14. Oza G, Pandey S, Shah R, Sharon M: **Extracellular fabrication of silver nanoparticles using** *Pseudomonas aeruginosa* **and its antimicrobial assay.** *Pelagia Res Lib Adv Appl Sci Res* 2012, **3**:1776–1783.
15. Ahmad I, Beg AZ: **Antimicrobial and phytochemical studies on 45 Indian medicinal plants against multiple drug resistant human pathogens.** *J Ethanopharmacol* 2001, **74**:113–123.
16. Sharma A: **Antibacterial activity of ethanolic extracts of some arid zone plants.** *Int J Pharm Tech Res* 2011, **3**:283–286.
17. Mazumder A, Mahato A, Mazumder R: **Antimicrobial potentiality of** *Phyllanthus amarus* **against drug resistant pathogens.** *Nat Prod Res* 2006, **20**:323–326.
18. Prabhu S, Poulose E: **Silver nanoparticles: mechanism of antimicrobial action, synthesis, medical applications, and toxicity effects.** *Int Nano Lett* 2012, **2**:32. doi:10.1186/2228-5326-2-32.
19. Yuandani, Ilangkovan M, Jantan I, Mohamad HF, Husain K, Abdul Razak AF: **Inhibitory effects of standardized extracts of** *Phyllanthus amarus* **and** *Phyllanthus urinaria* **and their marker compounds on phagocytic activity of human neutrophils.** *Evid Based Complement Alternat Med* 2013, **2013**:603634.
20. Jha AK, Prasad K, Prasad K, Kulkarni AR: **Plant system: nature's nanofactory.** *Colloids Surf B: Biointerfaces* 2009, **73**:219–223.
21. Bunghez IR, Barbinta Patrascu ME, Badea NM, Doncea SM, Popescu A, Ion RM: **Antioxidant silver nanoparticles green synthesized using ornamental plants.** *J Optoelectronics Adv Mater* 2012, **14**:1016–1022.

Green silver nanoparticles of Phyllanthus amarus: as an antibacterial agent against multi drug...

75

22. Kalainila P, Subha V, Ernest Ravindran RS, Sahadevan R: **Synthesis and characterization of silver nanoparticles from** *Erythrina indica*. *Asian J Pharm and Clin Res* 2014, **7**:39–43.

23. Sondi I, Salopek-Sondi B: **Silver nanoparticles as antimicrobial agent: a case study on E. coli as a model for Gram-negative bacteria.** *J Colloid Interface Sci* 2004, **275**:177–182.

24. Danilcauk M, Lund A, Saldo J, Yamada H, Michalik J: **Conduction electron spin resonance of small silver particles.** *Spectrochimaca Acta Part A* 2006, **63**:189–191.

25. Kim JS, Kuk E, Yu K, Kim JH, Park SJ, Lee HJ, Kim SH, Park YK, Park YH, Hwang CY, Kim YK, Lee YS, Jeong DH, Cho MH: **Antimicrobial effects of silver nanoparticles.** *Nanomedicine* 2007, **3**:95–101.

26. Feng QL, Wu J, Chen GQ, Cui FZ, Kim TN, Kim JO: **A mechanistic study of the antibacterial effect of silver ions on** *Escherichia coli* **and** *Staphylococcus aureus*. *J Biomed Mater Res* 2008, **52**:662–668.

27. Matsumura Y, Yoshikata K, Kunisaki S, Tsuchido T: **Mode of bacterial action of silver zeolite and its comparison with that of silver nitrate.** *Appl Environ Microbiol* 2003, **69**:4278–4281.

28. Shahverdi AR, Fakhimi A, Shahverdi HR, Minaian S: **Synthesis and effect of silver nanoparticles on the antibacterial activity of different antibiotics against Staphylococcus aureus and Escherichia coli Nanomed.** *Nanotechol Biol Med* 2007, **3**:168–171.

29. Sukhdeb P, Kyung TY, Myong SJ: **Does the antibacterial activity of silver nanoparticles depend on the shape of the nanoparticle? A study of the gram-negative bacterium** *Escherichia coli*. *Appl Environ Microbiol* 2007, **73**:1712–1720.

30. Sharma Virender K, Yngard RA, Yekaterina L: **Silver nanoparticles: green synthesis and their antimicrobial activities.** *Adv Colloid Interface Sci* 2009, **145**:83–96.

31. Humberto HL, Ayala-Nunez NV, del Carmen Ixtepan Turrent L, Padilla CR: **Bactericidal effect of silver nanoparticles against multidrug- resistant bacteria.** *World J Microbiol Biotechnol* 2010, **26**:615–621.

32. Kathireswari P, Gomathi S, Saminathan K: **Plant leaf mediated synthesis of silver nanoparticles using** *Phyllanthus niruri* **and its antimicrobial activity against multi drug resistant human pathogens.** *Int J Curr Microbiol App Sci* 2014, **3**:960–968.

33. Durairaj R, Amirulhusni AN, Palanisamy NK, Mohd-Zain Z, Ping LJ: **Antibacterial effect of silver nanoparticles on multi drug resistant pseudomonas aeruginosa.** *World Acad Sci Eng Technol* 2012, **6**:210–213.

34. Singh K, Panghal M, Kadyan S, Chaudhary U, Yadav JP: **Antibacterial activity of synthesized silver nanoparticles from** *Tinospora cordifolia* **against multi drug resistant strains of** *Pseudomonas aeruginosa* **isolated from burn patients.** *J Nanomed Nanotechnol* 2014, **5**:192. doi:10.4172/2157-7439.1000192.

35. Hawkey P, Law DA: *Medical Bacteriology: A Practical Approach*. New York: Oxford University Press; 2004.

36. Ryan KJ: **Normal Microbial flora.** In *Medical Microbiology*. 4th edition. Edited by Sherris JC, Ryan KJ, Ray GC. USA: McGraw Hill; 2004.

37. Pawar VB, Dutta D: **From Diagnostic Bacteriology.** In *A Procedure Manual for Routine Diagnostic Test*, Volume 2. Edited by Mukherjee KL. New Delhi: Tata MacGrew -Hill Publishing Company Limited; 2006:554–626.

38. Bauer AW, Kirby WM, Sherris JC, Turck M: **Antibiotic susceptibility testing by a standardized single disk method.** *Am J Clin Pathol* 1966, **45**:493–496.

39. Perez C, Pauli M, Bezevque P: **An antibiotic assay by agar well diffusion method.** *Acta Biologiae Med Experimentalis* 1990, **15**:113–115.

40. Sarker SD, Nahar L, Kumarasamy Y: **Microtitre plate-based antibacterial assay incorporating resazurin as an indicator of cell growth, and its application in the in vitro antibacterial screening of phytochemicals.** *Methods* 2007, **42**:321–324.

# 9

# Cell lysis-free quantum dot multicolor cellular imaging-based mechanism study for TNF-α-induced insulin resistance

Min Jung Kim, Sabarinathan Rangasamy, Yumi Shim and Joon Myong Song[*]

## Abstract

**Background:** TNF-α is an inflammatory cytokine that plays an important role in insulin resistance observed in obesity and chronic inflammation. Many cellular components involved in insulin signaling cascade are known to be inhibited by TNF-α. Insulin receptor substrate (IRS)-1 is one of the major targets in TNF-α-induced insulin resistance. The serine phosphorylation of IRS-1 enables the inhibition of insulin signaling. Until now, many studies have been conducted to investigate the mechanism of TNF-α-induced insulin resistance based on Western blot. Intracellular protein kinase crosstalk is commonly encountered in inflammation-associated insulin resistance. The crosstalk among the signaling molecules obscures the precise role of kinases in insulin resistance. We have developed a cell lysis-free quantum dots (QDots) multicolor cellular imaging to identify the biochemical role of multiple kinases (p38, JNK, IKKβ, IRS1$^{ser}$, IRS1$^{tyr}$, GSK3β, and FOXO1) in inflammation-associated insulin resistance pathway with a single assay in one run. QDot-antibody conjugates were used as nanoprobes to simultaneously monitor the activation/deactivation of the above seven intracellular kinases in HepG2 cells. The effect of the test compounds on the suppression of TNF-α-induced insulin resistance was validated through kinase monitoring. Aspirin, indomethacin, cinnamic acid, and amygdalin were tested.

**Results:** Through the measurement of the glycogen level in HepG2 cell treated with TNF-α, it was found that aspirin and indomethacin increased glycogen levels by almost two-fold compared to amygdalin and cinnamic acid. The glucose production assay proved that cinnamic acid was much more efficient in suppressing glucose production, compared with MAP kinase inhibitors and non-steroidal anti-inflammatory drugs. QDot multicolor cellular imaging demonstrated that amygdalin and cinnamic acid selectively acted via the JNK1-dependent pathway to suppress the inflammation-induced insulin resistance and improve insulin sensitivity.

**Conclusion:** The regulatory function of multiple kinases could be monitored concurrently at the cellular level. The developed cellular imaging assay provides a unique platform for the understanding of inflammation and insulin resistance signaling pathways in type II diabetes mellitus and how they regulate each other. The results showed that amygdalin and cinnamic acid inhibit serine phosphorylation of IRS-1 through targeting JNK serine kinase and enhance insulin sensitivity.

**Keywords:** Multicolor cellular imaging, Insulin resistance, Quantum dot, Inflammation

* Correspondence: jmsong@snu.ac.kr
College of Pharmacy, Seoul National University, Seoul 151-742, South Korea

## Background

The worldwide prevalence of diabetes has progressively risen over the past 30 years. According to the World Health Organization, the global number of people with diabetes is 371 million; of this population, around 90% suffer from type II diabetes [1]. Cardiovascular disease, obesity, kidney failure, diabetic retinopathy, and neuropathy are associated with type II diabetes mellitus (T2DM). Inflammation and insulin resistance play a vital role in the above T2DM-related diseases.

Perturbations in downstream proteins involved in insulin signaling pathways have been found in insulin resistance and inflammation-associated T2DM. Hundreds of protein molecules are intricately involved in the insulin signaling pathway. The insulin receptor substrate (IRS1-4) proteins, phosphatidylinositol 3 kinase (PI3K), and AKT/protein kinase B (PKB) are considered as the best junctions for potential crosstalk with other pathways [2]. IRS protein undergoes serine phosphorylation in response to such stimuli as TNF-α and negatively controls IRS signaling. In insulin-resistant states, the phosphorylation of IRS1 is elevated, and it activates many downstream kinases, such as extracellular signal-regulated kinase ERK, S6 kinase, and c-Jun-N-terminal kinase. TNF-α also functions through its receptor on the cell surface and targets multiple components, including the insulin receptor, the insulin receptor substrate (IRS), glucose synthesis through GSK3, gluconeogenesis via FOXO1, and glucose transporter 4 (Glut4) in insulin-signal transduction [3]. On the other hand, TNF-α is considered as one of the molecular targets for suppressing inflammation in insulin-resistant conditions. TNF-α induces the TAK kinase-IKKβ/p38/JNK kinase axis and finally promotes PPAR γ inhibition [4]. Common protein kinases located in the signaling cascade are responsible for crosstalk. In the case of inflammation-associated insulin resistance, there are several instances of crosstalk between insulin signaling composed of IRS1-4 proteins, PI3K, AKT/protein kinase B (PKB), and mitogen-activated protein kinases (MAPKs, i.e., p38, JNK, and IKKβ) of inflammatory signaling. The crosstalk intercommunication between the inflammation and insulin-resistant kinases complicates our understanding of signal propagation. Crosstalk creates a barrier to deciphering the biochemical function of individual protein kinases in metabolic disturbances. Consequently, inflammation-associated T2DM disease mechanisms are poorly understood. One of the most daunting challenges is to identify the function of individual signaling molecules in the presence of two disease conditions, such as inflammation and insulin resistance.

Until now, Western blot has been used as the main tool to monitor signaling transductions which lead to insulin resistance. The current approaches to evaluate signaling molecule activity are deficient in terms of sensing phosphorylated proteins, tracing the junctions of crosstalk, sensing variation in intensity level, and detecting morphological changes in cells, specifically to identify individual protein molecules in a cell population. Moreover, the current approaches are qualitative in nature. The quantification of the amount of specific proteins can be difficult. Pure acquisition of a particular protein from a pool of various proteins is not easy. Antibodies may exhibit some off-target binding, which can cause poor results. Performing a Western blot properly with good results can be challenging, and requires a well-trained staff. Moreover, during the entire procedure, the temperature and pH must be maintained properly. Loss of protein during the preparation of samples through many experimental steps, including cell lysis, is also possible. As a result, large numbers of cells are needed due to the degree of cell lysis. In spite of the large number of cells to be lysed, insensitivity of Western blot makes it difficult to correctly define activation or deactivation of the relevant proteins. In this work, cell lysis-free multicolor cellular imaging-based mechanism study for TNF-α-induced insulin resistance is introduced. Proteins involved in inflammation and insulin signaling were concurrently monitored without cell lysis. This approach is based on the use of quantum dot-antibody conjugates as nanoprobes for simultaneously observing relevant proteins. The nanoprobe can penetrate into the cellular membrane without cell lysis and bind to the target protein via its antibody. Several antibodies are capable of being attached to the surface of quantum dot by covalently bonding to 4-(maleimidomethyl)-1-cyclohexanecarboxylic acid N-hydroxysuccinimide ester (SMCC) compound. QDdots have superior optical properties, such as photostability, a high level of brightness, and a higher photobleaching threshold [5] than that of the organic dyes used in classic immunofluorescence. In fact, QDdots are 10–20 times brighter and have several thousand times more photobleaching resistance than organic dyes [6]. Additionally, QDots can be excited simultaneously at a particular excitation wavelength compared to organic dyes [7]. This property enables multicolor cellular imaging for simultaneous monitoring of many relevant proteins involved in TNF-α-induced insulin resistance. Biofunctionalized QDots have been actively used as optical probes for cell imaging. CdSe/ZnS QDots modified with dentate-like alkyl chains and multiple carboxyl groups were developed and conjugated with BRCAA1 and Her2 antibody. The QDots were used for *in vitro* MGC803 cell labeling and *in vivo* targeted imaging of gastric cancer cells [8]. A hydrophilic semiconductor quantum dot-peptide forster resonance energy transfer nanosensor was fabricated to monitor the activity of kallikrein, a key proteolytic enzyme functioning at the initiation of the blood clotting cascade [9]. Avian influenza H5N1 pseudotype virus (H5N1p) was labeled with NIR-emitting QDots by bioorthogonal chemistry. The prepared QDot-H5N1ps were used to visualize respiratory viral infections in mouse lung tissue in real-time [10]. QDot-tagged photonic crystal beads were successfully applied to the multiplex immunoassay of tumor markers [11]. Compared to Western blot, the present method consumes a much smaller number of cells because of the direct monitoring of proteins in the cytosol without cell lysis. First of all, direct monitoring of target proteins without lysis definitely increases the accuracy of the validations regarding the efficacy of test compounds for suppression of inflammatory signaling and enhancement of insulin signaling. High intensity, as well as lack of protein loss, leads to enhancement of accuracy level. As a result, the readouts are a closer reflection of physiological intracellular protein expression. Moreover, multicolor cellular imaging is more similar to *in vivo* results than biochemical assays, resulting in reducing failures in clinical trials. The entire procedure can be carried out faster than Western blot. In addition, more than one protein is easily monitored through a set of samples simultaneously. We have undertaken a quantitative approach and computational methodology to identify the components of two signaling pathways at the same time. Multicolor cellular imaging acts as a catalyst for the rational targeting of specific kinases, mainly focusing on their functional role in disease mechanisms. This assay can be considered as a fundamental tool for concurrently defining the biochemical functions of multiple kinases in multiple signaling pathways with a single assay in one run.

Herein, we propose a new set of multicolor cellular imaging to study biochemical cell-signaling networks which are convoluted, and contain different points of regulation, signal divergence, and crosstalk with other transduction pathways. Amygdalin and cinnamic acid were examined to elucidate their molecular mechanism on the suppression of TNF-α-induced insulin resistance using multicolor cellular imaging based on QDot nanoprobe. Seven kinases were monitored in HepG2 cells treated with TNF-α for the concurrent monitoring of inflammatory and insulin signaling. Serine kinases, such as JNK, IKK, and p38α were observed to verify their roles on serine phosphorylation of IRS-1. Furthermore, GSK3 and FOXO1 were monitored as target proteins for the enhancement of glycogen synthesis and suppression of gluconeogenesis induced by amygdalin and cinnamic acid.

## Results and discussion

Figure 1 shows a schematic model for TNF-α-induced insulin resistance. TNF-α is the most extensively studied cytokine from the point of view of insulin resistance. TNF-α acts by direct and indirect mechanisms to converge at multiple signaling nodes in the way of insulin action. Direct mechanisms include the stimulation of the serine phosphorylation of IRS-1 and decreasing the expression of IRS-1 and GLUT-4 [12]. Indirectly, TNF-α also interacts with muscle cells, liver cells, and adipose tissue to evoke insulin resistance. These stimuli may activate overlapping signal pathways via common upstream kinases in the insulin pathway, such as IRS1-4 proteins, PI3K and

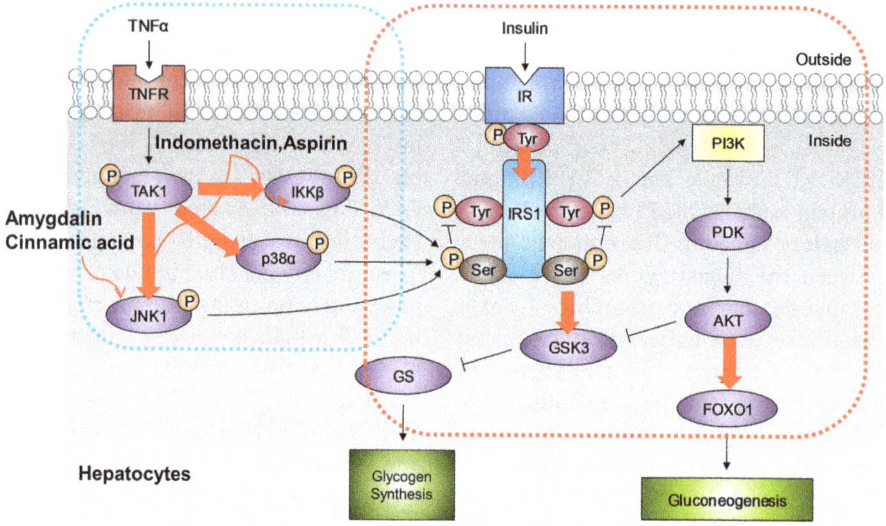

**Figure 1 Effect of four different chemicals on inflammation-associated insulin signaling pathway in HepG2 cells.** The QDot HCS assay was developed for various key kinases involved in inflammation-associated IR that are indicated with a red arrow and validated by specific inhibitors and anti-inflammatory drugs as shown. The p38α, JNK1, and IKKβ involved in the inflammatory pathway and IRS1[ser307], IRS1[tyr], FOXO1, and GSK3β associated with the insulin signaling pathway were simultaneously monitored by QDot multicolor cellular imaging.

AKT/protein kinase B (PKB), and the activation of several kinases, such as p38α, JNK1, and IKKβ in inflammatory signaling. The crosstalk between inflammation and insulin signaling is a major hurdle for understanding the molecular link between the two pathways. The present approaches to studying cellular signaling mechanisms suffer from fluctuation in the activities of intracellular kinases and reproducible results. Therefore, we developed a novel QDot-based quantitative multicolor cellular imaging for simultaneous analysis and monitoring of the activity of various kinases in both disease mechanisms. As shown in Figure 2(a), the phospho-p38α, phospho-JNK1, phospho-IKKβ, phospho-IRS1$^{ser307}$, phospho-IRS1$^{tyr}$, phospho-GSK3β, and phospho-FOXO1 antibodies were conjugated with 565, 565, 565, 605, 705, 525, and 655 QDots, respectively, using an antibody conjugation kit for deciphering the insulin resistance pathway. The conjugate between QDot and antibody was verified through a dynamic light scattering and zeta potential measurement. Figure 2(b) and (c) show particle sizes of QDot605 and QDot605-antibody conjugate measured with dynamic light scattering. As a result of conjugation, the size of QDot605-antibody conjugate increased compared to QDot605. Table 1 summarizes

particle sizes and zeta potential values of QDots and QDot-antibody conjugates used in this study. Antibodies conjugated to QDots have different structures and charges. As a result, the size of QDot-antibody conjugate was not proportional linearly to that of QDot. Zeta potential values of QDot-antibody conjugates were larger than those of QDots due to the conjugation between QDot and antibody. Zeta potential values of QDot-antibody conjugates were hardly changed three weeks after the conjugation. Emission spectra of five different QDots are very narrow (Figure 2[d]), which is appropriate for the elimination of crosstalk in high-content cell-based assay. In addition, acousto-optic tunable filter (AOTF) can contribute greatly to the spectral overlap-free high-content monitoring. AOTF allows cellular imaging at particular single wavelengths devoid of spectral overlap among QDot-antibody conjugates. The crosstalk-free high-content monitoring of inflammation and insulin signal transduction was attempted using QDot-antibody conjugates and AOTF in this work. We investigated the effect of various inflammatory kinase inhibitors acting on insulin signaling and evaluated the compound efficacies for the functional ability to inhibit gluconeogenesis and enhance glycogen

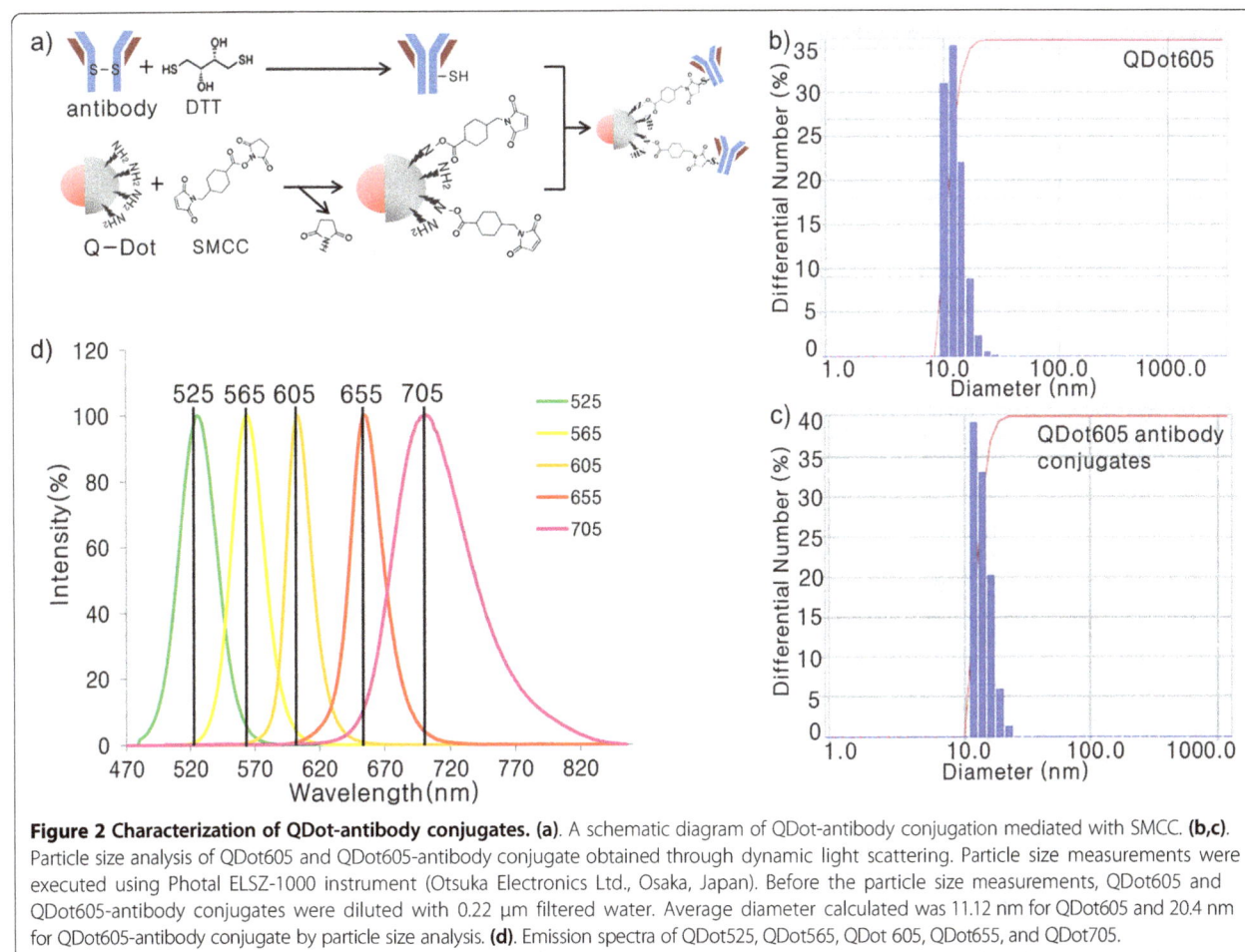

Figure 2 Characterization of QDot-antibody conjugates. (a). A schematic diagram of QDot-antibody conjugation mediated with SMCC. (b,c). Particle size analysis of QDot605 and QDot605-antibody conjugate obtained through dynamic light scattering. Particle size measurements were executed using Photal ELSZ-1000 instrument (Otsuka Electronics Ltd., Osaka, Japan). Before the particle size measurements, QDot605 and QDot605-antibody conjugates were diluted with 0.22 μm filtered water. Average diameter calculated was 11.12 nm for QDot605 and 20.4 nm for QDot605-antibody conjugate by particle size analysis. (d). Emission spectra of QDot525, QDot565, QDot 605, QDot655, and QDot705.

**Table 1 Summary of particle sizes and zeta potential values of QDots and QDot-antibody conjugates**

| Sample | Particle size (nm) | Zeta potential (mV) |
| --- | --- | --- |
| QDot525 | 9.1 | −2.1 |
| QDot525 antibody conjugate | 15.16 | −13.5 |
| QDot565 | 10.3 | −2.4 |
| QDot565 antibody conjugate | 20.3 | −11.98 |
| QDot605 | 13.7 | −3.72 |
| QDot605 antibody conjugate | 16.1 | −16.65 |
| QDot655 | 15.9 | −4.5 |
| QDot655 antibody conjugate | 20.4 | −17.6 |
| QDot705 | 17.1 | −5.54 |
| QDot705 antibody conjugate | 23.2 | −18.7 |

content, with the goal of identifying potential kinase for suppressing inflammation-induced insulin resistance. Our experiment also addresses the suitability of multicolor cellular imaging for studying kinase crosstalk operating in complex diseases, such as inflammation-associated insulin resistance, at a single shot in a single cell. Surprisingly, amygdalin and cinnamic acid acted selectively via the JNK1-dependent pathway to improve insulin sensitivity. The HepG2 cell line was chosen for this study as it is a perpetual, epithelial cell line derived from well-differentiated hepatocellular carcinoma. These cells solely depend upon exogenous growth factors for survival and respond to stimuli, such as TNF-α, adiponectin, leptin, etc. To study the causal role of elevated cytokines levels and MAP kinase inhibitors in hepatic insulin resistance, HepG2 cells were treated with inhibitors 30 min prior to stimulation with 10 ng/ml TNF-α for 5 h. The cells were then treated with 100 nM insulin for 10 min. Past studies using the obese

TNF-α[+/+] mice model have shown disturbances in insulin signaling in response to TNF-α [13]. Therapies that have successfully targeted TNF-α, including genetic silencing of the TNF-α or TNF receptor in mice, have demonstrated significant efficacy in the treatment of obesity-related insulin resistance. Therefore, we established the insulin resistance model *in vitro* using TNF-α stimulation of HepG2 cells. The glycogen amount decreased in the TNF-α treated group, suggesting compromised insulin sensitivity. The MAP kinase inhibitors suppressed the effect of TNF-α on the insulin transduction pathway and consequently resulted in elevated levels of glycogen content (Figure 3a). The inflammatory signaling inhibitors, such as p38α kinase inhibitors (SB203580), JNK1 inhibitors (SP600125), IKKβ inhibitors, aspirin, and indomethacin increased glycogen levels by almost two-fold in comparison to amygdalin and cinnamic acid. Glycogen content in HepG2 cells treated with p38, JNK1, IKKβ inhibitors, aspirin, and indomethacin were four to five times higher than that of the control; whereas, glycogen content in amygdalin or cinnamic acid-treated HepG2 cells were two to three times higher than that of the control [14]. As shown by a glucose production assay, exposure of HepG2 cells to inhibitors reduced gluconeogenesis in comparison to the control group (Figure 3b). Cinnamic acid was much more potent in suppressing glucose production than MAP kinase inhibitors and non-steroidal anti-inflammatory drugs. The rate of hepatic glucose production by amygdalin was similar to that of aspirin.

Crosstalk among the common signaling molecules complicates our understanding of the relation between inflammation and insulin resistance. Our next goal was to develop novel QDot-based multicolor cellular imaging for simultaneous monitoring of inflammatory and insulin signaling pathway kinases. For the first time, the QDot

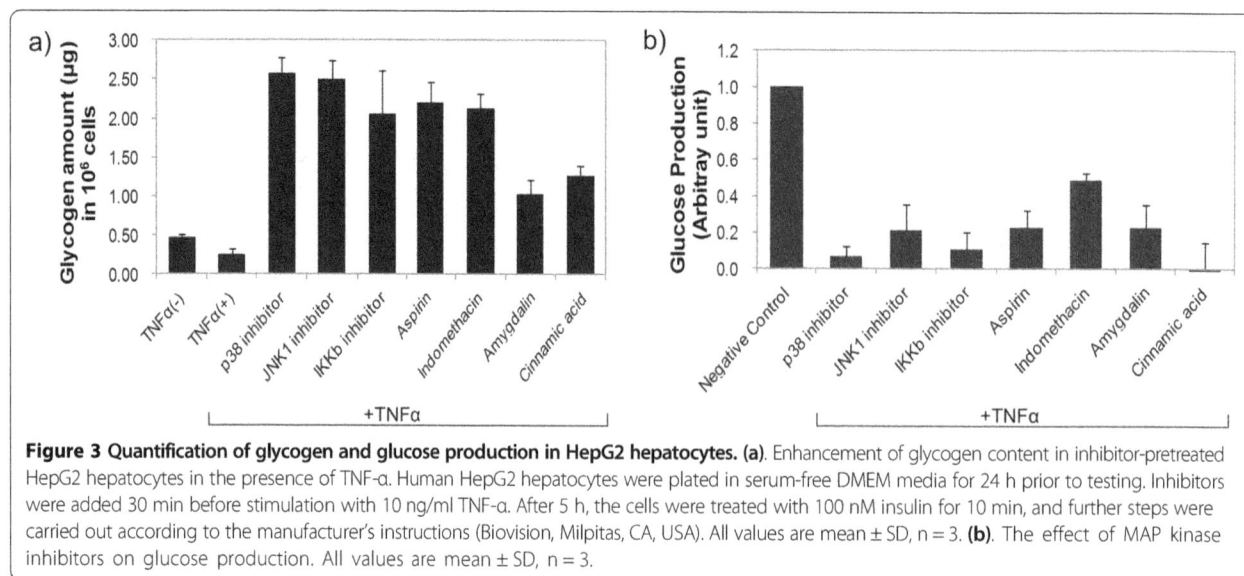

**Figure 3 Quantification of glycogen and glucose production in HepG2 hepatocytes. (a)**. Enhancement of glycogen content in inhibitor-pretreated HepG2 hepatocytes in the presence of TNF-α. Human HepG2 hepatocytes were plated in serum-free DMEM media for 24 h prior to testing. Inhibitors were added 30 min before stimulation with 10 ng/ml TNF-α. After 5 h, the cells were treated with 100 nM insulin for 10 min, and further steps were carried out according to the manufacturer's instructions (Biovision, Milpitas, CA, USA). All values are mean ± SD, n = 3. **(b)**. The effect of MAP kinase inhibitors on glucose production. All values are mean ± SD, n = 3.

immunoassay was developed for understanding of TNF-α-induced insulin resistance using the quantitative multicolor cellular imaging. The insulin signaling and one of three inflammatory MAP kinases (p38α, JNK1, and IKKβ) were simultaneously observed. Selective binding of QDot-antibody conjugates to targeted proteins is essential for the successful observation of intracellular signal transduction related to TNF-α-induced insulin resistance. This novel assay is quite useful in tracing kinases without morphological changes in the cell being investigated. The inflammatory pathways via MAP kinases (p38α, JNK1, and IKKβ) were not activated in the negative control group free of any TNF-α stimulation, as shown in Figure 4. In the positive control group, the HepG2 cells were treated

with TNF-α to mimic the inflammation-induced insulin-resistant conditions. TNF-α stimulated the phosphorylation of MAP kinases (p38α, JNK1, and IKKβ) and IRS1-$^{ser307}$, and inhibited insulin downstream kinases (GSK3β, FOXO1, and IRS1$^{tyr}$) (Figure 4).

To further elucidate the role of p38α in relation to insulin resistance, we tested insulin signaling kinases, such as GSK3β, FOXO1, IRS1$^{ser307}$, and IRS1$^{tyr}$ in TNF-α-stimulated HepG2 cells pretreated with a 5 μM p38-specific inhibitor SB203580 for 30 min. As shown in Figure 4a, TNF-α-stimulated HepG2 cells show the phosphorylation of p38α along with IRS1$^{ser307}$ in comparison to the negative control group. The SB203580 inhibitor suppressed the activation of p38α and IRS1$^{ser307}$; whereas, the activated

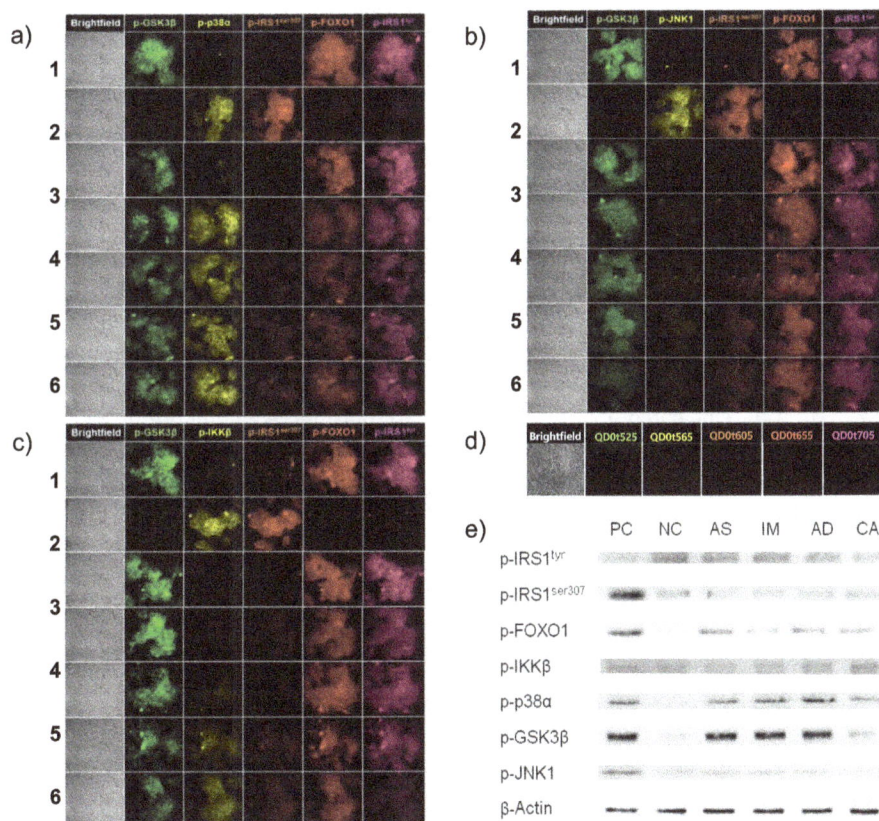

Figure 4 High-content cellular images of kinases. (a,b,c). Multicolor cellular imaging showing simultaneous monitoring of the upregulation/downregulation of five kinases in HepG2 cells. Five kinases: p-GSK3β, p-p38α, p-IRS1$^{ser307}$, p-FOXO1, and p-IRS1$^{tyr}$. (a) The positive control group was stimulated with TNF-α; whereas, in the negative control, TNF-α treatment was absent. For inhibitor studies, HepG2 cells were plated in serum-free DMEM media for 24 h prior to testing. P38 inhibitor was added 30 min before stimulation with 10 ng/ml TNF-α (for 5 h), and the cells were treated with 100 nM insulin. The cells were treated with formaldehyde for fixing the cells following permeability enhancement using saponin. The QDot-antibody conjugate (p-p38α, p-JNK1, p-IKKβ, p-IRS1$^{ser}$, p-IRS1$^{tyr}$, p-GSK3β, and p-FOXO1) treatment was done. Quantitative estimation and monitoring of the phosphorylation of the five kinases were simultaneously carried out according to emission wavelengths mentioned in the experimental section. 1: Positive Control, 2: Negative Control, 3: p38 inhibitor (SB203580), 4: Aspirin treatment, 5: Indomethacin treatment, 6: Amygdalin treatment, 7: Cinnamic acid treatment. (b) 1: Positive Control, 2: Negative Control, 3: JNK-1 inhibitor (SP600125), 4: Aspirin treatment, 5: Indomethacin treatment, 6: Amygdalin treatment, 7: Cinnamic acid treatment. (c) 1: Positive Control, 2: Negative Control, 3: IKKβ inhibitor, 4: Aspirin treatment, 5: Indomethacin treatment, 6: Amygdalin treatment, 7: Cinnamic acid treatment. (d) Cellular images of HepG2 cells treated with non-conjugated QDots (QDot525, QDot565, QDot605, QDot655, QDot705). (e) Western blot analysis of upregulation/downregulation of seven different kinases in HepG2 cells. TNF-α induction was absent in the negative control (NC). The positive control (PC) was stimulated with TNF-α. AS: Aspirin, IM: Indomethacin, AD: Amygdalin, CA: Cinnamic acid.

phosphor-protein levels of GSK3β, FOXO1, and IRS1$^{tyr}$ were similar to those of the negative control group and had a favorable effect on insulin sensitivity, similar to previous studies using Western blot [15]. To explore the application of the developed assay for pathway studies, we further screened the activities of NSAIDs, such as aspirin and indomethacin, along with two herbal active constituents, such as amygdalin and cinnamic acid. The above four molecules have not been shown to inhibit the p38 inflammatory pathway, but they still inhibited the phosphorylation of IRS1$^{ser307}$ responsible for insulin resistance by acting through other signaling kinases (Figure 4a). We next investigated whether these four molecules can act via the JNK1 pathway. The experimental conditions were similar to those of the p38 screening, except for the use of specific JNK inhibitor SP600125 (4 μM). Positive-controlled HepG2 cells cause activation of IRS1$^{ser307}$ by the JNK1 pathway (Figure 4b). The JNK1-specific inhibitor completely inhibited the phosphorylation of JNK1 and IRS1$^{ser307}$. The four inhibitor molecules inhibited the JNK1 pathway to almost the same extent and enhanced insulin sensitivity, as shown in the restored extent of phosphorylation of GSK3β, FOXO1, and IRS1$^{tyr}$ (Figure 5b). There are several reports of the hypoglycemic effects of naturally-derived active components which have anti-inflammatory activity, such as phenolic acid (cinnamic acid) and cyanogenic glycosides amygdalin. The cellular and molecular mechanism of action of cinnamic acid and amygdalin has not been well elucidated in conditions mimicking inflammation-associated insulin resistance. Although cinnamic acid and amygdalin were expected to act through inhibition of the IKKβ and NF-κB pathway, they acted via the JNK1-dependent pathway to improve insulin sensitivity. Our results are congruent with past studies

conducted on mouse liver FL83B cells using phenolic acid, such as cinnamic acid. Cinnamic acid up-regulates the expression of insulin signal associated proteins, including phosphatidylinositol-3 kinase, glycogen synthase, and insulin receptor; it also increases the uptake of glucose, and abates insulin resistance [16]. Our results agree with the JNK1 pathway studies conducted on hepatocytes and mouse liver cells [17]. Finally, we used the specific IKKβ inhibitor (2 μM) to find the relation to the insulin signaling. The IKKβ inhibitor also inhibited IRS1$^{ser307}$ via suppression of IKKβ kinase. Among the four molecules, aspirin substantially inhibited IKKβ kinase activation followed by indomethacin; whereas, amygdalin and cinnamic acid showed moderate inhibition (Figures 4c and 5c). Figure 4e is a Western blot analysis to show suppression of TNF-α-induced insulin resistance induced by the four test molecules. Activations/deactivations of seven different kinases were observed to compare the results obtained with QDot multicolor cellular imaging. Although detection sensitivity of Western blot is poorer than that of QDot multicolor cellular imaging, the results by Western blot were matched with those by QDot multicolor cellular imaging. Figure 5 represents the quantification of cellular images in Figure 4. Our results are in line with past studies supporting the major role of IKKβ in insulin resistance [18].

In insulin resistance-free conditions, insulin phosphorylates Forkhead box-containing O subfamily-1(FOXO1), resulting in the inhibition of transcriptional activity, leading to reduced glucose production. Moreover, insulin phosphorylates GSK-3, thereby leading to an increase in glycogen synthase activity. The glycogen synthesis is controlled by glycogen synthase kinase-3 (GSK-3). On the other hand, TNF-α stimulation inhibits the phosphorylation of FOXO1 kinase and increases glucose production.

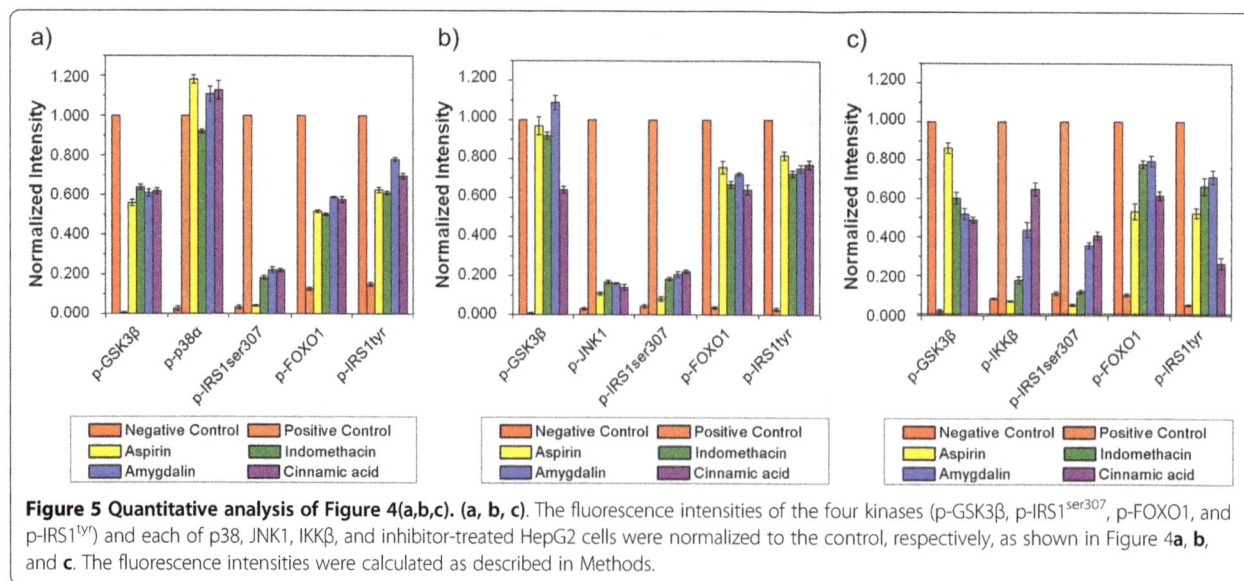

**Figure 5 Quantitative analysis of Figure 4(a,b,c). (a, b, c)**. The fluorescence intensities of the four kinases (p-GSK3β, p-IRS1$^{ser307}$, p-FOXO1, and p-IRS1$^{tyr}$) and each of p38, JNK1, IKKβ, and inhibitor-treated HepG2 cells were normalized to the control, respectively, as shown in Figure 4**a**, **b**, and **c**. The fluorescence intensities were calculated as described in Methods.

TNF-α is known to inhibit the activities of many components involved in insulin signaling cascade. Insulin receptor, IRS, and glucose transporter 4 (Glut4) are representative proteins to be inhibited by TNF-α. Particularly, IRS has received great attention as a major target in TNF-α-induced insulin resistance. Insulin signaling is suppressed by an increase of serine phosphorylation of IRS proteins caused by TNF-α. A few mechanisms have been reported to be involved in serine phosphorylation of IRS proteins, such as inhibition of tyrosyl phosphorylation of IRS-1 [19] and proteasome-mediated degradation of IRS-1 [20]. Interaction between insulin receptor and IRS-1 is interfered by the inhibition of tyrosyl phosphorylation of IRS-1; as a result, IRS-mediated insulin signaling is suppressed. Serine phosphorylation of IRS-1 by TNF-α can be achieved through activation of several serine kinases, including kinases related to the inflammatory pathway, such as JNK. The suppression of IRS-mediated insulin signaling leads to reduced GSK-3 and FOXO1 phosphorylation, followed by decreased glycogen synthesis and increased gluconeogenesis. Our results showed that cinnamic acid and amygdalin enhanced the phosphorylation level of GSK-3 and FOXO1. As a result, glycogen synthesis was increased and glucose production was reduced.

## Conclusion

The above results corroborate that QDot multicolor cellular imaging can be applied to investigate the molecular pathogenesis and inhibitor studies of multiple signaling pathways (i.e., insulin signaling and the inflammatory pathway) which share common intracellular proteins. Compared to Western blot, QDot multicolor cellular imaging enabled direct and concurrent accesses to intracellular target proteins related to TNF-α-induced insulin resistance. The designed monitoring proved that cell lysis-free QDot multicolor cellular imaging was a powerful tool for identifying novel molecular targets for suppressing inflammation in insulin resistance. The developed assay successfully verified that cinnamic acid and amygdalin suppressed TNF-α-induced insulin resistance mainly via the inhibition of JNK.

## Methods
### Materials
General chemicals, including a glucose assay kit and TNF-α, were obtained from Sigma-Aldrich (St. Louis, MO, USA) and were of the highest purity available. The glycogen assay kit was purchased from BioVision (Milpitas, CA, USA). The phospho-p38α, phospho-JNK1, phospho-IKKβ, phospho-IRS1$^{ser307}$, phospho-IRS1$^{tyr}$, phospho-GSK3β, and phospho-FOXO1 antibodies were obtained from Santa Cruz Biotechnology (Dallas, TX, USA) and conjugated with 565, 565, 605, 705, 525, and 655 QDots,

respectively, using an antibody conjugation kit from Invitrogen (Carlsbad, CA, USA).

### Cell culture
HepG2 cells were obtained from the Korean Cell Line Bank (Seoul, South Korea) and cultured in Dulbecco's modified Eagle's medium supplemented with 10% fetal bovine serum, 100 μg/ml penicillin, and 100 μg/ml streptomycin. All of the cells were cultured in 25 cm$^2$ cell culture flasks at 37°C in a humidified atmosphere of 5% $CO_2$.

For inhibitor studies, HepG2 cells were plated in serum-free DMEM media for 24 h prior to testing. Inhibitors were added 30 min before stimulation with 10ng/ml TNF-α. After 5-h stimulation with TNF-α, the cells were treated with 100 nM insulin for 10 min.

### Analysis of glycogen content
Glycogen content in various inhibitor-treated HepG2 cells was measured with a glycogen assay kit according to the manufacturer's instructions.

### Glucose production assay
Cells were washed three times with PBS to remove glucose, incubated for 16 h in 1 ml of glucose production medium (glucose and phenol red-free DMEM, containing gluconeogenic substrates, 20 mm sodium lactate, and 2 mm sodium pyruvate), and in the presence of 1 nm insulin during the last 3 h. 300 μl of the medium was sampled for the measurement of glucose concentration using a glucose assay kit.

### QDot conjugation with specific antibody
The p38α, JNK1, IKKβ, IRS1$^{ser307}$, IRS1$^{tyr}$, GSK3β, and FOXO1 antibodies were conjugated with 565, 565, 565, 605, 705, 525, and 655 QDots, respectively, using an antibody conjugation kit. The used QDots are semiconductor materials that consisted of core, shell, and polymeric coating. The core is made up of cadmium selenide and passivated with zinc sulfide as the shell. The QDot composed of core-shell is highly hydrophobic. In order to enhance water solubility and conjugate efficiently to biomolecules, QDots surfaces were modified with the amine-functionalized polyethylene glycol (PEG) linker. Conjugation steps were carried out according to the manufacturer's instructions. QDots were activated with SMCC used as an amine-to-thiol crosslinker to the maleimide-nanocrystal surface. To break the disulfide bond in antibodies and to expose free sulfhydryls, the antibodies were treated with dithiothreitol (DTT). Size exclusion chromatography was performed to remove excess SMCC and DTT. Maleimide-QDots were incubated with the reduced antibodies for 1 h. By this reaction, antibodies were covalently bound to QDots. The excess maleimide groups were removed by β-mercaptoethanol. A separation media

column supplied in the kit was used to eliminate un-bounded QDots and antibodies. The maximum emission wavelengths of phospho-GSK3β, phospho-IKKβ, phospho-p38α, phospho-JNK1, phospho-IRS$^{Ser307}$, phospho-FOXO1, and phospho-IRS$^{tyr}$ are 525, 565, 565, 565, 605, 655, and 705 nm, respectively.

## QDot immunoassay using QDot multicolor cellular imaging

HepG2 cells were separately seeded into 12 well culture plates ($5 \times 10^5$ cells/well). After 24 h, the cells were washed twice with 1× phosphate-buffered saline (PBS), treated with accutase and incubated at 37°C for 10–15 min. The detached cells from the culture plates were centrifuged at 220 $g$ for 3 min. After removing the supernatant, the cells were treated with 3.7% formaldehyde for 15 min. The cells were then rinsed twice with 1 × PBS and centrifuged at 220 $g$ for 3 min. The cells were treated with 0.2% saponin for 15 min to increase the pore size of the cell membrane, followed by washing twice with 1 × PBS and centrifugation at 220 $g$ for 3 min. After the QDot-antibody conjugate, its concentration was determined to be 2 μM using an absorption spectrophotometer. QDot-antibody conjugates (p38α, JNK1, IKKβ, IRS1$^{ser}$, IRS1$^{tyr}$, GSK3β, and FOXO1) were diluted (1/200) in 100 μl of blocking buffer (1% BSA in 1 × PBS). The HepG2 cell pellet was immersed in the diluted QDot-antibody solution of 100 μl and kept for 1 h at room temperature. The cells were then washed twice with 1 × PBS and centrifuged at 220 $g$ for 3 min. Intracellular monitoring of the five different kinases were simultaneously carried out at 525 nm, 565 nm, 625 nm, 655 nm, and 705 nm emission wavelengths to observe their phosphorylations induced by tested drugs [21-23]. The fixed cell formed by formaldehyde treatment is a kind of dead cell that maintains its morphology. The fixed dead HepG2 cells were treated with Qdot-antibody probes for the immunostaining. Accordingly, toxicity inherent to Qdots does not affect drug-induced up-regulation or down-regulation of intracellular target proteins. Imaging analysis was performed using commercially available software (MetaMorph, Version 7.1.3.0, Molecular Devices, Sunnyvale, CA, USA).

## Calculation of normalized intensity

Figure 5(a-c) shows the quantification of fluorescence intensities in the cell images obtained with QDot multicolor cellular imaging. Fluorescence intensities of p-GSK3β, p-FOXO1, and p-IRS$^{tyr}$ were normalized according to the following equation:

$$\text{Normalized Intensity} = (I_s/I_n),$$

The fluorescence intensity of the inhibitor-treated cells is represented by $I_s$, and $I_n$ represents the fluorescence intensity of cells in the negative control group.

The normalized fluorescent intensities of p-p38, p-JNK, p-IKKβ, and p-IRS$^{ser307}$ were calculated according to the following equation:

$$\text{Normalized Intensity} = (I_s/I_p),$$

The fluorescence intensity of the inhibitor-treated cells is represented by $I_s$, and $I_p$ is the fluorescence intensity of cells in the positive control. All of the intensities in Figure 5 were the averaged value of cellular intensities obtained from three different cellular regions. The standard deviation was represented as the error bar in Figure 5.

## Western blotting

HepG2 cells ($1 \times 10^6$) were lysed using Lysis-M solution (Roche, Manheim, Germany). Electrophoresis was performed on 12% sodium dodecyl sulfate-polyacrylamide gel (SDS-PAGE) by loading 60 μg of protein from HepG2 cells. The proteins were transferred to a polyvinylidene difluoride (PVDF) membrane (BioRad, Hercules, CA, USA) after the electrophoresis. Appropriate primary antibodies were used for Western blot analysis. Membranes were blocked overnight at 4°C in 1 × PBS, containing 0.05% TWEEN® 20 and 5% bovine serum albumin. Each specific antibody at a dilution of 1:1,000 was used in the Western blot analysis. Similarly, beta actin antibody at a dilution of 1:1,000 was used for the detection of beta actin (positive control). Primary antibodies were detected via a secondary peroxidase-conjugated antibody at a dilution of 1:10,000 (Dako Ltd., High Wycombe, Bucks, UK). An enhanced chemiluminescence detection kit (Roche, Basel, Switzerland) was used for signal detection.

### Abbreviations
TNF: Tumor necrosis factor; JNK: c-Jun N-terminal kinase; IKKβ: Ikappaβ kinase; IRS1: Insulin receptor substrate-1; GSK3β: Glycogen synthase kinase 3β; FOXO1: Forkhead box O1.

### Competing interests
The authors declare that they have no competing interests.

### Authors' contributions
JMS supervised the study, and contributed to the drafting of this article, selection of methodology, and finalized the manuscript. MJK executed all the experimental studies, analyzed the data, and drafted the manuscript. All authors read and approved the final manuscript.

### Acknowledgements
This work was supported by the National Research Foundation of Korea (NRF) grant funded by the Ministry of Education, Science and Technology (MEST) (2010–0017903). We are grateful to the Research Institute of Pharmaceutical Sciences at Seoul National University for providing some experimental equipment.

### References
1.  WHO Diabetes [http://www.who.int/mediacentre/factsheets/fs312/en/]
2.  Taniguchi CM, Emanuelli B, Kahn CR. Critical nodes in signaling pathways: insights into insulin action. Nat Rev Mol Cell Biol. 2006;7:85–96.

3. Feinstein R, Kanety H, Papa MZ, Lunenfeld B, Karasik A. Tumor necrosis factor-alpha suppresses insulin-induced tyrosine phosphorylation of insulin receptor and its substrates. J Biol Chem. 1993;268:26055–8.

4. Hirabara SM, Gorjao R, Vinolo MA, Rodrigues AC, Nachbar RT, Curi R. Molecular targets related to inflammation and insulin resistance and potential interventions. J Biomed Biotechnol. 2012;2012:16.

5. Han MY, Gao XH, Su JZ, Nie S. Quantum-dot-tagged microbeads for multiplexed optical coding of biomolecules. Nat Biotechnol. 2001;19:631–5.

6. Gao X, Yang L, Petros JA, Marshall FF, Simons JW, Nie S. In vivo molecular and cellular imaging with quantum dots. Curr Opin Biotechnol. 2005;16:63–72.

7. Alivisatos AP, Gu W, Larabell C. Quantum dots as cellular probes. Annu Rev Biomed Eng. 2005;7:55–76.

8. Chao L, Yang J, Can W, Shujing L, Fei P, Chunlei Z, et al. BRCAA1 antibody- and Her2 antibody-conjugated amphiphilic polymer engineered CdSe/ZnS quantum dots for targeted imaging of gastric cancer. Nanoscale Res Lett. 2014;9:244.

9. Joyce C, Breger Kim E, Sapsford Jessica G, Kimihiro S, Michael H, Stewart Igor M. Detecting kallikrein proteolytic activity with peptide-quantum dot nanosensors. ACS Appl Mater Interfaces. 2014;6:11529–35.

10. Hong P, Pengfei Z, Duyang G, Yijuan Z, Ping L, Lanlan L, et al. Noninvasive visualization of respiratory viral infection using bioorthogonal conjugated near-infrared-emitting quantum dots. ACS Nano. 2014;8:5468–77.

11. Li J, Wang H, Dong S, Zhu P, Diao G, Yang Z. Quantum-dot-tagged photonic crystal beads for multiflex detection of tumor markers. Chem Commun. 2014;50:14589–92.

12. Ruan H, Hacohen N, Golub TR, Van PL, Lodish HF. Tumor necrosis factor-alpha suppresses adipocyte-specific genes and activates expression of preadipocyte genes in 3T3-L1 adipocytes: nuclear factor-kappaB activation by TNF-alpha is obligatory. Diabetes. 2002;51:1319–36.

13. Uysal KT, Wiesbrock SM, Marino MW, Hotamisligil GS. Protection from obesity-induced insulin resistance in mice lacking TNF-alpha function. Nature. 1997;389:610–4.

14. Huang DW, Shen SC, Wu JS. Effects of caffeic acid and cinnamic acid on glucose uptake in insulin-resistant mouse hepatocytes. J Agric Food Chem. 2009;57:7687–92.

15. Zhenqi L, Wenhong C. p38 Mitogen-activated protein kinase: a critical node linking inflammation resistance and cardiovascular diseases in type 2 diabetes mellitus. Endocr Metab Immune Disord Drug Targets. 2009;9:38–46.

16. Hwang HJ, Lee HJ, Kim CJ, Shim I, Hahm DH. Inhibitory effect of amygdalin on lipopolysaccharide-inducible TNF-α and IL-1β mrna expression and carrageenan-induced rat arthritis. J Microbiol Biotechnol. 2008;18:1641–7.

17. Nakatani Y, Kaneto H, Kawamori D, Hatazaki M, Miyatsuka T, Matsuoka T. Modulation of the JNK pathway in liver affects insulin resistance status. J Biol Chem. 2004;279:45803–9.

18. Yuan M, Konstantopoulos N, Lee J, Hansen L, Li ZW, Karin M. Reversal of obesity and diet-induced insulin resistance with salicylates or targeted disruption of Ikkβ. Science. 2001;293:1673–7.

19. Aguirre V, Werner ED, Giraud J, Lee Y, Shoelson SE, White MF. Phosphorylation of Ser307 in insulin receptor substrate-1 blocks interactions with the insulin receptor and inhibits insulin action. J Biol Chem. 2002;277:1531–7.

20. Zhande R, Mitchell JJ, Wu J, Sun XJ. Molecular mechanism of insulin-induced degradation of insulin receptor substrate 1. Mol Cell Biol. 2002;22:1016–26.

21. Tak YK, Naoghare PK, Kim BJ, Kim MJ, Lee ES, Song JM. High-content quantum dot-based subtype diagnosis and classification of breast cancer patients using hypermulticolor quantitative single cell imaging cytometry. Nano Today. 2012;7:231–44.

22. Kim JA, Han E, Eun CJ, Tak YK, Song JM. Real-time concurrent monitoring of apoptosis, cytosolic calcium, and mitochondria permeability transition for hypermulticolor high-content screening of drug-induced mitochondrial dysfunction-mediated hepatotoxicity. Toxicol Lett. 2012;214:175–81.

23. Tak YK, Naoghare PK, Han E, Song JM. VEGF inhibitor (Iressa) arrests histone deacetylase expression: single-cell cotransfection imaging cytometry for multi-target-multi-drug analysis. J Cell Physiol. 2011;226:2115–22.

# 10

# In vitro assessment of antibody-conjugated gold nanorods for systemic injections

Sonia Centi[1], Francesca Tatini[2], Fulvio Ratto[2*], Alessio Gnerucci[1], Raffaella Mercatelli[3], Giovanni Romano[1], Ida Landini[4], Stefania Nobili[4], Andrea Ravalli[3], Giovanna Marrazza[3], Enrico Mini[5], Franco Fusi[1] and Roberto Pini[2]

## Abstract

**Background:** The interest for gold nanorods in biomedical optics is driven by their intense absorbance of near infrared light, their biocompatibility and their potential to reach tumors after systemic administration. Examples of applications include the photoacoustic imaging and the photothermal ablation of cancer. In spite of great current efforts, the selective delivery of gold nanorods to tumors through the bloodstream remains a formidable challenge. Their bio-conjugation with targeting units, and in particular with antibodies, is perceived as a hopeful solution, but the complexity of living organisms complicates the identification of possible obstacles along the way to tumors.

**Results:** Here, we present a new model of gold nanorods conjugated with anti-cancer antigen 125 (CA125) antibodies, which exhibit high specificity for ovarian cancer cells. We implement a battery of tests *in vitro*, in order to simulate major nuisances and predict the feasibility of these particles for intravenous injections. We show that parameters like the competition of free CA125 in the bloodstream, which could saturate the probe before arriving at the tumors, the matrix effect and the interference with erythrocytes and phagocytes are uncritical.

**Conclusions:** Although some deterioration is detectable, anti-CA125-conjugated gold nanorods retain their functional features after interaction with blood tissue and so represent a powerful candidate to hit ovarian cancer cells.

**Keywords:** Gold nanorods, Cancer antigen 125, Active targeting, Competitive assay, Matrix effect, Blood compatibility

## Background

Cancer remains one of the leading causes of death. The majority of patients suffering from cancer undergo invasive treatments, such as surgery, radiation therapy and chemotherapy. Radiation therapy is based on the use of ionizing radiation to exterminate malignant cells via the production of free radicals that damage cellular DNA [1]. However, radio-toxicity to healthy tissue is a critical factor, because ionizing radiation does not well discriminate between malignant and normal cells [2,3]. Also chemotherapeutics do not exclusively act on malignant cells and exhibit side effects, mainly due to their poor specificity [4]. In this context, the hope for more selective alternatives has been revived by the advent of nanotechnology. In particular, gold nanoparticles (GNPs) have received considerable attention. In addition to their good biocompatibility, ease of preparation and stability, their optical features are ideal for applications in biomedical optics [5-10]. Their capacity to scatter and, more significantly, to absorb light results from localized plasmonic resonances [11-16].

Among the various shapes of GNPs, so-called gold nanorods (GNRs) exhibit two plasmonic bands, i.e. a weaker transversal band at ~ 520 nm, similar to that of gold nanospheres, and a more intense longitudinal band that moves from the visible to the near infrared (NIR) domains, say from 600 to 1100 nm, with increasing their aspect ratios [17-20]. Since tissue and skin components do not significantly absorb NIR light, GNRs are being proposed as contrast agents for many applications *in vivo* [21-24].

While polyethylene glycol (PEG) imparts very low cellular uptake [10], PEGylated GNRs tend to accumulate into tumours after intravenous injection much more than they do into normal tissue, because the vascular and lymphatic networks of neoplastic tissue are abnormal. This passive accumulation is known as the enhanced permeability and retention (EPR) effect. However, the fraction

* Correspondence: f.ratto@ifac.cnr.it
[2]Istituto di Fisica Applicata 'Nello Carrara', Consiglio Nazionale delle Ricerche, Via Madonna del Piano 10, 50019 Sesto Fiorentino, Italy
Full list of author information is available at the end of the article

of GNRs that reaches tumours is quite low, say around 10%, while their entrapment in vital organs, such as the liver and the spleen, is substantial [25-29].

Various targeting units, such as antibodies [30-32], aptamers [33-35], peptides [36-38] and small molecules [39], have been anchored to the surface of GNRs, in an attempt to enhance their specificity for tumors. The interaction between these targeting units and their receptors on the membranes of malignant cells activates pathways of active uptake. The choice of molecular targets is critical. Popular receptors, such as folate [40-42] and growth factor receptors [43-45], are also found in most normal cells, and cause some undeliberate uptake from these non-targeted cells [46]. Nonspecific binding and specific binding to non-targeted cells are common nuisances. Some authors have proposed a dual-ligand approach to gain more specificity, especially when one of the molecular targets is rather unspecific [47-49]. In spite of all this effort, the classification of problems and bottlenecks in the systemic delivery of GNRs is hard, due to the extreme complexity of the biological interface.

In this paper, we propose an analytical approach to model in vitro some of the most critical issues that arise from the interaction between GNRs and the bloodstream. We focus on a single-ligand strategy, because the molecular target of our choice is Cancer Antigen 125 (CA125), which is very specific for ovarian cancers. CA125, also known as mucin 16, is the most reliable biomarker to confirm the diagnosis and the management of ovarian cancers, which is one of the most lethal gynaecological malignancies, and is a large molecular weight transmembrane glycoprotein.

We describe the preparation and the application of GNRs conjugated with anti-CA125 antibodies to detect cells overexpressing CA125 and mediate their selective photothermal ablation. The design of our probe starts from the PEGylation of GNRs with heterobifunctional PEG strands that confer biocompatibility, colloidal stability [10] and an easy dock for anti-CA125 antibodies. We place a special emphasis on the compatibility of these particles with intravenous injections, both in terms of their performances of molecular recognition and their interactions with erythrocytes and phagocytes. As for the formers, the threat of biological environments providing for competition and passivation is analyzed in solution by complementary tests with a quantitative profile. The qualitative translation of these findings into the cellular arena is confirmed by the specificity of anti-CA125 particles for HeLa cells, which are CA125- positive, even after incubation in biological fluids containing physiological levels of this antigen. Moreover, we address their haemolytic activity and their detection from macrophages, in an attempt to mimic the interactions occurring in the blood, liver, kidneys and spleen and exacerbating their blood clearance

and organ sequestration. In Additional file 1, we provide evidence for the photothermal ablation of HeLa cells, thus confirming the efficacy and selectivity of the treatment.

Our results demonstrate that anti-CA125 GNRs are non-toxic, retain much of their ability of molecular recognition after incubation in biological fluids, do not compromise the erythrocytes and are not detected by the macrophages. For these reasons, bio-conjugated GNRs represent a promising platform for systemic delivery, in view of mini invasive imaging or therapeutic options based on concepts of photothermal or photoacoustic conversion.

## Results and discussion

### CTAB-capped GNRs

As it is described in Methods, the preparation of our particles began with the synthesis of GNRs stabilized by hexadecyltrimethylammonium bromide (CTAB). TEM images of CTAB-capped GNRs revealed average lengths and widths of $(43 \pm 7)$ and $(10 \pm 3)$ nm, respectively (see Figure 1A). These particles exhibited a longitudinal plasmonic band around 800 nm (see Figure 1B).

### Anti-CA125-conjugated GNRs

Due to the toxicity of CTAB, the initial coating was substituted with a mixture of mono- and bi-functional PEG strands (methoxylated PEG, or mPEG, and carboxylated PEG, or cPEG), which are nontoxic polyether compounds in common use to improve the biocompatibility

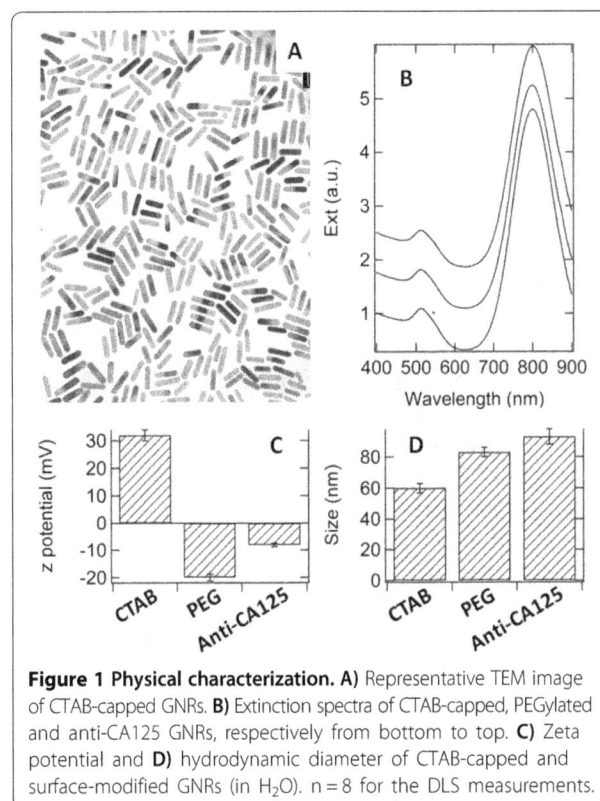

**Figure 1 Physical characterization. A)** Representative TEM image of CTAB-capped GNRs. **B)** Extinction spectra of CTAB-capped, PEGylated and anti-CA125 GNRs, respectively from bottom to top. **C)** Zeta potential and **D)** hydrodynamic diameter of CTAB-capped and surface-modified GNRs (in H$_2$O). n = 8 for the DLS measurements.

and systemic circulation of many particles [10,50,51]. The carboxy-terminals of GNRs were conjugated with antibodies anti-CA125, using the zero-length crosslinker 1-ethyl-3-(3-dimethylaminopropyl)carbodiimide (EDC) stabilized by N-hydroxysuccinimide (NHS) [52]. The reaction mechanism between cPEG and antibodies anti-CA125 involves the activation of the carboxy moieties of cPEG with EDC and NHS to form an unstable succinimide ester, which is prone to react with the amino moieties of antibodies to form a stable amide bond. As a confirmation of their successive modifications, zeta potential and hydrodynamic size measurements were performed by dynamic light scattering (DLS) on CTAB-capped GNRs, GNRs after immobilization of mPEG and cPEG mixtures and GNRs after conjugation with antibodies. The results are reported in Figure 1C and D. Their zeta potentials revealed the cationic [53], anionic and zwitteronic profiles of CTAB-capped, PEGylated and anti-CA125 GNRs, respectively. Likewise, their hydrodynamic radii underwent a progressive increase, which may be expected from the replacement of CTAB with PEG and then the addition of antibodies. On the other hand, the optical extinction of CTAB-capped, PEGylated and anti-CA125 GNRs showed negligible variations (Figure 1B), thus suggesting that these modifications preserved their plasmonic features.

## Cytotoxicity

In order to gain some preliminary insight into the biocompatibility of anti-CA125 GNRs, cell viability was evaluated *in vitro* in the presence of different doses of PEGylated or anti-CA125 GNRs on HeLa cells (see Figure A1 in Additional file 1). Anti-CA125 GNRs proved to be slightly more cytotoxic than PEGylated GNRs, probably because of their active targeting or the effect of antibodies per se. However, also anti-CA125 GNRs exerted little effect up to 100 μM Au.

## Specificity and environmental competition

A direct dot immunoassay was performed using GNRs with different modifications. The essential steps of this test involved the immobilization of CA125 on nitrocellulose membranes and its detection with anti-CA125 GNRs. This assay was developed to mimic an *in vitro* scenario, where CA125 is overexpressed on the surface of certain malignant cells and anti-CA125 GNRs are brought into contact with them. Staining occurred both with monoclonal antibody (mAb) anti-CA125 GNRs and polyclonal antibody (pAb) anti-CA125 GNRs, whereas GNRs conjugated with anti-rabbit immunoglobulins G (IgGs) did not adhere to the membranes, thus demonstrating the active role of the molecular recognition.

Furthermore, a dot immunoassay based on a competitive scheme was developed using mAb anti-CA125 GNRs. This assay was carried out to understand whether mAb

anti-CA125 GNRs retain their ability to target their analyte even in the presence of free CA125. This circumstance mimics the *in vivo* conditions, where CA125 is present in the bloodstream, besides that on the surface of the malignant cells. In this case, the main steps of the assay involved the immobilization of CA125 on nitrocellulose membranes (at one given concentration), the incubation of a certain amount of anti-CA125 GNRs with standard solutions of CA125 (at different concentrations) and finally their interaction with the membranes. Staining of the membranes was found to decrease with an increase of free CA125 (Figure 2, on the right), consistent with the trend of a competitive assay. A dose–response curve for CA125 was retrieved by darkfield microscopy, from a quantitative measurement of the intensity of optical scattering from the particles (Figure 2, on the right). The average coefficient of variation among the various concentrations of free CA125 was found to be 10%. The signal began to decrease for CA125 concentrations higher than ~ 50 ppm and nicely followed a logistic behavior. The detection limit of this assay, i.e. the lowest concentration of free CA125 that was distinguishable from the absence of the analyte beyond statistical fluctuations, was ~ 90 ppm.

In practice, our immunoassay is unsuitable to discriminate healthy patients (CA125 in the range of 0 – 35 ppm) from those with pathological levels of CA125 (≥ 35 ppm). We note that the concentration of bio-conjugated GNRs

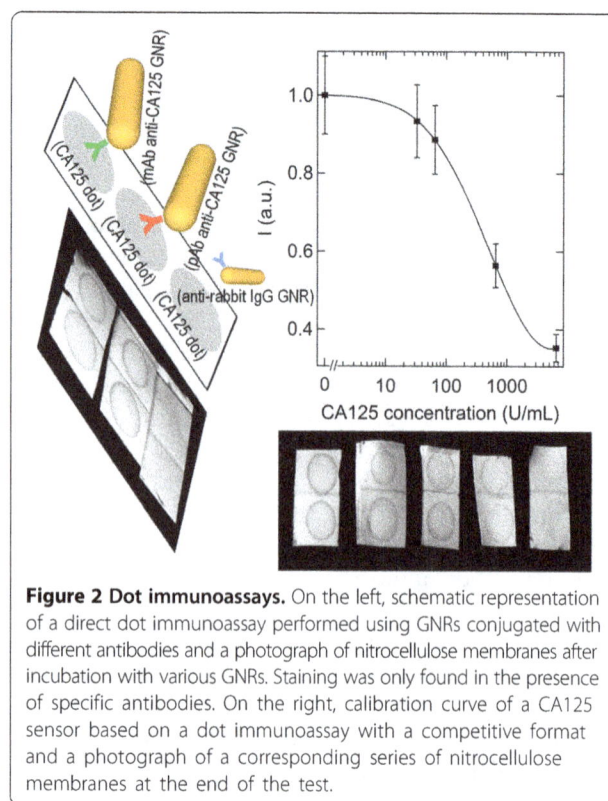

**Figure 2 Dot immunoassays.** On the left, schematic representation of a direct dot immunoassay performed using GNRs conjugated with different antibodies and a photograph of nitrocellulose membranes after incubation with various GNRs. Staining was only found in the presence of specific antibodies. On the right, calibration curve of a CA125 sensor based on a dot immunoassay with a competitive format and a photograph of a corresponding series of nitrocellulose membranes at the end of the test.

that we used is not higher than the typical doses that are injected in the bloodstream for tests *in vivo* (say at least 10 mg Au per Kg animal [27,54-56] or 50 g blood, i.e. 1 mM Au in the blood). Therefore, our findings imply that the potential of anti-CA125 GNRs to target tumors is retained even in a regime of pathological conditions. In other words, our load of antibodies per particles is far from saturation even in a pathological environment. This result is not obvious, when it is considered that 400 μM Au amount to ~ 2 nM particles and 35 ppm CA125 corresponds to 40 – 150 nM CA125. At a glance, a lower limit for the number of recognition sites per particle must be ~ 20. In essence, anti-CA125 GNRs are good candidates to bind ovarian cancer cells *in vitro* and *in vivo*.

### Specificity and the matrix effect

Another source of criticalities is the matrix effect. This effect was evaluated by a sandwich assay with an enzymatic label. A schematic representation of this assay is shown in the left panel of Figure 3. The rate of appearance of the enzymatic product (r) is proportional to the number of fundamental events of molecular recognition. Optical measurements in buffer solution and plasma were recorded over time (0 – 60 minutes), in order to quantify the enzymatic product. The kinetics of the enzymatic reactions are reported in the right panel of Figure 3. The slopes of the curves are similar in the cases when the analyte was dissolved in a standard solution (r ~ $(6.0 \pm 0.6)*10^{-2} \, s^{-1}$) or contained in a complex matrix such as plasma (r ~ $(3.3 \pm 0.3)*10^{-2} \, s^{-1}$). When CA125 was dissolved in the buffer solution, the kinetics was somewhat higher, which may be ascribed to various factors, including that the plasma could contain less than 30 ppm CA125 or also suppress any aspecific signal, due to the passivation given by the adsorption of plasmatic proteins. Anyway, the comparison between these two kinetics suggests that the matrix effect is not critical for these particles. The standard solution of CA125 was also incubated with

GNRs modified with anti-bovine IgGs and the sandwich assay was run in order to gain an estimate of the extent of aspecific signal. In the right panel of Figure 3, this kinetics is compared with those obtained in the case of GNRs conjugated with specific antibodies. The incidence of aspecific signal (r ~ $(3 \pm 3)*10^{-5} \, s^{-1}$) proved to be negligible with respect to its specific counterpart.

### Specificity *in vitro* and the effect of biological fluids

The cellular uptake of GNRs was evaluated by darkfield microscopy, silver staining and spectrophotometry. The results of these three methods agreed on the effect of the surface modification on the uptake of GNRs by HeLa cells: PEGylated GNRs exhibited the lowest uptake, while anti-CA125 GNRs featured the highest uptake and specificity.

#### Darkfield microscopy

The plasmonic features of the GNRs are useful to reveal their cellular uptake by darkfield microscopy, which exploits the modulation of the optical scattering from a thin sample. This method has become a popular approach to identify GNRs in vitro [41,57], because of its noninvasive profile and suitability for dynamic inspections of living cells. After a preliminary characterization of the coefficients of optical scattering from the GNRs, the method described in refs. [57,58] was used. For each field of view, two darkfield images were acquired, spectrally filtered in and off the principal plasmonic resonance of the GNRs (780 nm high-pass and 510 nm bandpass filters). Then, after background subtraction, a pixel by pixel operation was performed to give a ratio image ($R = I_{780 \, nm}/I_{510 \, nm}$, where I is the intensity at the named wavelength). This ratio proved to be sensitive to the presence of GNRs. Three samples of HeLa cells were prepared, i.e. with overnight incubation of anti-CA125 GNRs or PEGylated GNRs and a blank sample without particles. In order to keep a focus on the cells, a mean value of $R$ was calculated from

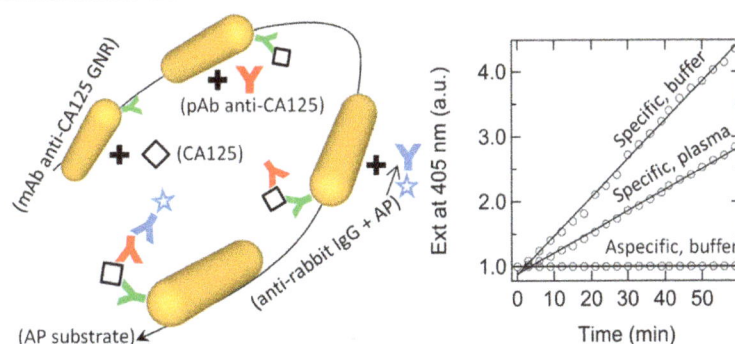

**Figure 3 Sandwich assays.** Left: schematic representation of the sandwich assay with enzymatic label performed on GNRs. Right: kinetics of the enzymatic reactions when GNRs modified with specific antibodies were incubated with a standard solution of CA125 (steepest line), human plasma (second steepest line) or when GNRs conjugated with aspecific antibodies (flattest line) were incubated with the same standard solution of CA125.

individual cells or cell clusters ( ≈ 300) in each field of view and from various fields of view (≈ 10).

Results are plotted in Figure 4. The mean value of $R$ associated with the anti-CA125 GNRs sample (red circles, upper panel) was higher than those of the blank as well as the PEGylated GNRs samples (black and blue circles, respectively). A Student's t-test was performed to qualify this observation, with the following results: $p < 10^{-5}$ for both anti-CA125 GNRs – blank and anti-CA125 GNRs – PEGylated GNRs pairs; $p = 0.53$ in the case of the blank – PEGylated GNRs pair (~ 300 points for each sample). These figures are consistent with an accumulation of anti-CA125 GNRs and an absence of PEGylated GNRs.

### Silver staining

Silver staining has become an option of choice for a qualitative assessment of the specificity of various gold nanoparticles in vitro, because of its convenience and sensitivity [36,43,59-65]. Here, metal particles nucleate the specific deposition of silver from an appropriate silver salt (silver acetate), in the presence of a suitable reducing agent (hydroquinone). Silver-coated particles then catalyze more silver deposition and so the silver grains grow in size and eventually become visible under a standard microscope. This principle was used to highlight the cellular uptake of anti-CA125 GNRs.

HeLa and HCT 116 cells were treated with PEGylated GNRs or anti-CA125 GNRs. Figure 5 shows that only the specific GNRs/cell combination produced a significant precipitation of silver and thus a significant accumulation of particles. For HCT 116 cells, no deposition of silver was observed for either kind of GNRs. Instead, for HeLa cells, a high precipitation of silver was only observed in the case of anti-CA125 GNRs and this was well confined within the cells. The comparison between anti-CA125 GNRs and PEGylated GNRs was corroborated with a quantitative spectrophotometric analysis [60], which gave a ratio between the extent of specific to aspecific uptake from HeLa cells in the order of $6 \pm 3$ (see Figure A2 in Additional file 1).

Finally, we verified the translation of our findings on the interplay of environmental competition and matrix effect *in vitro*. Particles were incubated with critical examples of biological fluids (serum, plasma or ascitic fluid from mice bearing ovarian cancers, at a representative rate of 400 μM Au) for one hour and then left to interact with HeLa cells. Even after this treatment, only anti-CA125 GNRs were found to retain a significant uptake from HeLa cells, although some attenuation of the pristine contrast with their PEGylated counterpart is visible. This result confirms that the interaction with free analyte in biological tissue does not saturate the antibodies on the surface of the particles, consistent with the outcome from our dot immunoassays. In addition, the specificity of anti-CA125 GNRs without and with preincubation in biological fluids was found to correlate well with the efficiency of a hyperthermic effect based on an optical treatment, as it is discussed in Additional file 1 (see Figure A3).

### Haemolysis and detection from macrophages

In order to complement our analysis on the suitability of anti-CA125 GNRs for an intravenous administration, we

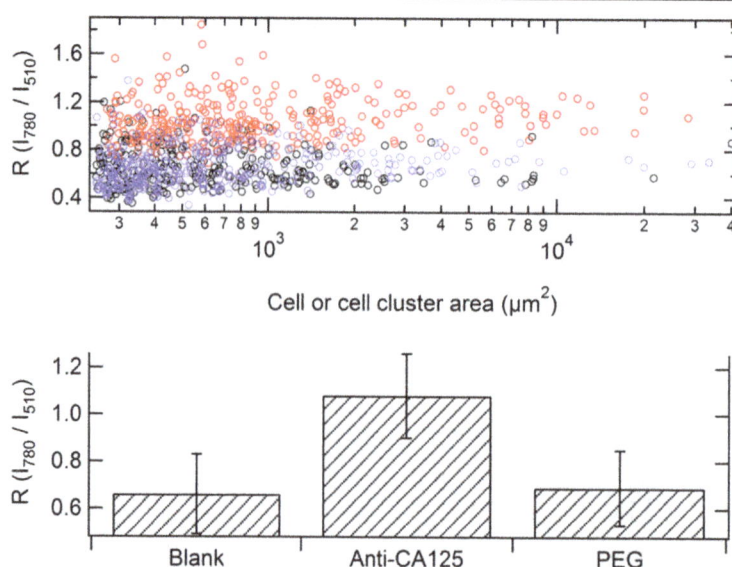

**Figure 4 Darkfield microscopy analysis.** Topmost panel: $R$ value for each cell or cell cluster for each of the three samples as a function of the area of the cell or cell cluster (black, red and blue for the blank, anti-CA125 GNRs and PEGylated GNRs samples, respectively). Bottommost panel: the mean values of $R$ for each of the three samples with their standard deviations.

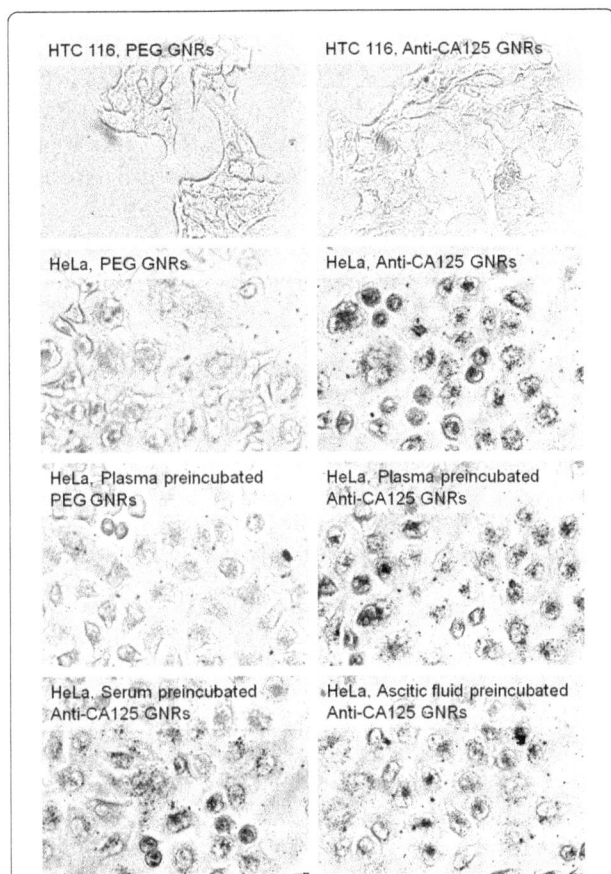

Figure 5 Silver enhancement. Evidence of targeting of CA125 via silver staining, using HCT 116 and HeLa cells as negative and positive models, respectively. Some samples of GNRs were preincubated with serum, plasma and ascitic fluid before their administration into the culture media.

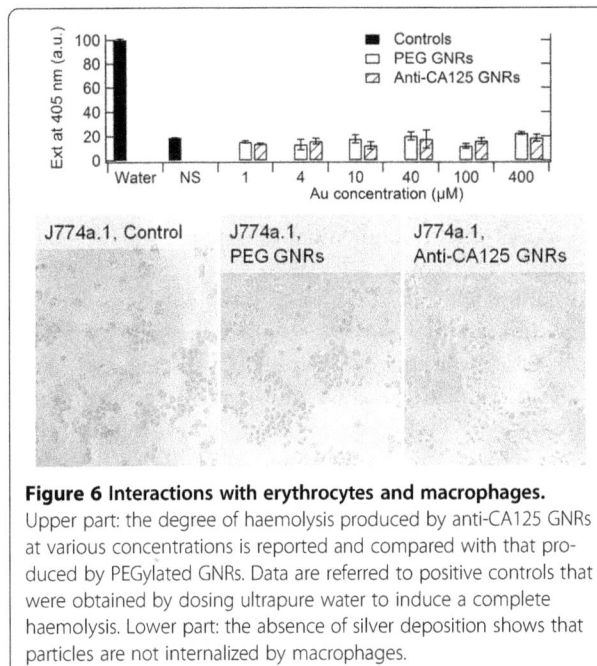

Figure 6 Interactions with erythrocytes and macrophages. Upper part: the degree of haemolysis produced by anti-CA125 GNRs at various concentrations is reported and compared with that produced by PEGylated GNRs. Data are referred to positive controls that were obtained by dosing ultrapure water to induce a complete haemolysis. Lower part: the absence of silver deposition shows that particles are not internalized by macrophages.

assessed their haemolytic activity. Erythrocytes were incubated with a positive control (ultrapure water), a negative control (normal saline) or various concentrations of anti-CA125 GNRs or PEGylated GNRs. According to the topmost panel of Figure 6, anti-CA125 GNRs exhibited the same behavior as PEGylated GNRs and both types of particles displayed no haemolytic activity, even at their highest concentrations. Data are referred to positive controls obtained by dosing ultrapure water to induce a complete haemolysis.

Moreover, we implemented a phagocytosis assay, because this parameter may impair the ability of anti-CA125 GNRs to remain in the bloodstream by their sequestration from phagocytes. The amount of gold internalized by macrophages exposed to anti-CA125 GNRs or PEGylated GNRs at a concentration of 100 μM Au was probed by silver staining after an overnight incubation. Here, 12 – 18 hours are regarded as an upper limit for the persistence of bioconjugated GNRs in the bloodstream [44]. As shown in the bottommost panel of Figure 6, on visual inspection, no

precipitation of silver was found for the PEGylated GNRs sample, as it is expected from the literature [10,28], but also for the anti-CA125 GNRs sample. Therefore, the addition of anti-CA125 antibodies did not jeopardize the stealth profile imparted by the PEG portion.

## Conclusions

In conclusion, we have presented a model of anti-CA125-conjugated gold nanorods that are intended to target ovarian cancer cells after intravenous injection. We have combined a battery of tests to understand their specificity for surfaces and cells overexpressing CA125, as well as possible issues that may arise from their interface with a bloodstream, both in terms of their performances of molecular recognition and their compatibility with erythrocytes and phagocytes. We have found that both the competition from free CA125 in biological fluids and the matrix effect affected the ability of our particles to detect their biochemical target to a moderate extent. This modulation was analytically quantified in solution and qualitatively confirmed in cells. In addition, our particles were not harmful to erythrocytes and did not suffer from massive phagocytosis and sequestration from macrophages, such as those residing in the liver, kidneys and spleen.

With these premises, our particles are a meaningful candidate for future investigations with animal tissue ex vivo and in vivo. While this analysis does not intend to replace animal testing, we are confident that our approach may inspire additional efforts to enhance the preliminary screening of functional particles that are directed to systemic administration. Our future work will aim to refine the dependability of our models and the quantitative profile of our predictions on the interactions between particles and their biological targets in the presence of a circulatory system.

## Methods

### Materials

HAuCl$_4$ (hydrogen tetrachloroaurate (III) hydrate), CTAB (hexadecyltrimethylammonium bromide), NaBH$_4$ (sodium borohydride), ascorbic acid, silver nitrate, NHS (N-hydroxysuccinimide), EDC (1-ethyl-3-(3-dimethylaminopropyl) carbodiimide), polysorbate 20, paraformaldehyde, silver acetate, hydroquinone, trypsin, trypan blue, anti-rabbit IgG labelled with alkaline phosphatase, 4-nitrophenyl phosphate bis(cyclohexylammonium) salt, milk powder, human serum, human plasma and MTT (3-(4,5-dimethylthiazol-2-yl)-2,5-diphenyltetrazolium bromide) assay kit as well as all chemicals for the various buffer solutions were purchased from Sigma Aldrich. Monoclonal mouse antibody anti-CA125 (mAb anti-CA125), polyclonal rabbit antibody anti-CA125 (pAb anti-CA125) and CA125 partial recombinant protein were purchased from Novus Biologicals. Alpha-methoxy-omega-mercapto-poly(ethylene glycol) (mPEG-SH) and alpha-carboxy-omega-mercapto-poly(ethylene glycol) (cPEG-SH), M$_w$ $\approx$ 5000 gmol$^{-1}$, were provided by Iris Biotech. All cell culture media, fetal calf serum and antibiotics (penicillin and streptomycin) were purchased from Gibco. All chemicals were of analytical grade. Nitrocellulose membranes with pore size of 0.45 μm were purchased from Whatman.

### Cell lines and culture conditions

Human colon colorectal carcinoma cells (HCT 116) (negative line, i.e. not expressing CA125), human cervix carcinoma cells (HeLa) (positive line, i.e. overexpressing CA125) and murine macrophages were used. All cell lines were maintained in Dulbecco Modified Eagle Medium (DMEM) supplemented with fetal bovine serum, 100 units/mL penicillin, and 100 μg/mL streptomycin and kept under standard culture conditions (37°C, 5% CO$_2$, 95% air and 100% relative humidity).

### Instrumentation

Optical spectra of aqueous suspensions of GNRs were measured by a UV-NIR spectrophotometer (V-560, Jasco, Japan). Their zeta potential and hydrodynamic size were characterized by Dynamic Light Scattering (DLS, Zetasizer Nano-ZS90, Malvern Instruments, UK). Imaging was performed by Transmission Electron Microscopy (TEM, CM12, Philips, the Netherlands) or optical microscopy operated in darkfield or standard conditions. For TEM, GNRs were left to dry on carbon-coated films and imaged at 100 kV. The darkfield microscope consisted of a Nikon (Japan) Eclipse TE-2000 platform equipped with a Nikon darkfield condenser (immersion oil, min NA = 1.2, max

NA = 1.4), a Nikon 10 × objective (NA = 0.3), a set of optical filters (510 nm, 40 nm FWHM passband filter XF3043, Omega Optical, USA and 780 nm highpass filter OG780, Schott AG, Germany) and a CCD camera (Coolsnap-HQ2, Roper Scientific, USA). Cells were also observed with a Leica (Germany) DMI3000B inverted microscope. The optical excitation described in Additional file 1 was performed with a low power 810 nm diode laser (Weld 800, El.En., Italy).

### Synthesis of GNRs

CTAB-capped GNRs were synthesized by the autocatalytic reduction of HAuCl$_4$ with ascorbic acid, according to the method proposed by Nikoobakht et al. [66], with the variant and overgrowth by Ratto et al. [18].

### PEGylation of GNRs

After purification by two cycles of centrifugation and decantation with a dead volume ratio of ~ 1/200, GNRs were transferred at a concentration of 1.6 mM Au into a 100 mM acetate buffer at pH 5 containing 500 μM cetrimonium bromide and 5 μM cPEG-SH. This suspension was left to react at 37°C for 30 minutes and then 50 μM mPEG-SH was added and kept at rest for another 90 minutes. After purification, GNRs were transferred at a concentration of 1.6 mM Au into a 10 mM MES buffer at pH 6 containing 120 mM NaCl and 0.005% (v/v) polysorbate 20. The M$_w$ of PEG of $\approx$ 5000 gmol$^{-1}$ was chosen to provide for high colloidal stability, low aspecific interactions with cells [10] and so the perspective to take full advantage of the EPR effect [67].

### Preparation of anti-CA125-conjugated GNRs

An equal volume of a solution containing 12 mM NHS and 48 mM EDC was added to a suspension of GNRs at a concentration of 1.6 mM Au in 10 mM MES buffer at pH 6. After 15 minutes of activation, this suspension was incubated with a double volume of 20 ppm Ab anti-CA125 in MES buffer at pH 6 containing 120 mM NaCl and 0.005% (v/v) polysorbate 20. After one hour, 10 mM 2-methoxyethylamine was dosed for 30 minutes, in order to block any unreacted succinimide ester. After purification by two cycles of centrifugation and decantation with a dead volume ratio of ~ 1/200, GNRs were transferred at a concentration of 4.0 mM Au into sterile PBS.

### Dot immunoassay

Dot immunoassays were performed using 0.45 μm pore size nitrocellulose membranes. In a typical protocol of a direct assay, 1 μL of 1000 ppm CA125 partial recombinant protein in carbonate buffer at pH 9.6 was spotted onto a membrane. Then, the spot was left to dry in an oven at 37°C for 20 minutes. Nonspecific binding was inhibited by incubation of the membrane for 40 minutes at room temperature in a blocking PBS buffer containing 3% (w/v) milk powder. Then, the membrane was incubated for one hour at room temperature and under gentle stirring with 500 μL of a suspension of 400 μM Au mAb anti-CA125 GNRs, pAb anti-CA125 GNRs or anti-rabbit IgG GNRs. Finally, the membrane was washed twice with a PBS buffer containing 0.1% (v/v) polysorbate 20 and left to dry at room temperature.

For a competitive assay, nitrocellulose membranes were spotted with CA125 and blocked, as in the case of a direct assay. Meanwhile, 400 μM Au mAb anti-CA125 GNRs were incubated for one hour with standard solutions containing variable concentrations of CA125, in the range 0 – 5000 ppm. After purification, GNRs were resuspended at a concentration of 400 μM Au in 1 mL of PBS buffer and incubated with the membranes for one hour at room temperature and under gentle stirring. Finally, the membranes were rinsed with abundant PBS buffer containing 0.1% (v/v) polysorbate 20 and left to dry at room temperature. The readout was devised as a quantitative light scattering measurement by darkfield microscopy, which reflects the amount of GNRs bound to the membranes.

## Sandwich assay

50 μL of mAb anti-CA125 GNRs at a concentration of 4.0 mM Au in PBS buffer were added to 450 μL of PBS buffer supplemented with 30 ppm CA125 or 450 μL of human serum or plasma containing their physiological level of CA125. After one hour of incubation at 37°C, GNRs were purified and resuspended at a concentration of 4.0 mM Au in 50 μL of PBS buffer and incubated for one hour at 37°C with 450 μL of PBS buffer containing 20 ppm pAb anti-CA125 that had formerly been left to react for 30 minutes with anti-rabbit IgG labelled with alkaline phosphatase (1/20000 of its stock solution). After purification, 50 μL of GNRs at a concentration of 4.0 mM Au were transferred into 450 μL of 2.4 mM 4-nitrophenyl phosphate bis(cyclohexylammonium) salt in DEA buffer. The alkaline phosphatase enzyme catalyzed the formation of a soluble end product that was bright yellow. This reaction was monitored with a spectrophotometer at 405 nm.

## Measurement of cellular uptake

Cellular uptake of the mAb anti-CA125 GNRs was evaluated using three different techniques, i.e. darkfield microscopy, silver staining and spectrophotometry. HeLa and HCT 116 cells were seeded and allowed to grow for 24 hours in 24-well culture plates or on glass coverslips. Cells were then treated overnight with mPEG GNRs (non-targeted particles) and mAb anti-CA125 GNRs (targeted particles) at a concentration of 100 μM Au in culture medium. Untreated cells served as a background

control. Alternatively, some aliquots of mPEG GNRs and mAb anti-CA125 GNRs at a concentration of 400 μM Au were exposed to human serum, plasma or murine ascitic fluid for one hour, centrifuged and decanted, prior to their incubation with the cells at a concentration of 100 μM Au in culture medium. The day after, cells were washed with abundant PBS in order to remove all unbound GNRs.

For darkfield microscopy and silver staining, cells were fixed in a solution of 3.6% paraformaldehyde in PBS buffer for 5 minutes and washed with PBS buffer to remove the excess of reagents. For a qualitative inspection by silver staining, samples were incubated for 5 minutes with 23 mM hydroquinone in citrate buffer at pH 3.8 and then for 4 – 18 minutes with the same solution supplemented with 6 mM silver acetate. All solutions were as fresh as possible. Samples were observed with a standard microscope. For a quantitative optical analysis, cells were counted, centrifuged and suspended in 120 μL of DI water, before inspection with a spectrophotometer (see Figure A2 in Additional file 1).

## Measurement of interactions with erythrocytes and macrophages

For the evaluation of haemolysis, informed signed consent was obtained and human whole blood was collected from healthy volunteers. Test tubes containing 1.8 mg/mL EDTA were used to collect the whole blood. Samples were centrifuged at 3000 rpm for 20 minutes and the buffy coat was collected and washed with normal saline. 100 μl of samples diluted with normal saline to a 50% hematocrit were added to 3 mL of normal saline (as a negative control), ultrapure water (as a positive control) and suspensions of anti-CA125 GNRs in PBS buffer at different concentrations. All samples were incubated at 37°C for one hour and haemolysis was stopped by the addition of 50 μl of 2.5% glutaraldehyde, prior to centrifugation at 3000 rpm for 15 minutes. Supernatants were collected in 96-well microplates. Their absorbance was measured at 405 nm by an automated plate reader.

The uptake of anti-CA125 GNRs from macrophages was visualized by silver staining.

## Additional file

Additional file 1: Cytotoxicity, quantitative measurement of cellular uptake, optical hyperthermia in vitro. This file contains additional information on the biological profiles and functional properties of anti-CA125 GNRs [68-71].

### Competing interests
The authors declare that they have no competing interests.

### Authors' contributions
SC prepared the particles, performed the dot immunoassays, the sandwich assays and drafted the manuscript, FT performed all experiments with cells, FR coordinated and conceived of the work, AG and RM performed the

darkfield analyses, GR devised all procedures for the darkfield analyses, IL and SN selected the biological model and molecular target and prepared the HeLa cells, AR consolidated the protocols for the conjugation of anti-CA125 antibodies to the gold nanorods, GM supervised the work by AR, EM supervised the work by IL and SN, FF supervised the work by SC, AG, RM and GR and RP supervised the work by FT and FR. All authors read and approved the final manuscript.

## Acknowledgments

This work has been partially supported by the Projects of the Health Board of the Tuscan Region "NANOTREAT" and "NANO-CHROM".

## Author details

[1]Dipartimento di Scienze Biomediche Sperimentali e Cliniche 'Mario Serio', Università degli Studi di Firenze, Viale Pieraccini 6, 50139 Firenze, Italy. [2]Istituto di Fisica Applicata 'Nello Carrara', Consiglio Nazionale delle Ricerche, Via Madonna del Piano 10, 50019 Sesto Fiorentino, Italy. [3]Dipartimento di Chimica 'Ugo Shiff', Università degli Studi di Firenze, Via della Lastruccia 3, 50019 Sesto Fiorentino, Italy. [4]Dipartimento di Scienze della Salute, Università degli Studi di Firenze, Viale Pieraccini 6, 50139 Firenze, Italy. [5]Dipartimento di Medicina Sperimentale e Clinica, Università degli Studi di Firenze, Largo Brambilla 3, 50134 Firenze, Italy.

## References

1. Mladenov E, Magin S, Soni A, Iliakis G: **DNA double-strand break repair as determinant of cellular radiosensitivity to killing and target in radiation therapy.** *Front Oncol* 2013, **10**:113.
2. Paulides MM, Stauffer PR, Neufeld E, Maccarini PF, Kyriakou A, Canters RA, Diederich CJ, Bakker JF, Van Rhoon GC: **Simulation techniques in hyperthermia treatment planning.** *Int J Hyperthermia* 2013, **19**:346–357.
3. Hainfeld JF, Dilmanian FA, Slatkin DN, Smilowitz HM: **Radiotherapy enhancement with gold nanoparticles.** *J Pharm Pharmacol* 2008, **60**:977–985.
4. Ibsen S, Schutt CE, Esener S: **Microbubble-mediated ultrasound therapy: a review of its potential in cancer treatment.** *Drug Des Devel Ther* 2013, **7**:375–388.
5. Tiwari PM, Vig K, Dennis VA, Singh SR: **Functionalized gold nanoparticles and their biomedical applications.** *Nanomaterials* 2011, **1**:31–63.
6. Alkilany AM, Murphy CJ: **Toxicity and cellular uptake of gold nanoparticles: what we have learned so far?** *J Nanopart Res* 2010, **12**:2313–2333.
7. Jeong EH, Jung G, Hong CA, Lee H: **Gold nanoparticle (AuNP)-based drug delivery and molecular imaging for biomedical applications.** *Arch Pharm Res* 2014, **37**:53–59.
8. Khan MS, Vishakante GD, Siddaramaiah H: **Gold nanoparticles: a paradigm shift in biomedical applications.** *Adv Colloid Interface Sci* 2013, **199–200**:44–58.
9. Papasani MR, Wang G, Hill RA: **Gold nanoparticles: the importance of physiological principles to devise strategies for targeted drug delivery.** *Nanomed Nanotech Biol Med* 2012, **8**:804–814.
10. Tatini F, Landini I, Scaletti F, Massai L, Centi S, Ratto F, Nobili S, Romano G, Fusi F, Messori L, Mini E, Pini R: **Size dependent biological profiles of PEGylated gold nanorods.** *J Mater Chem B* 2014, **2**:6072–6080.
11. Fang J, Chen YC: **Nanomaterials for photohyperthermia: a review.** *Curr Pharm Des* 2013, **19**:6622–6634.
12. Melancon MP, Zhou M, Li C: **Cancer theranostics with near-infrared light-activatable multimodal nanoparticles.** *Acc Chem Res* 2011, **44**:947–956.
13. Jain PK, Huang X, El-Sayed IH, El-Sayed MA: **Noble metals on the nanoscale: optical and photothermal properties and some applications in imaging, sensing, biology, and medicine.** *Acc Chem Res* 2008, **41**:1578–1586.
14. Young JK, Figueroa ER, Drezek RA: **Tunable nanostructures as photothermal theranostic agents.** *Ann Biomed Eng* 2012, **40**:438–459.
15. Choi KY, Liu G, Lee S, Chen X: **Theranostic nanoplatforms for simultaneous cancer imaging and therapy: current approaches and future perspectives.** *Nanoscale* 2012, **4**:330–342.
16. Ghosh P, Han G, De M, Kim CK, Rotello VM: **Gold nanoparticles in delivery applications.** *Adv Drug Deliv Rev* 2008, **60**:1307–1315.
17. Chen H, Shao L, Li Q, Wang J: **Gold nanorods and their plasmonic properties.** *Chem Soc Rev* 2013, **42**:2679–2724.
18. Ratto F, Matteini P, Rossi F, Pini R: **Size and shape control in the overgrowth of gold nanorods.** *J Nanopart Res* 2010, **12**:2029–2036.
19. Li N, Zhao P, Astruc D: **Anisotropic gold nanoparticles: synthesis, properties, applications, and toxicity.** *Angew Chem Int Ed Engl* 2014, **53**:1756–1789.
20. Alkilany AM, Thompson LB, Boulos SP, Sisco P, Murphy CJ: **Gold nanorods: their potential for photothermal therapeutics and drug delivery, tempered by the complexity of their biological interactions.** *Adv Drug Deliv Rev* 2012, **64**:190–199.
21. Zhang Z, Wang J, Chen C: **Gold nanorods based platforms for light-mediated theranostics.** *Theranostics* 2013, **3**:223–238.
22. Choi WI, Sahu A, Kim YH, Tae G: **Photothermal cancer therapy and imaging based on gold nanorods.** *Ann Biomed Eng* 2012, **40**:534–546.
23. Wang Y, Black KCL, Luehmann H, Li W, Zhang Y, Cai X, Wan D, Liu SY, Li M, Kim P, Li ZY, Wang LV, Liu Y, Xia Y: **Comparison study of gold nanohexapods, nanorods, and nanocages for photothermal cancer treatment.** *ACS Nano* 2013, **7**:2068–2077.
24. Jokerst JV, Cole AJ, Van de Sompel D, Gambhir SS: **Gold nanorods for ovarian cancer detection with photoacoustic imaging and resection guidance via raman imaging in living mice.** *ACS Nano* 2012, **6**:10366–10377.
25. Kennedy LC, Bear AS, Young JK, Lewinski NA, Kim J, Foster AE, Drezek RA: **T cells enhance gold nanoparticle delivery to tumors in vivo.** *Nanoscale Res Lett* 2011, **6**:283.
26. Perrault SD, Walkey C, Jennings T, Fischer HC, Chan WC: **Mediating tumor targeting efficiency of nanoparticles through design.** *Nano Lett* 2009, **9**:1909–1915.
27. Von Maltzahn G, Park JH, Agrawal A, Bandaru NK, Das SK, Sailor MJ, Bhatia SN: **Computationally guided photothermal tumor therapy using long-circulating gold nanorod antennas.** *Cancer Res* 2009, **69**:3892–3900.
28. Niidome T, Yamagata M, Okamoto Y, Akiyama Y, Takahashi H, Kawano T, Katayama Y, Niidome Y: **PEG-modified gold nanorods with a stealth character for in vivo applications.** *J Control Release* 2006, **114**:343–347.
29. Rayavarapu RG, Petersen W, Hartsuiker L, Chin P, Janssen H, van Leeuwen FWB, Otto C, Manohar S, van Leeuwen TG: **In vitro toxicity studies of polymer-coated gold nanorods.** *Nanotechnology* 2010, **21**:145101.
30. Joshi PP, Yoon SJ, Hardin WG, Emelianov S, Sokolov KV: **Conjugation of antibodies to gold nanorods through Fc portion: synthesis and molecular specific imaging.** *Bioconjug Chem* 2013, **19**:878–888.
31. Lee E, Hong Y, Choi J, Haam S, Suh JS, Huh YM, Yang J: **Highly selective CD44-specific gold nanorods for photothermal ablation of tumorigenic subpopulations generated in MCF7 mammospheres.** *Nanotechnology* 2012, **23**:465101.
32. Charan S, Sanjiv K, Singh N, Chien FC, Chen YF, Nergui NN, Huang SH, Kuo CW, Lee TC, Chen P: **Development of chitosan oligosaccharide-modified gold nanorods for in vivo targeted delivery and noninvasive imaging by NIR irradiation.** *Bioconjug Chem* 2012, **23**:2173–2182.
33. Wang J, Sefah K, Altman MB, Chen T, You M, Zhao Z, Huang CZ, Tan W: **Aptamer-conjugated nanorods for targeted photothermal therapy of prostate cancer stem cells.** *Chem Asian J* 2013, **10**:2417–2422.
34. Wang J, Zhu G, You M, Song E, Shukoor MI, Zhang K, Altman MB, Chen Y, Zhu Z, Huang CZ, Tan W: **Assembly of aptamer switch probes and photosensitizer on gold nanorods for targeted photothermal and photodynamic cancer therapy.** *ACS Nano* 2012, **6**:5070–5077.
35. Yang X, Liu X, Liu Z, Pu F, Ren J, Qu X: **Near-infrared light-triggered, targeted drug delivery to cancer cells by aptamer gated nanovehicles.** *Adv Mater* 2012, **24**:2890–2895.
36. Heidari Z, Sariri R, Salouti M: **Gold nanorods-bombesin conjugate as a potential targeted imaging agent for detection of breast cancer.** *J Photochem Photobiol B* 2013, **130**:40–46.
37. Bartneck M, Ritz T, Keul HA, Wambach M, Bornemann J, Gbureck U, Ehling J, Lammers T, Heymann F, Gassler N, Lüdde T, Trautwein C, Groll J, Tacke F: **Peptide-functionalized gold nanorods increase liver injury in hepatitis.** *ACS Nano* 2012, **6**:8767–8777.
38. Wang J, Dong B, Chen B, Jiang Z, Song H: **Selective photothermal therapy for breast cancer with targeting peptide modified gold nanorods.** *Dalton Trans* 2012, **41**:11134–11144.

39. Yang X, Liu Z, Li Z, Pu F, Ren J, Qu X: Near-infrared-controlled, targeted hydrophobic drug-delivery system for synergistic cancer therapy. Chemistry 2013, 19:10388–10394.

40. Huff TB, Tong L, Zhao Y, Hansen MN, Cheng JX, Wei A: Hyperthermic effects of gold nanorods on tumor cells. Nanomedicine 2007, 2:125–132.

41. Tong L, Wei QS, Wei A, Cheng JX: Gold nanorods as contrast agents for biological imaging: optical properties, surface conjugation and photothermal effects. Photochem Photobiol 2009, 85:21–32.

42. Lu W, Zhang GD, Zhang R, Flores LG, Huang Q, Gelovani JG, Li C: Tumor site-specific silencing of NF-kappa B p65 by targeted hollow gold nanosphere-mediated photothermal transfection. Cancer Res 2010, 70:3177–3188.

43. Eghtedari M, Liopo AV, Copland JA, Oraevsky AA, Motamedi M: Engineering of hetero-functional gold nanorods for the in vivo molecular targeting of breast cancer cells. Nano Lett 2009, 9:287–291.

44. Huang XH, Peng XH, Wang YQ, Wang YX, Shin DM, El-Sayed MA, Nie SM: A reexamination of active and passive tumor targeting by using rod-shaped gold nanocrystals and covalently conjugated peptide ligands. ACS Nano 2010, 4:5887–5896.

45. Ungureanu C, Kroes R, Petersen W, Groothuis TAM, Ungureanu F, Janssen H, van Leeuwen FWB, Kooyman RPH, Manohar S, van Leeuwen TG: Light interactions with gold nanorods and cells: implications for photothermal nanotherapeutics. Nano Lett 2011, 11:1887–1894.

46. Weitman SD, Lark RH, Coney LR, Fort DW, Frasca V, Zurawski VR, Karmen BA: Distribution of the folate receptor GP38 in normal and malignant cell lines and tissues. Cancer Res 1992, 52:3396–3401.

47. Saul JM, Annapragada AV, Bellamkonda RV: A dual-ligand approach for enhancing targeting selectivity of therapeutic nanocarriers. J Control Rel 2006, 114:277–287.

48. Ying X, Wen H, Lu WL, Du J, Guo J, Tian W, Men Y, Zhang Y, Li RJ, Yang TY, Shang DW, Lou JN, Zhang LR, Zhang Q: Dual-targeting daunorubicin liposomes improve the therapeutic efficacy of brain glioma in animals. J Control Rel 2010, 141:183–192.

49. Kluza E, van der Schaft DWJ, Hautvast PAI, Mulder WJM, Mayo KH, Griffioen AW, Strijkers GJ, Nicolay K: Synergistic targeting of alpha(v)beta(3) integrin and galectin-1 with heteromultivalent paramagnetic liposomes for combined MR imaging and treatment of angiogenesis. Nano Lett 2010, 10:52–58.

50. Qian X, Peng XH, Ansari DO, Yin-Goen Q, Chen GZ, Shin DM, Yang L, Young AN, Wang MD, Nie S: In vivo tumor targeting and spectroscopic detection with surface-enhanced Raman nanoparticle tags. Nature Biotechnology 2008, 26:83–90.

51. Shah NB, Vercellotti GM, White JG, Fegan A, Wagner CR, Bischof JC: Blood–nanoparticle interactions and in vivo biodistribution: impact of surface PEG and ligand properties. Mol Pharmaceutics 2012, 9:2146–2155.

52. Grabarek Z, Gergely J: Zero-length crosslinking procedure with the use of active esters. Anal Biochem 1990, 185:131–135.

53. Das M, Mordoukhovski L, Kumacheva E: Sequestering gold nanorods by polymer microgels. Adv Mater 2008, 20:2371–2375.

54. Dickerson EB, Dreaden EC, Huang X, El-Sayed IH, Chu H, Pushpanketh S, McDonald JF, El-Sayed MA: Gold nanorod assisted near-infrared plasmonic photothermal therapy (PPTT) of squamous cell carcinoma in mice. Cancer Lett 2008, 269:57–66.

55. Choi WI, Kim JY, Kang C, Byeon CC, Kim YH, Tae G: Tumor regression in vivo by photothermal therapy based on gold-nanorod-loaded, functional nanocarriers. ACS Nano 2011, 5:1995–2003.

56. Bagley AF, Hill S, Rogers GS, Bhatia SN: Plasmonic photothermal heating of intraperitoneal tumors through the use of an implanted near-infrared source. ACS Nano 2013, 7:8089–8097.

57. Mercatelli R, Romano G, Ratto F, Matteini P, Centi S, Cialdai F, Monici M, Pini R, Fusi F: Quantitative measurement of scattering and extinction spectra of nanoparticles by darkfield microscopy. Appl Phys Lett 2011, 99:131113.

58. Mercatelli R, Ratto F, Centi S, Soria S, Romano G, Matteini P, Quercioli F, Pini R, Fusi F: Quantitative readout of optically encoded gold nanorods using an ordinary dark-field microscope. Nanoscale 2013, 5:9645.

59. Tatini F, Ratto F, Centi S, Landini I, Nobili S, Witort E, Fusi F, Capaccioli S, Mini E, Pini R: Specific markers, micro-environmental anomalies and tropism: opportunities for gold nanorods targeting tumors in laser-induced hyperthermia. Proc. SPIE 2014, 8955:895519.

60. Ratto F, Witort E, Tatini F, Centi S, Lazzeri L, Carta F, Lulli M, Vullo D, Fusi F, Supuran CT, Scozzafava A, Capaccioli S, Pini R: Plasmonic particles that hit hypoxic cells. Adv Funct Mater 2014, doi:10.1002/adfm.201402118.

61. Rayavarapu RG, Petersen W, Ungureanu C, Post JN, van Leeuwen TG, Manohar S: Synthesis and bioconjugation of gold nanoparticles as potential molecular probes for light-based imaging techniques. Int J Biomed Imag 2007, 2007:29817.

62. Kim D, Jeong YY, Jon S: A drug-loaded aptamer-gold nanoparticle bioconjugate for combined CT imaging and therapy of prostate cancer. ACS Nano 2010, 4:3689–3696.

63. Carpin LB, Bickford LR, Agollah G, Yu TK, Schiff R, Li Y, Drezek RA: Immunoconjugated gold nanoshell-mediated photothermal ablation of trastuzumab-resistant breast cancer cells. Breast Cancer Res Treat 2011, 125:27–34.

64. England CG, Priest T, Zhang G, Sun X, Patel DN, McNally LR, van Berkel V, Gobin AM, Frieboes HB: Enhanced penetration into 3D cell culture using two and three layered gold nanoparticles. Int J Nanomed 2013, 8:3603–3617.

65. Yao L, Daniels J, Moshnikova A, Kuznetsov S, Ahmed A, Engelman DM, Reshetnyak YK, Andreev OA: pHLIP peptide targets nanogold particles to tumors. Proc Natl Acad Sci USA 2013, 110:465–470.

66. Nikoobakht B, El-Sayed MA: Preparation and growth mechanism of gold nanorods (NRs) using seed-mediated growth method. Chem Mater 2003, 15:1957–1962.

67. Zhang G, Yang Z, Lu W, Zhang R, Huang Q, Tian M, Li L, Liang D, Li C: Influence of anchoring ligands and particle size on the colloidal stability and in vivo biodistribution of polyethylene glycol-coated gold nanoparticles in tumor-xenografted mice. Biomater 2009, 30:1928–1936.

68. Pérez-Juste J, Pastoriza-Santos I, Liz-Marzán LM, Mulvaney P: Gold nanorods: synthesis, characterization and applications. Coord Chem Rev 2005, 249:1870–1901.

69. Ratto F, Matteini P, Cini A, Centi S, Rossi F, Fusi F, Pini R: CW laser-induced photothermal conversion and shape transformation of gold nanodogbones in hydrated chitosan films. J Nanopart Res 2011, 13:4337–4348.

70. Matteini P, Ratto F, Rossi F, de Angelis M, Cavigli L, Pini R: Hybrid nanocomposite films for laser-activated tissue bonding. J Biophotonics 2012, 5:868–877.

71. Etchegoin PG, Le Ru EC, Meyer M: An analytic model for the optical properties of gold. J Chem Phys 2006, 125:164705.

# 11

# Collagen-based silver nanoparticles for biological applications: synthesis and characterization

Vinicius S Cardoso[1,2], Patrick V Quelemes[1], Adriany Amorin[1], Fernando Lucas Primo[3], Graciely Gomides Gobo[3], Antonio C Tedesco[3], Ana C Mafud[4], Yvonne P Mascarenhas[4], José Raimundo Corrêa[5], Selma AS Kuckelhaus[6], Carla Eiras[7], José Roberto SA Leite[1], Durcilene Silva[1] and José Ribeiro dos Santos Júnior[8*]

## Abstract

**Background:** Type I collagen is an abundant natural polymer with several applications in medicine as matrix to regenerate tissues. Silver nanoparticles is an important nanotechnology material with many utilities in some areas such as medicine, biology and chemistry. The present study focused on the synthesis of silver nanoparticles (AgNPs) stabilized with type I collagen (AgNPcol) to build a nanomaterial with biological utility. Three formulations of AgNPcol were physicochemical characterized, antibacterial activity *in vitro* and cell viability assays were analyzed. AgNPcol was characterized by means of the following: ultraviolet–visible spectroscopy, dynamic light scattering analysis, Fourier transform infrared spectroscopy, atomic absorption analysis, transmission electron microscopy and of X-ray diffraction analysis.

**Results:** All AgNPcol showed spherical and positive zeta potential. The AgNPcol at a molar ratio of 1:6 showed better characteristics, smaller hydrodynamic diameter ($64.34 \pm 16.05$) and polydispersity index ($0.40 \pm 0.05$), and higher absorbance and silver reduction efficiency (0.645 mM), when compared with the particles prepared in other mixing ratios. Furthermore, these particles showed antimicrobial activity against both *Staphylococcus aureus* and *Escherichia coli* and no toxicity to the cells at the examined concentrations.

**Conclusions:** The resulted particles exhibited favorable characteristics, including the spherical shape, diameter between 64.34 nm and 81.76 nm, positive zeta potential, antibacterial activity, and non-toxicity to the tested cells (OSCC).

**Keywords:** Silver nanoparticles, Collagen, Antimicrobial activity, Cell viability

## Background

Collagen is the most abundant protein constituting to the 30% of total protein and 6% of animal body weight [1,2]. Type I collagen, a natural polymer, is a major extracellular matrix protein in mammals and exhibits favorable characteristics for promoting cell proliferation [3-5]. It can influence the cell physiology and morphology [4,6], create a good matrix for endothelial cells *in vitro*, induce platelet aggregation, promote blood clotting, and consequently accelerate the healing of skin wounds [7].

Since 1980s, some scientists have been using collagen as a matrix to regenerate tissues for repairing skin [8], bone [9], knee meniscal [10], joint cartilage [11], esophagus [12], dura mater [13], muscle [14] and nervous system [15]. The use of collagen combined with glycosaminoglycans as a skin implant has been already tested [16,17]. The ability of collagen gel to regenerate cornea and nerves has been also demonstrated by recent animal studies and clinical trials [18,19]. Furthermore, it has been shown that the combined collagen and hyaluronic acid can promote the revascularization of tissues in animal models [20].

In the field of nanotechnology, collagen scaffold has been widely used in biological experiments for introducing chemical and pharmaceutical substances. Bakare et al. [21] proposed a method for constructing a film by using poly(hydroxybutyrate valerate) (PHBV) grafted

* Correspondence: jribeiro@ufpi.edu.br
[8]Department of Chemistry, Campus Teresina, Federal University of Piauí, 64049-550 Teresina, Piauí, Brazil
Full list of author information is available at the end of the article

with scaffold tipo I collagen to support silver nanoparticles (AgNPs). Jithendra et al. [22] suggested a blend of *Aloe Vera* with collagen and chitosan scaffold for tissue engineering applications.

Metal nanoparticle, especially those made of noble metals, show excellent properties for biotechnology applications [23–25]. In particular, AgNPs have established a broad range of applications in the majority of biomedical studies [26], due to their antibacterial ability and selective toxicity to microorganisms [27].

In addition, AgNPs are widely used in various medical and industrial fields for venous catheters coating; vascular prostheses manufacturing; wound dressing manufacturing; treatment for chronic wounds and ulcers [25]; or as a constituent incorporated into cement for the realignment of bone fractures [27], in to water purification filter [28] and into wall paint for providing an aseptic environment to hospital patients [29].

The ability of AgNPs to control bacterial activity relies on the interactions with three major structural components of the bacteria: namely peptidoglycan in the cell wall, DNA, and proteins, by mainly affecting the enzymes involved in the electron transport chain [30–33].

The ideal properties of AgNPs for biomedical applications include prolonged effectiveness, high levels of bactericidal and bacteriostatic activity, ability to prevent a broad spectrum of bacteria, high biocompatibility, and low toxicity *in vivo* [33]. In particular, the shape and concentration of AgNPs in solutions are important factors in ensuring the effective contact of the particles with the bacterial membranes and in determining the amount of AgNPs for effectively inhibiting the targeting bacteria [34].

Some literatures reported the application of AgNPs for treating the wounds of mice, and these particles showed excellent tensile properties and resulted in improved alignment of fibers for skin repair [35,36].

Based on the previously discussed properties and applications of collagen and AgNPs, we designed and synthesized three types of AgNPs stabilized with type I collagen (AgNPcols) by using a chemical synthesis route in the present study. This article presents their chemical synthesis, physicochemical characterization, analysis of activity against gram-positive and gram-negative bacteria, and *in vitro* cell viability assays.

## Results and discussion

Type I collagen is the most abundant protein in mammals and is present during tissue repair [1–5,7]. Although collagen has been used in biomedical research for several years, AgNPs stabilized with collagen, as well as their biocompatibility and antibacterial properties, have been recently reported by Alarcon et al. [37]. The authors used a photochemical route for fabricating AgNPs from silver nitrate ($AgNO_3$), and this route was different from the chemical route employed in this study, where a reducing agent, sodium borohydride ($NaBH_4$), was involved. Because $NaBH_4$ is unstable when being in contact with water at room temperature, it is necessary to stabilize $NaBH_4$ by using ultra-pure water at low temperature (4°C) and keep the solution refrigerated until use. In addition, Sun et al. [38] reported the use of $NaBH_4$ for the synthesis AgNPs associated to a trisodium citrate solution. Thereafter, a multilayer film consisting of AgNPs and collagen in a layer-by-layer (LbL) configuration is generally constructed for stabilizing the particles.

An exclusive study on AgNPs stabilized by collagen has been reported [37]. Based on this study, we designed and synthesized three different formulations of AgNPs, at $AgNO_3$ to $NaBH_4$ molar ratios of 1:1, 1:6, and 1:15, by varying the concentration of $NaBH_4$ to obtain the best silver ($Ag^0$) reduction result in solution. The solution at the $AgNO_3/NaBH_4$ molar ratio of 1:6 resulted in a final $Ag^0$ concentration of 0.64 mM (Table 1), as confirmed by the atomic absorption test. In the ratio of 1:1 between $AgNO_3$ and $NaBH_4$, the amount of reducer was not sufficient to reduce all molecules of silver. At ratio of 1:6 was obtained the best concentration for the chemical reaction, probably the molecules amount of $AgNO_3$ and $NaBH_4$ reached an optimum value for reduction. However, the ratio was 1:15 excess $NaBH_4$ causing release of ions in solution and forming nanoparticles with hydrodynamic diameter higher by aggregation [39].

All synthesized solutions were characterized in terms of particle size, zeta potential, and polydispersity index (PDI) by dynamic light scattering (DLS) analysis. A positive potential (19.9–31.8 mV) was obtained for all AgNPcols (Table 1). This occurs due to amino group carries a positive charge and is present in AgNPcol [40,41] (Figure 1D). The hydrodynamic diameter of the nanoparticles was between 64.34 nm and 81.76 nm and PDI value was between

**Table 1 Diameter, zeta potential, PDI of AgNPcols (mean ± standard deviation) and molar concentration of silver in the solution**

|  | Diameter (nm) | Zeta Potential (mv) | PDI* | [Ag] (mM) |
| --- | --- | --- | --- | --- |
| AgNPcol (1:1) | 78.87 ± 12.89 | 31.8 ± 0.62 | 0.60 ± 0.02 | 0.434 |
| AgNPcol (1:6) | 64.34 ± 16.05 | 24.9 ± 0.79 | 0.10 ± 0.05 | 0.645 |
| AgNPcol (1:15) | 81.76 ± 18.22 | 19.9 ± 0.4 | 0.77 ± 0.17 | 0.345 |

*PDI: polydisperity index.

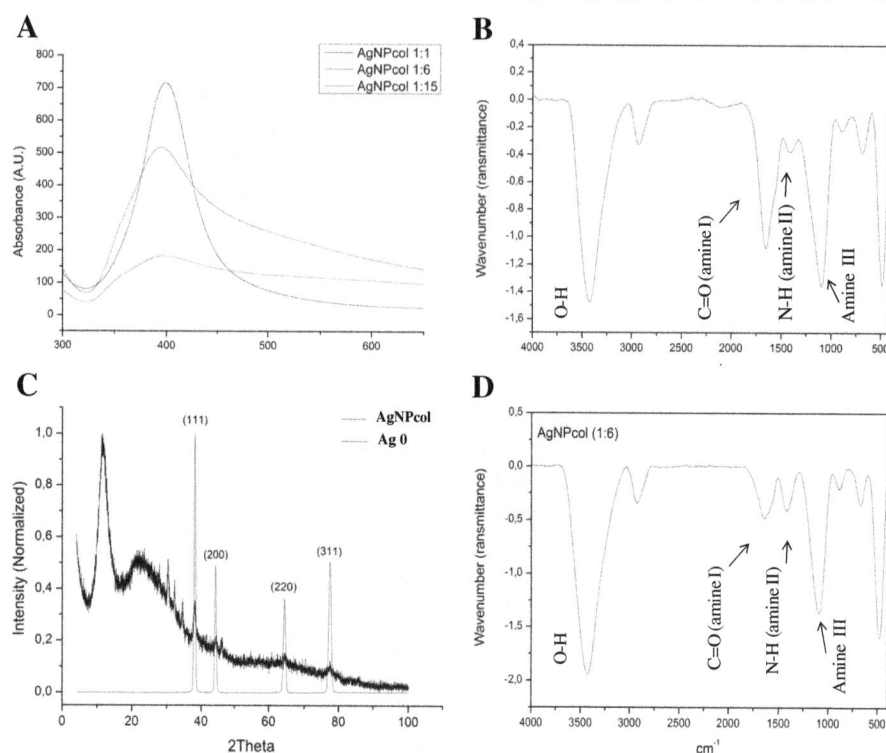

**Figure 1 AgNPcol characterization. (A)** Absorbance spectra of AgNPcols at three different NaBH$_4$ to AgNO$_3$ molar ratios; **(B)** FTIR spectra of collagen; **(C)** XDR patterns of AgNPcol (1:6 molar ratio); **(D)** FTIR spectra of AgNPcol (1:6 molar ratio).

0.40 and 0.77. The AgNPs associated with titanium dioxide synthesized by Desai and Kowshik [42] showed PDI value of 0.47, which was very close to the result obtained from this study, although other PDI values were also reported [43–45]. The value of PDI is one of the major parameters used for selecting a low-polydispersity solution for the subsequent cell viability test.

The presence of a positive zeta potential favors the interaction between the particles and Gram-negative and Gram-positive bacteria [46]. The efficiency of ionic silver against bacteria with negatively charged membranes is related to the electrostatic attraction caused by the positive potentials of the particles [47]. In the present study, the positive zeta potential of AgNPcols is one of the aspects that may explain the favorable result of its acting against *E. coli* and *S. aureus*. Hamouda and Baker [48] reported that the opposite surface charges could promote the interactions between the bacterial membranes and AgNPs. They also mentioned that, due to the small size of nanoparticles, the tested solutions could easily permeate the membranes of the bacteria and promote their death [34,49]. Furthermore, Baker et al. [50] reported that small particles with large contact areas showed increased efficiency against bacteria, as compared with the particles with large sizes. Saptarshi et al. [51] suggests that associate protein with nanoparticle,

there are better cell absorption because the protein favors interaction with cell membrane facilitating interaction to nanoparticle with bacteria and another live cells.

The increase in the proportion of NaBH$_4$ during particle synthesis could reduce the zeta potential of the resulting particles. Zhang and Wu [39] reported the same behavior of gold nanoparticles and claimed that this was due to the aggregation of metal particles. The AgNPcols produced in our study demonstrated similar behaviors, as indicated by the decrease in the amount of nanoparticles in the solution. This is because that the aggregated Ag$^0$ formed larger particles, resulting in a polydisperse solution and precipitation during centrifugation. The relationship between the increases of the ratio of NaBH$_4$ in relation to the increase in diameter of the nanoparticles is due to the release of electrons caused by NaBH$_4$. Because when an increase occurs in the concentration of NaBH$_4$ increases the number of free electrons in the solution and decreases the zeta potential favors the aggregation of silver [39].

After synthesis, all solutions were characterized by using ultraviolet–visible (UV–vis) spectroscopy analysis, which was efficient for detecting the sensitive AgNPs that could display a strong absorption peak [52,53]. In this study, we found a wider plasmon band and lower absorption peak intensity for the solution at a higher $NaBH_4$ to $AgNO_3$ molar ratio, as compared with the solutions at lower molar ratios (Figure 1A). It is believed that this is due to the aggregation of $Ag^0$ molecules [53,54], as indicated by the values of zeta potential described above and the presence of large particles in AgNPcol at molar ratio of 1:15. We can also notice the presence of the plasmon band between 380 nm and 450 nm, and this is indicative of the spherical shape of AgNPs [55], which can be further confirmed by transmission electron microscopy (TEM) analysis (Figure 2). Some researchers [35,56] reported that the spherical shape is the optimal morphology for nanoparticles against bacteria, as it can facilitate the interaction between the particles and the bacterial membranes.

The difference in size AgNPcol found between the results of Table 1 (DLS) and Figure 2 (MET) occurs because the DLS diameter is measured in solution (hydrodynamic diameter value). Already in the TEM, the nanoparticle is no in solution and the result is a projected estimate of the diameter of the nanoparticle. The hydrodynamic diameter of the nanoparticles (DLS) was

highlight, because this nanoparticle was developed for use in a biological environment and will be in solution [57].

From the Fourier transform infrared spectra (FTIR) of collagen and AgNPcol (1:6 molar ratio) (Figure 1B and D), we can observe the presence of $C = O$ (amine I at $1652.84$ cm$^{-1}$) and NH bands (amine II at $1571.64$ cm$^{-1}$) in both samples of collagen and AgNPcol. However, the band due to $C = O$ (amine I at $1652.84$ cm$^{-1}$) in the spectrum of AgNPcol showed a low intensity, indicating that this group was possibly involved in the reduction and stabilization of AgNPs. Sun et al. [38] suggested that these changes were due to the association of collagen molecules (i.e., amines) with AgNPs.

The phases of the samples were determined by X-ray powder diffraction (XDR) analysis by searching against databases. In Figure 1C, it can see the silver peaks (ICSD: 44387-Ag0), with reflections identified. Traces of silver oxides (ICSD: 35540-Ag2O, 27659-AgO, 15999/59193-Ag2O3, 202218-Ag3O4) were also identified from the sample. Silver oxides reflections can be found in [Additional file 1]. This result is consistent with our expectation that oxidation products can be formed on the

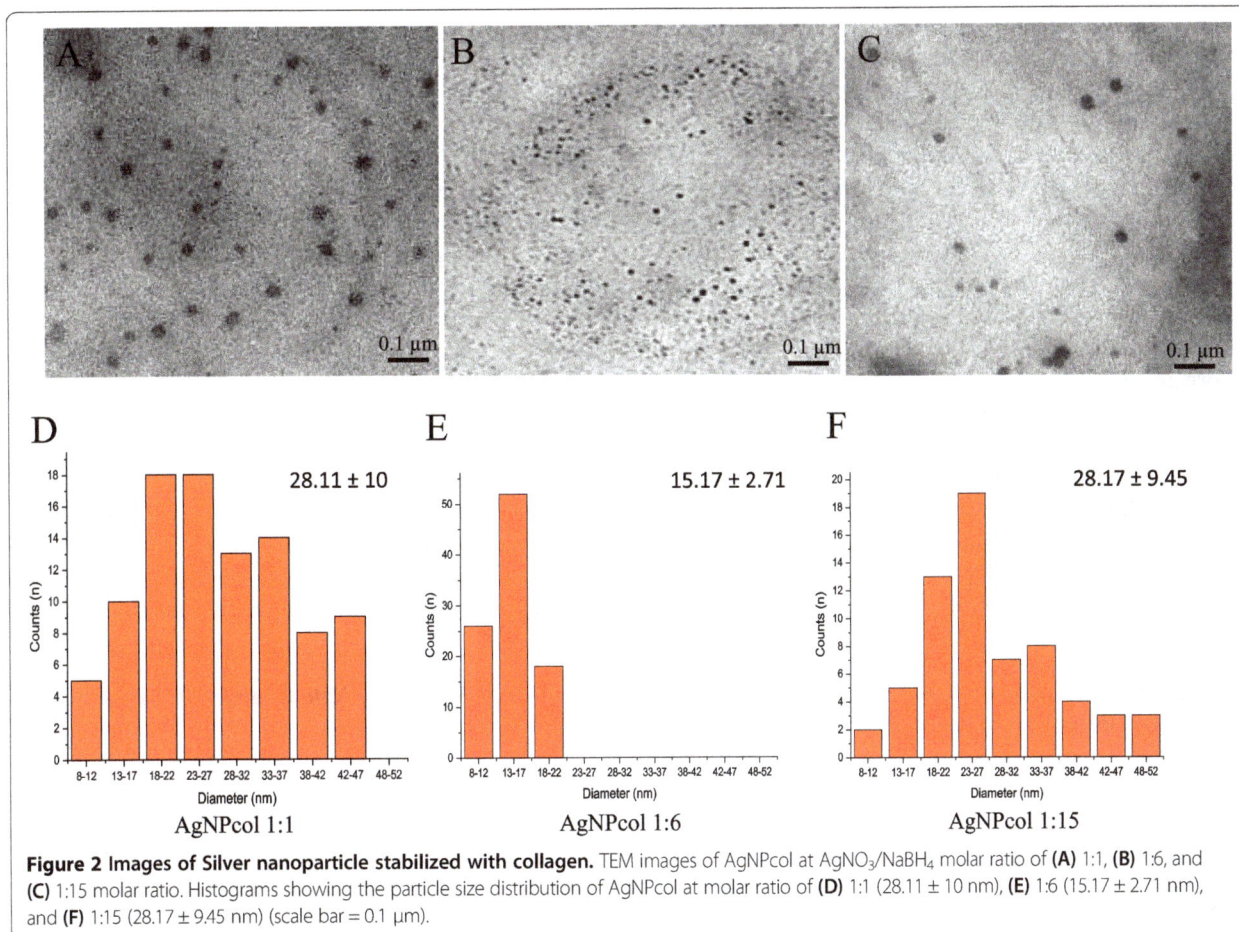

**Figure 2 Images of Silver nanoparticle stabilized with collagen.** TEM images of AgNPcol at $AgNO_3/NaBH_4$ molar ratio of **(A)** 1:1, **(B)** 1:6, and **(C)** 1:15 molar ratio. Histograms showing the particle size distribution of AgNPcol at molar ratio of **(D)** 1:1 (28.11 ± 10 nm), **(E)** 1:6 (15.17 ± 2.71 nm), and **(F)** 1:15 (28.17 ± 9.45 nm) (scale bar = 0.1 μm).

surface of pure silver. In addition, we found that the amorphous phase of collagen affected the sample's crystallinity, resulting in its semi-crystalline state.

The activity of AgNPcols against the gram-positive bacterium, *Staphylococcus aureus* (ATCC 29213), and gram-negative bacterium, *E. coli* (ATCC 25922), was tested by using an AgNO$_3$ solution as control. Based on the results of the atomic absorption spectrometric study, the concentration of AgNPcols was corrected for the antimicrobial assays. It was found that the behavior of AgNPcol (1:6 molar ratio) for inhibiting the growth of bacteria was comparable to that of AgNO$_3$ (Table 2). Thus, we may assume that the silver particle can maintain its antimicrobial property when being incorporated into the collagen-stabilized nanoparticles. In Alarcon's study [37] about AgNPs stabilized with collagen, was lower than that of AgNO$_3$ used as control.

For the cell viability test, we chose only one synthesized solution by analyzing the relevant characterization data. AgNPcol at the molar ratio of 1:6 was chosen for the test, due to its smaller particle size, lower PDI, and a higher percentage of Ag$^0$ than those of other samples, as determined by atomic absorption spectroscopy. The results (Figure 3) indicated that the AgNPcol solution at the tested concentrations did no cause significant differences in cell viability as compared with the control (CT). In addition, AgNO$_3$ and collagen (Col) were also used for comparison. It is known that collagen does not show any cytotoxicity towards cells, as this can be evidenced by its abundance in animals and the human body. Although AgNO$_3$ solution was reported to be toxic to cells, the AgNPcol at the approximate Ag concentration as that of AgNO$_3$ did not show any toxicity to the cells tested in this study. We attempted to use higher concentrations of AgNPcol to evaluate its cytotoxicity; however, precipitation occurred in the solution before incubation under the physiological pH and ambient temperature conditions.

Gurunathan et al. [58] performed the cell viability test by using breast cancer cells (MDA-MB-23) and AgNP at 5 µg/ml, which did not exhibit cytotoxicity as compared with the control. In addition, Prokopovich et al. [59] synthesized the AgNPs by using NaBH$_4$, and the produced nanoparticles were incorporated into the bone

cement, which did not show cytotoxicity to osteoblast cells (MC 3TC) either.

The results of the present study showed that the synthesized AgNPcol was effective against the tested bacteria and was non-toxic to the examined cells. Further tests will be conducted to evaluate the *in vivo* cytotoxicity and healing ability of AgNPcol by using biological tissues and animal samples.

## Conclusion

In the present study, we demonstrated the synthesis of an AgNP solution stabilized with type I collagen by using NaBH$_4$ as a reducing agent. The resulted particles exhibited favorable characteristics, including the spherical shape, diameter between 64.34 nm and 81.76 nm, positive zeta potential, antibacterial activity, and non-toxicity to the tested cells (OSCC). It is found that the activity against bacterium is facilitated by the electrostatic interaction between the positively charged AgNPcols and the negatively charged bacterial membranes. Probably the shape, size and positive zeta potential of AgNPcols facilitates the activity against gram negative bacterium and gram positive bacterium. Furthermore, the cell viability test provides the basics for the future study that aims to investigate the *in vivo* behaviors of AgNPcols by using biological tissues.

## Methods

### Synthesis of collagen-based silver nanoparticles (AgNPcols)

A solution of silver nitrate (AgNO$_3$) at a concentration of 108 µgAg/mL, a collagen type I from rat tail (Santa Cruz Biotechnology) solution at a concentration of 0.1 mg/ml and a solution of borohydride (NaBH$_4$) at 3.78 mg/ml, prepared using ultrapure water at 4°C were used to carry out the synthesis of nanoparticles.

The AgNO$_3$ solution was added to the collagen, both with the same volume and remained under agitation to homogenize for 10 min. The NaBH$_4$ solution was added later, in the form of jet, for any solution of NaBH$_4$, came in contact with the Beker solutions quickly and completely. This solution was stirred for 10 minutes to homogenize. Subsequently, the reaction mixture was centrifuged at 3600 rpm for 15 minutes and finally

**Table 2 Minimum inhibitory concentrations (MICs) of AgNPcol (µg Ag/mL), AgNO$_3$ (µg Ag/mL), and standard antibiotics (µg/mL) for inhibiting *Staphylococcus aureus* and *Escherichia coli***

| | AgNPcol (µgAg/mL) | | | Controls | |
|---|---|---|---|---|---|
| Bacterial strains | 1:1 | 1:6 | 1:15 | AgNO$_3$ (µgAg/mL) | Antibiotic (µg/mL) |
| *S. aureus* | 11.7 | 17.4 | 11.7 | 13.5 | <0.5[a] |
| *E. coli* | 11.7 | 8.7 | 11.7 | 6.75 | <0.5[b] |

[a]Oxacilin.
[b]Meropenen.

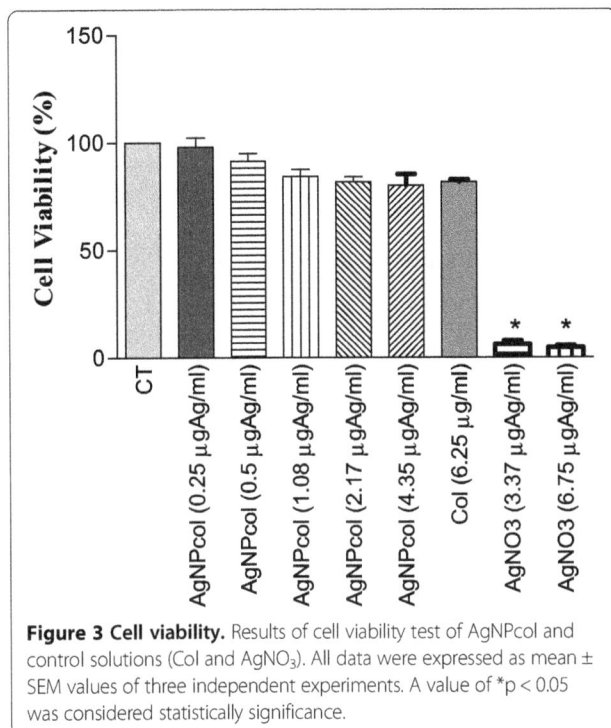

**Figure 3 Cell viability.** Results of cell viability test of AgNPcol and control solutions (Col and AgNO₃). All data were expressed as mean ± SEM values of three independent experiments. A value of *p < 0.05 was considered statistically significance.

separated from the supernatants of the final solution present in the container. In the present study three different proportions of borohydride solution regarding Silver Nitrate (AgNO₃) (molar ratio: 1:1, 1:6 e 1:15) were selected.

### Physicochemical characterization of AgNPcols

The AgNPcols were characterized by UV–vis spectroscopy using a Shimadzu (UV 1800) spectrophotometer. Were subsequently characterized according to their size, electrical potential and PDI using the DLS (Malvern Zetasizer Nano ZS Model 3600) with laser with a wavelength of 633 nm and scattering angle of 90° all measurements were performed in triplicate. To verify the shape and confirm the diameter of the nanoparticles non-diluted samples were placed on two screens (20 µL) for transmission electron microscopy (TEM) previously coated with Formvar. After drying for 2 h at room temperature (25 ± 2°C) screens were analyzed in a Jeol JEM-1010 electron microscope and photomicrographed by an UltraScan® with Digital Micrograph 3.6.5 software (Gatan/USA) [25].

In order to quantify the percentage of silver in solution, the atomic absorption spectroscopy (Varian - Model AA240FS) was used, with a wavelength of 328.1 nm and multielement lamp (Varian No. 5610108700). The reading was held in atomic absorption flame with Oxygen and Acetylene gases.

XRD data were obtained at the Laboratory of X-ray Crystallography of IFSC/USP using a Rigaku Rotaflex diffractometer equipped with graphite monochromator and rotating anode tube, operating with Cu Ka, 50 kV and 100 mA. Powder diffraction patterns were obtained in step scanning mode, $2\theta = 5–100°$, step of 0.02° and 5 s/step. Peak Fitting Module program [60] was used for the peak decomposition of the semicrystalline pattern and determination of area due to the amorphous phase.

### Evaluation of antibacterial activity of AgNPcols

To study the antibacterial properties of *AgNPcols*, by the determination of Minimum Inhibitory Concentration (MIC), two bacterial strains were selected: *Staphylococcus aureus* ATCC 29213 (Gram-positive) and *Escherichia coli* ATCC 25922 (Gram-negative). The microorganisms were cultured in Mueller-Hinton agar at 37°C for 24 hours in aerobic conditions. Then a suspension of bacterial strains with an optical density of McFarland of 0.5 ($1 \times 10^8$ CFU/mL) was made in an isotonic sodium chloride 0.85% solution. Later in time, this solution was diluted ten times ($1 \times 10^7$ CFU/mL) and used as inoculum in the experiment. MIC was determined according to protocols previously described [61–63] using 96-well microdilution plate with Mueller-Hinton broth where the strains (concentration of $5 \times 10^5$ CFU/mL) were exposed to twofold dilution series of the AgNPcols with concentrations ranging from 34,8 to 0,36 µgAg/mL. The same procedure was used to determine the MIC of the following controls: collagen, AgNO₃, and standard antibiotics effective against the tested bacterial strains with concentrations ranging from 27 to 0.42 µgAg/mL for AgNO₃; 50 to 3,12 µg/mL for collagen and 32 to 0.5 µg/mL for antibiotics. Sterile Mueller-Hinton broth was used as the negative control and inoculated broth was used as the positive control. MIC was defined as the lowest concentration of agent that restricted the visual bacterial growth in the culture media.

### Cell viability

For the study of cell viability, the AgNPcol 1:6 was diluted four times with the ratio of two, starting at a concentration of 4.35 µgAg/ml. The cell lines used in this study was oral squamous cell carcinoma (OSCC) obtained from American Type Culture Collection (ATCC, Manassas, VA). Cells were grown in 75 cm² flasks and maintained in Dulbecco's modified Eagle medium (DMEM) supplemented with 10% fetal bovine serum, streptomycin/penicillin antibiotics and non-essential aminoacids. For the experiment the cells were seeded in a 96-well plate (5,000 cel./Well) and kept in an incubator (atmosphere at 37°C and humidified 5% CO₂) for 24 hours. In a 96-well plate was added 5 different concentrations AgNPcol solutions and control solutions (medium, collagen - 6.25 µg/ml, AgNO3 - 3.37 µgAg/ml and AgNO3 - 6.75 µgAg/ml). The plates were kept in an incubator for 3 hours. Subsequently, the added solutions were removed and placed in Hank's buffer for 5 minutes. The buffer was removed and fresh medium was added. After 24 hours the medium was removed and added to a solution of DMEM without phenol and MTT ([3-(4,5-dimethyl thiazol-2-yl)-2,5-*diphenyl tetrazolium bromide*) (15%) to each well. The plates were incubated for 4 hours. Thereafter all the medium with MTT was removed with care to do not remove formazam produced by living cells. Finally, isopropanol was added to each well to solubilize the formazam and taken to review the reader Safire (TECAN EUA Inc., Durham, NC). Statistical analysis was performed using Prism 5.0 (GraphPad Software) by ANOVA and Tukey test. All data were expressed as mean and standard deviation of three independent experiments. We used the statistical significance of $p < 0.05$ for this study [64].

## Additional file

Additional file 1: Additional information about XRD result.

### Abbreviations

AgNPs: Silver nanoparticles; AgNPcols: Silver nanoparticles stabilized with type I collagen; $AgNO_3$: Silver nitrate; $NaBH_4$: Sodium borohydride; LbL: Layer-by-layer; $Ag^0$: Silver; mM: Millimolar; PDI: Polydispersity index; UV–vis: Ultraviolet–visible; DLS: Dynamic light scattering; TEM: Transmission electron microscopy; FTIR: Fourier transform infrared spectra; XDR: X-ray powder diffraction; MICs: Minimum inhibitory concentrations; CT: Control; Col: Collagen.

### Competing interests

The authors declare that they have no competing interests.

### Authors' contributions

VSC contributed to the organization and drafting of this article. PVQ, AA, FLP, GGG, ACT, ACM, YPM, JRC, SASK, CE, JRSA, DS and JRSJ contributed to the selection of methodology, analysis and discussion of the results. All authors read and approved the final manuscript.

### Acknowledgements

We thank the Laboratory of Photobiology and Photomedicine of University of São Paulo, the Laboratory of Microscopy of University of Brasília and the Institute of Physics of São Carlos to contribute with this paper. ACM are grateful to FAPESP (2014/02282-6). YPM are grateful to CAPES (AUX-PERM-705/2009).

### Author details

[1]Research Center in Biodiversity and Biotechnology (Biotec), Campus Parnaíba, Federal University of Piauí, Av São Sebastian 2819, 64202-020 Parnaíba, Piauí, Brazil. [2]Physiotherapy Department, Campus Parnaíba, Federal University of Piauí, Av. São Sebastião 2819, 64202-020 Parnaíba, Piauí, Brazil. [3]Departamento de Química, Laboratório de Fotobiologia e Fotomedicina, Faculdade de Filosofia, Ciências e Letras de Ribeirão Preto, Universidade de São Paulo, 14040-901, Ribeirão Preto, SP, Brazil. [4]Institute of Physics of São Carlos (IFSC), University of São Paulo (USP), 13566-590 São Carlos, SP, Brazil. [5]Laboratory of Microscopy, Institute of Biology, University of Brasília, 70910900 Brasília, DF, Brazil. [6]Area of Morphology, Faculty of Medicine, University of Brasília, Brasília 70910900DF, Brazil. [7]Interdisciplinary Laboratory for Advanced Materials (LIMAV), Federal University of Piauí, 64049-550 Teresina, PI, Brazil. [8]Department of Chemistry, Campus Teresina, Federal University of Piauí, 64049-550 Teresina, Piauí, Brazil.

### References

1. Dornelles C, Costa S: **Estudo comparativo da dissolução de três diferentes marcas de colágeno utilizadas em técnicas cirúrgicas otológicas.** *Rev Bras Otorrinolaringol* 2003, **69:**744–751.
2. Tonhi E, Plepis AMG: **Obtenção e caracterização de blendas colágeno-quitosana.** *Qim nova* 2002, **25:**943–948.
3. Lin YC, Tan FJ, Marra KG, Jan SS, Liu DC: **Synthesis and characterization of collagen/hyaluronan/chitosan composite sponges for potential biomedical applications.** *Acta Biomater* 2009, **5:**2591–2600.
4. Wang XH, Li DP, Wang WJ, Feng QL, Cui FZ, Xu YX, Song XH, Van der Werf M: **Crosslinked collagen/chitosan matrix for artificial livers.** *Biomaterials* 2003, **24:**3213–3220.
5. Nehrer S, Breinan HA, Ramappa A, Young G, Shortkroff S, Louie LK, Sledge CB, Yannas IV, Spector M: **Matrix collagen type and pore size influence behaviour of seeded canine chondrocytes.** *Biomaterials* 1997, **18:**769–776.
6. Nishikawa AK, Taira T, Yoshizato K: **In vitro maturation of collagen fibrils modulates spreading, DNA synthesis, and collagenolysis of epidermal cells and fibroblasts.** *Exp Cell Res* 1987, **171:**164–177.
7. Heimbach D, Luterman A, Burke J, Cram A, Herndon D, Hunt J, Jordan M, McManus W, Solem L, Warden G, Zawacki B: **Artificial dermis for major burns.** *Ann Surg* 1988, **208:**313–320.
8. De Vries HJC, Middelkoop E, Mekkes JR, Dutrieux RP, Wildevuur CHR, Westerhof W: **Dermal regeneration in native noncross-linked collagen sponges with diferent extracellular matrix molecules.** *Wound Repair Regen* 1994, **2:**37–47.
9. Nevins M, Kirkerhead C, Nevins M, Wozney JA, Palmer R: **Bone formation in the goat maxillary sinus induced by absorbable collagen sponge implants impregnated with recombinant human bone morphogenetic protein-2.** *Int J Periodont Restorative Dent* 1996, **16:**9–19.
10. Stone KR, Steadman JR, Rodkey WG, Li ST: **Regeneration of a meniscal cartilage with use of a collagen scaffold: analysis of preliminary data.** *J Bone Jt Surg* 1997, **79A:**1770–1777.
11. Speer DP, Chvapil M, Volz RG, Holmes MD: **Enhancement of healing in osteochondral defects by collagen sponge implants.** *Clin Orthop Relat Res* 1979, **144:**326–335.
12. Natsume T, Ike O, Okada T, Takimoto N, Shimizu Y, Ikada Y: **Porous collagen sponge for esophageal replacement.** *J Biomed Mater Res* 1993, **27:**867–875.
13. Narotam PK, Van Dellen JR, Bhoola KD: **A clinicopathological study of collagen sponge as a dural graft in neurosurgery.** *J Neurosurg* 1995, **82:**406–412.
14. Van-Wachem PB, Van-Luyn MJA, Costa MLP: **Myoblast seeding in a collagen matrix evaluated in vitro.** *J Biomed Mater Res* 1996, **30:**353–360.
15. Ding T, Lu WW, Zheng Y, Li ZY, Pan HB, Luo Z: **Rapid repair of rat sciatic nerve injury using a nanosilver-embedded collagen scaffold coated with laminin and fibronectin.** *Regen Med* 2011, **6:**437–447.
16. Matsuda K, Suzuki S, Isshiki N, Yoshioka K, Okada T, Ikada Y: **Influence of glycosaminoglycans on the collagen sponge component of a bilayer artificial skin.** *Biomaterials* 1990, **11:**351–355.
17. Srivastava S, Gorham SD, French DA, Shivas AA, Courtney JM: **In vivo evaluation and comparison of collagen, acetylated collagen and collagen/glycosaminoglycan composite films and sponges as candidate biomaterials.** *Biomaterials* 1990, **11:**155–161.
18. Liu W, Deng C, McLaughlin CR, Fagerholm P, Lagali NS, Heyne B, Scaiano JC, Watsky MA, Kato Y, Munger R, Shinozaki N, Li F, Griffith M: **Collagen-phosphorylcholine interpenetrating network hydrogels as corneal substitutes.** *Biomaterials* 2009, **30:**1551–1559.
19. Fagerholm P, Lagali NS, Merrett K, Jackson WB, Munger R, Liu Y, Polarek JW, Söderqvist M, Griffith M: **A biosynthetic alternative to human donor tissue for inducing corneal regeneration: 24-month follow-up of a phase 1 clinical study.** *Sci Transl Med* 2010, **2:**46ra61.
20. Perng CK, Wang YJ, Tsi CH, Ma H: **In vivo angiogenesis effect of porous collagen scaffold with hyaluronic acid oligosaccharides.** *J Surg Res* 2011, **168:**9–15.
21. Bakare RA, Bhan C, Raghavan D: **Synthesis and characterization of collagen grafted Poly(hydroxybutyrate-valerate) (PHBV) scaffold for loading of bovine serum albumin capped silver (Ag/BSA) nanoparticles**

in the potential use of tissue engineering application. *Biomacromolecules* 2014, 15:423–435.

22. Jithendra P, Rajam AM, Kalaivani T, Mandal AB, Rose C: **Preparation and characterization of aloe vera blended collagen-chitosan composite scaffold for tissue engineering applications.** *ACS Appl Mater Interfaces* 2013, 5:7291–7298.

23. Hackenberg S, Scherzed A, Kessler M, Hummel S, Technau A, Froelich K, Ginzkey C, Koehler C, Hagen R, Kleinsasser N: **Silver nanoparticles: evaluation of DNA damage, toxicity and functional impairment in human mesenchymal stem cells.** *Toxicol Lett* 2011, 201:27–33.

24. Shang L, Wang Y, Huang L, Dong S: **Preparation of DNA-silver nanohybrids in multilayer nanoreactors by in situ electrochemical reduction, characterization, and application.** *Langmuir* 2007, 23:7738–7744.

25. Dipankar C, Murugan S: **The green synthesis, characterization and evaluation of the biological activities of silver nanoparticles synthesized from Iresine herbstii leaf aqueous extracts.** *Colloids Surf B* 2012, 98:112–119.

26. Neto EAB, Ribeiro C, Zucolotto V: **Síntese de nanopartículas de prata para aplicação na sanitização de embalagens.** In *Embrapa*. 2008. http://www.clickciencia.ufscar.br/portal/edicao19/Artigo.pdf.

27. Wong KKY, Liu X: **Silver nanoparticles-the real "silver bullet" in clinical medicine?** *Med Chem Commun* 2010, 1:125–131.

28. Chaloupka K, Malam Y, Seifalian AM: **Nanosilver as a new generation of nanoproduct in biomedical applications.** *Trends Biotechnol* 2010, 28:580–588.

29. Ahamed M, Alsalhi MS, Siddiqui MKJ: **Silver nanoparticle applications and human health.** *Clin Chim Acta* 2010, 411:1841–1848.

30. Lok C, Ho C, Chen R, He Q, Yu W, Sun H, Tam PK, Chiu J, Che C: **Proteomic analysis of the mode of antibacterial action of silver research articles.** *J Proteome Res* 2006, 5:916–924.

31. Shahverdi AR, Fakhimi A, Shahverdi HR, Minaian S: **Synthesis and effect of silver nanoparticles on the antibacterial activity of different antibiotics against Staphylococcus aureus and Escherichia coli.** *Nanomedicine* 2007, 3:168–171.

32. Panáček A, Kvítek L, Prucek R, Kolář M, Večeřová R, Pizúrová N, Sharma VK, Nevěcná TJ, Zbořil R: **Silver colloid nanoparticles: synthesis, characterization, and their antibacterial activity.** *J Phys Chem B* 2006, 110:16248–16253.

33. Gnanadhas DP, Ben Thomas M, Thomas R, Raichur AM, Chakravortty D: **Interaction of silver nanoparticles with serum proteins affects their antimicrobial activity in vivo.** *Antimicrob Agents Chemother* 2013, 57:4945–4955.

34. Pal S, Tak YK, Song JM: **Does the antibacterial activity of silver nanoparticles depend on the shape of the nanoparticle? A study of the Gram-negative bacterium Escherichia coli.** *Appl Environ Microbiol* 2007, 73:1712–1720.

35. Morones JR, Elechiguerra JL, Camacho A, Holt K, Kouri JB, Ramírez JT, Yacaman MJ: **The bactericidal effect of silver nanoparticles.** *Nanotechnology* 2005, 16:2346–2353.

36. Kwan KHL, Liu X, To MKT, Yeung KWK, Ho C, Wong KKY: **Modulation of collagen alignment by silver nanoparticles results in better mechanical properties in wound healing.** *Nanomedicine* 2011, 7:497–504.

37. Alarcon EI, Udekwu K, Skog M, Pacioni NL, Stamplecoskie KG, González-Béjar M, Polisetti N, Wickham A, Richter-Dahlfors A, Griffith M, Scaiano JC: **The biocompatibility and antibacterial properties of collagen-stabilized, photochemically prepared silver nanoparticles.** *Biomaterials* 2012, 33:4947–4956.

38. Sun Y, Wang L, Sun L, Guo C, Yang T, Liu Z, Xu F, Li Z: **Fabrication, characterization, and application in surface-enhanced Raman spectrum of assembled type-I collagen-silver nanoparticle multilayered films.** *J Chem Phys* 2008, 128:074704.

39. Zhang Z, Wu Y: **Investigation of the NaBH4-induced aggregation of Au nanoparticles.** *Langmuir* 2010, 26:9214–9223.

40. Li Y, Douglas EP: **Effects of various salts on structural polymorphism of reconstituted type I collagen fibrils.** *Colloids Surf B* 2013, 112:42–50.

41. Sano S, Kato K, Ikada Y: **Introduction of functional groups onto the surface of polyethylene for protein immobilization.** *Biomaterials* 1993, 14:817–822.

42. Desai V, Kowshik M: **Synthesis and characterization of fumaric acid functionalized AgCl/titania nanocomposite with enhanced antibacterial activity.** *J Nanosci Nanotechnol* 2013, 13:2826–2834.

43. Prasad RY, McGee JK, Killius MG, Suarez DA, Blackman CF, DeMarini DM, Simmons SO: **Investigating oxidative stress and inflammatory responses elicited by silver nanoparticles using high-throughput reporter genes in HepG2 cells: effect of size, surface coating, and intracellular uptake.** *Toxicol In Vitro* 2013, 27:2013–2021.

44. Stevanović M, Bračko I, Milenković M, Filipović N, Nunić J, Filipič M, Uskoković DP: **Multifunctional PLGA particles containing poly(l-glutamic acid)-capped silver nanoparticles and ascorbic acid with simultaneous antioxidative and prolonged antimicrobial activity.** *Acta Biomater* 2014, 10:151–162.

45. Hebeish A, El-Rafie MH, El-Sheikh MA, Seleem AA, El-Naggar ME: **Antimicrobial wound dressing and anti-inflammatory efficacy of silver nanoparticles.** *Int J Biol Macromol* 2014, 65:509–515.

46. Silva T, Pokhrel LR, Dubey B, Tolaymat TM, Maier KJ, Liu X: **Particle size, surface charge and concentration dependent ecotoxicity of three organo-coated silver nanoparticles: comparison between general linear model-predicted and observed toxicity.** *Sci Total Environ* 2014, 468–469:968–976.

47. Kim JS, Kuk E, Yu KN, Kim JH, Park SJ, Lee HJ, Kim SH, Park YK, Park YH, Hwang CY, Kim YK, Lee YS, Jeong DH, Cho MH: **Antimicrobial effects of silver nanoparticles.** *Nanomedicine* 2007, 3:95–101.

48. Hamouda T, Baker JR: **Antimicrobial mechanism of action of surfactant lipid preparations in enteric Gram-negative bacilli.** *J Appl Microbiol* 2000, 89:397–403.

49. Shang L, Nienhaus K, Nienhaus GU: **Engineered nanoparticles interacting with cells: size matters.** *J Nanobiotechnol* 2014, 12:5.

50. Baker C, Pradhan A, Parkstis L, Pochan DJ, Shah SI: **Synthesis and antibacterial properties of silver nanoparticles.** *J Nanosci Nanotechnol* 2005, 5(2):244–249.

51. Saptarshi SR, Duschl A, Lopata AL: **Interaction of nanoparticles with proteins: relation to bio-reactivity of the nanoparticle.** *J Nanobiotechnol* 2013, 11:26.

52. Gao X, Gu G, Hu Z, Guo Y, Fu X, Song J: **A simple method for preparation of silver dendrites.** *Colloids Surfaces A Physicochem Eng Asp* 2005, 254:57–61.

53. Sileikaitė A, Prosyčevas I, Puišo J, Juraitis A, Guobienč A: **Analysis of silver nanoparticles produced by chemical reduction of silver salt solution.** *Mater Sci (Medziagotyra)* 2006, 12(4):287–291.

54. Yamamoto SY, Ujiwara KF, Atarai HW: **Surface-enhanced Raman scattering from oleate-stabilized silver colloids at a liquid/liquid interface.** *Anal Sci* 2004, 20(September):1347–1352.

55. Zaheer K, Shaeel AA, Abdullah YO, Ziya AK, Abdulrahman AOA: **Shape-directing role of cetyltrimethylammonium bromide in the preparation of silver nanoparticles.** *J Colloid Interface Sci* 2012, 367:101–108.

56. Lara HH, Garza-Treviño EN, Ixtepan-Turrent L, Singh DK: **Silver nanoparticles are broad-spectrum bactericidal and virucidal compounds.** *J Nanobiotechnol* 2011, 9:30.

57. Kato H, Nakamura A, Takahashi K, Kinugasa S: **Accurate size and size-distribution determination of polystyrene latex nanoparticles in aqueous medium using dynamic light scattering and asymmetrical flow field flow fractionation with multi-angle light scattering.** *Nanomaterials* 2012, 2:15–30.

58. Gurunathan S, Han JW, Eppakayala V, Jeyaraj M, Kim JH: **Cytotoxicity of biologically synthesized silver nanoparticles in MDA-MB-231 human breast cancer cells.** *Biomed Res Int* 2013, 2013:535796.

59. Prokopovich P, Leech R, Carmalt CJ, Parkin IP, Perni S: **A novel bone cement impregnated with silver – tiopronin nanoparticles: its antimicrobial, cytotoxic, and mechanical properties.** *Int J Nanomed* 2013, 8:2227–2237.

60. *PEAK Fitting Module.* Northampton: OriginLab Corporation, One Roundhouse Plaza; 2002.

61. CLSI-Clinical Laboratory Standards Institute: *Methods for Dilution Antimicrobial Susceptibility Test for Bacteria that Grow Aerobically.* Available online: http://antimicrobianos.com.ar/ATB/wp-content/uploads/2012/11/03-CLSI-M07-A9-2012.pdf (accessed on 18 September 2013).

62. Quelemes PV, Araruna FB, de Faria BEF, Kuckelhaus SAS, da Silva DA, Mendonça RZ, Eiras C, Soares MJS, Leite JRSA: **Development and**

antibacterial activity of cashew gum-based silver nanoparticles. *Int J Mol Sci* 2013, **14**:4969–4981.

63. Guzman M, Dille J, Godet S: **Synthesis and antibacterial activity of silver nanoparticles against gram-positive and gram-negative bacteria.** *Nanomedicine* 2012, **8**:37–45.

64. Falqueiro AM, Siqueira-Moura MP, Jardim DR, Primo FL, Morais PC, Mosiniewicz-Szablewska E, Suchocki P, Tedesco AC: **In vitro cytotoxicity of Selol-loaded magnetic nanocapsules against neoplastic cell lines under AC magnetic field activation.** *J Appl Phys* 2012, **111**:07B335.

# 12

# Dual-imaging model of SQUID biosusceptometry for locating tumors targeted using magnetic nanoparticles

Jen-Jie Chieh[1*], Kai-Wen Huang[2,3], Yi-Yan Lee[1] and Wen-Chun Wei[1]

**Abstract**

**Background:** For intraoperative imaging in operating theaters or preoperative imaging in clinics, compact and economic integration rather than large and expensive equipment is required to coregister structural and functional imaging. However, current technologies, such as those integrating optical and gamma cameras or infrared and fluorescence imaging, involve certain drawbacks, including the radioactive biorisks of nuclear medicine indicators and the inconvenience of conducting measurements in dark environments.

**Methods:** To specifically and magnetically label liver tumors, an anti-alpha-fetoprotein (AFP) reagent was synthesized from biosafe iron oxide magnetic nanoparticles (MNPs) coated with anti-AFP antibody and solved in a phosphate buffered saline solution. In addition, a novel dual-imaging model system integrating an optical camera and magnetic scanning superconducting-quantum-interference device (SQUID) biosusceptometry (SSB) was proposed. The simultaneous coregistration of low-field magnetic images of MNP distributions and optical images of anatomical regions enabled the tumor distribution to be determined easily and in real time. To simulate targeted MNPs within animals, fewer reagents than the injected dose were contained in a microtube as a sample for the phantom test. The phantom test was conducted to examine the system characteristics and the analysis method of dual images. Furthermore, the animal tests were classified into two types, with liver tumors implanted either on the backs or livers of rats. The tumors on the backs were to visually confirm the imaging results of the phantom test, and the tumors on the livers were to simulate real cases in hepatocellular carcinoma people.

**Results:** A phantom test was conducted using the proposed analysis method; favorable contour agreement was shown between the MNP distribution in optical and magnetic images. Consequently, the positioning and discrimination of liver tumors implanted on the backs and livers of rats were verified by conducting in vivo and ex vivo tests. The results of tissue staining verified the feasibility of using this method to determine the distribution of liver tumors.

**Conclusion:** The results of this study indicate the clinical potential of using anti-AFP-mediated MNPs and the dual-imaging model SSB for discriminating and locating tumors.

**Keywords:** Magnetic nanoparticle, Tumor, Dual imaging, Scanning superconducting-quantum-interference device

* Correspondence: jjchieh@ntnu.edu.tw
[1]Institute of Electro-Optical Science and Technology, National Taiwan Normal University, Taipei 116, Taiwan
Full list of author information is available at the end of the article

## Background

Tumor imaging is a crucial medical practice that is performed after positive tumor screening results have been confirmed by blood tests. By using medical imaging, clinicians can analyze the phase and distribution of tumors to determine treatment options such as surgery. Medical imaging procedures are classified into structural or functional imaging. Structural imaging is developed on the basis of the physical characteristics of the tissues, whereas functional imaging is developed on the basis of the biological features of tumors or characteristics of bioprobe-mediated nanoparticles, which is an image contrast medium. Hence, simultaneous positioning and discrimination of tumors can be achieved by incorporating structural imaging and functional imaging. For example, structural imaging methods, such as computed tomography (CT) [1] or magnetic resonance imaging (MRI) [2], can be combined with functional imaging methods, such as radioactive positron emission tomography (PET). However, for biosafety, bioprobe-mediated magnetic nanoparticles (MNPs) without radioactive risks are increasingly adopted as a contrast medium in functional imaging [3] for MRI.

In addition, sensitive imaging methodologies such as MRI, CT, or PET are generally difficult to implement in both general medical clinics and clinical practices, particularly because the equipment is expensive to install and maintain. For example, using MRI devices is restricted to preoperative diagnosis because of the high cost of constructing a shielding room with few metal objects, and also the expense involved in maintaining liquid helium coolants. Hence, for the intraoperative positioning of tumors, alternate navigation surgery methodologies involve using robotic or hand-held probes in integrated systems composed of a gamma camera and ultrasound [4] or an optical video [5].

To conform to the requirements of the diverse imaging technologies used in various clinical practices such as preoperative diagnosis and intraoperative positioning of tumors, various functional contrast media have been developed as multimodal contrast media, such as MNPs coated with radioactive or fluorescent [6] indicators in addition to bioprobes [7]. However, using such complex contrast media is costly, and using multimodal nanoparticles involves high biorisk. Hence, simple contrast mediums with biosafety and economic viability, such as gadolinium and iron-oxide MNPs without coated radioactive or fluorescent materials, are approved by the USA Food and Drug Administration [8,9]. According to a previous study, iron-oxide MNPs are superior to gadolinium because gadolinium MNPs induce kidney disease [10]. An imaging technique for intraoperative positioning of tumors must therefore be developed to expand the application of iron-oxide MNPs beyond MRI preoperative diagnosis.

Recently, developments for noninvasively examining MNP distributions have been focused on the magnetic characteristics of MNPs. For example, to examine the remanent properties of MNPs, a static superconducting-quantum-interference device (SQUID) sensor or a pickup coil in a shielded sensing unit detects the magnetized and moved sample from distant magnetization coils or magnets [11,12]. This method is suitable for in vitro tests because of the fast sample movement. The biomedical application of SQUID relaxometry based on MNP relaxation [13-15] is limited to in vitro or ex vivo tests because in addition to the requirement of the shielding environment, the involved signals are sensitive to the dynamic and size distribution, hydrodynamic size, and temperature of MNPs in animals. Furthermore, magnetic particle imaging technologies based on the nonlinear characteristics of MNPs under high field gradients can be used to image the three-dimensional distribution of MNPs. However, the practical application of such technologies is limited because they are difficult to integrate with other real-time structural imaging methods (e.g., MRI) [16].

Conversely, because of the alternate-current (AC) susceptibility of MNPs under low magnetic fields, scanning SQUID biosusceptometry (SSB) examinations of dynamic MNP distributions in the liver, heart, and tumors of animals for pharmacokinetics [17], metabolism [18], and tumor targeting [19] have yielded satisfactory agreement with other biological examinations. The earliest SSB technologies enabled magnetic functional measurement, but an optical video camera was not incorporated. SSB is advantageous because it does not require a shielded environment, animal torsos can be scanned easily because the device can be handled similarly to an ultrasound probe, and liquid nitrogen involves low maintenance costs. Moreover, the AC susceptibility of the MNPs employed in this study has certain advantages. The AC excitation field contributed the centrifugal force to bioprobe-coating MNPs; nontargeted molecules were then removed. Based on this unique characteristic, immunomagnetoreduction (IMR) assays required no complex and washing steps in in vitro blood tests, unlike the enzyme-linked immunosorbent assay currently used in clinics [20,21]. Similarly, the utility of the centrifugal force in in vivo tests, such as in this study, could improve the targeting specificity of bioprobe-coating MNPs for the correctness of tumor label. Furthermore, AC-susceptibility technology can be operated in an unshielded environment by using a general lock-in amplifier, which is superior in comparison with remanent- or relaxation-based technologies that require an expensive shielded environment.

This study proposed a novel SSB method that integrates an optical video camera into the vertical pickup coils, which is in contrast to the planar pickup coils of early SSB technologies. In addition, the integrated and compact probe can scan arbitrarily along an animal torso in an unshielded environment as an ultrasound probe. Novel SSB methods can be used to immediately fuse magnetic and optical images. Thus, SSB is a powerful tool for preoperative diagnosis and the intraoperative positioning of tumors. Although the spatial resolutions of 2-dimensional SSB fusion images are less accurate than those of three-dimensional MRI images for preoperative diagnosis, using 2-dimensional SSB fusion images is adequate for tumor positioning and safer than using gamma cameras or fluorescence imaging for intraoperative positioning. To verify the feasibility of using the proposed SSB technique for surgical navigation, simple anti-alpha-fetoprotein (AFP)-mediated MNPs were employed to conduct both phantom and animal tests, in which AFP was used as a biomarker in rats with tumors of the liver.

## Results and discussion

### Phantom test

The dual-imaging model SSB shown in Figure 1 was used to capture optical and magnetic images of microtest tubes filled with the anti-AFP reagents. The injection dose for animals in this study was 0.9 g with anti-AFP reagents at a concentration of 0.3 emu/g. Figure 2A shows dual-images of the microtest tube filled with 0.3 emu/g and 0.25 g, which is approximately 28% of the injection dose, as well as the overlaid images. In Figure 2A, the optical image shows a top-down view of one of the microtest tubes, as well as magnetic images of the same test tube. In the magnetic images, the upper red spot indicates the raw signal intensity I, whereas the lower magnetic image indicates filtered signals where I is higher than 50% of the peak signal intensity $I_{max}$ in each red spot, not in the entire image. In other words, the upper magnetic spot has more signals with I lower than 50% of $I_{max}$ compared with the lower one.

The magnetic signals were distributed spherically from the sample; therefore, the red spot in the raw magnetic image covers a larger area than that indicated by the optical image. However, the red spot in the filtered magnetic image is similar to the distribution shown in the optical image. The spatial contour error between the red spot in the filtered magnetic image and the brown circle in the optical image is within 3 mm. Hence, the red spot in the filtered magnetic image indicates the MNP distribution shown in the optical image.

Consequently, the sensitivity of this system was studied by using the maximum detectable distance of the same phantom sample. The line graph in Figure 2B shows that the $I_{max}$ of the red spots in the magnetic image decreased as the sample distance between the top surface of the anti-AFP reagents and the bottom surface of the scanning probe unit was increased from 31 to 66 mm. Furthermore, $I_{max}$ decreased as the reagent

concentration was reduced from 0.3 to 0.005 emu/g, with Fe concentration ranging from 1.95 mg/g to 32.5 µg/g. This shows that the detectable distance was approximately 56 mm for the samples with a concentration of 0.1–0.3 emu/g, whereas that for the samples with a concentration of 0.005–0.01 emu/g was approximately 44 mm, which is sufficient for detecting MNPs in tumors implanted in the livers or grafted onto the backs of animals [22,23]. In other words, the sensitivity to the amount of Fe in the MNPs was approximately 250 µg at 56 mm and 12.5 µg at 44 mm. Although these discussed distances between the sample and sensing probe were tens of millimeters in this study, and the measurement was performed in an unshielded environment, the minimal detection of MNPs was tens of pictograms at the short distance of 2 mm; this is similar to the results reported by previous research [12]. Furthermore, the detectable distance can be increased for clinical applications involving humans by simply modifying the equipment, such as by increasing the product of the area and current of the cylindrical excitation coil, rather than by injecting more MNPs, which would increase toxicity. For example, the expected detection distance can be increased to approximately 15 cm, which is approximately the half thickness of a general belly, if this product increases tens of times; this reason is the excitation field increases with this product while the sample distance is much larger than the radius of excitation coil based on Biot-Savart law. In addition, if the imaged tumor is large, the detection limit improves because of increased target MNPs.

Figure 2C shows that the integral of I, which represents the product of the sum of I values greater than 50% of $I_{max}$ and the pixel spacing, decreased with the distance between the sample and the scanning probe, but increased with the sample magnetism, which is the product of the reagent concentration and weight. The minimal value was observed at approximately 0.05 Volt. $mm^2$, which can be considered as the sensitivity of the integral of I. Moreover, evaluating the level of magnetism in the sample (i.e., MNP amount) was feasible by using the integral of I as a reference.

### Animal test of exterior liver tumors

Figure 3 shows the results of locating a tumor in the back of one of the rats. The figure shows that at 0 h, before injection of the MNPs, the integral of I was low, but it was higher than the background level because of the presence of weakly paramagnetic materials in the tissue, such as red blood cells. The tumor region generally expressed high I values because it was close to the scanning probe, causing it to dominate the integral of I at 0 h. At 24 h, most of the I of the red spot were high because of the high accumulation of anti-AFP MNPs on the back tumors [19]. Moreover, by 24 h, the anti-AFP

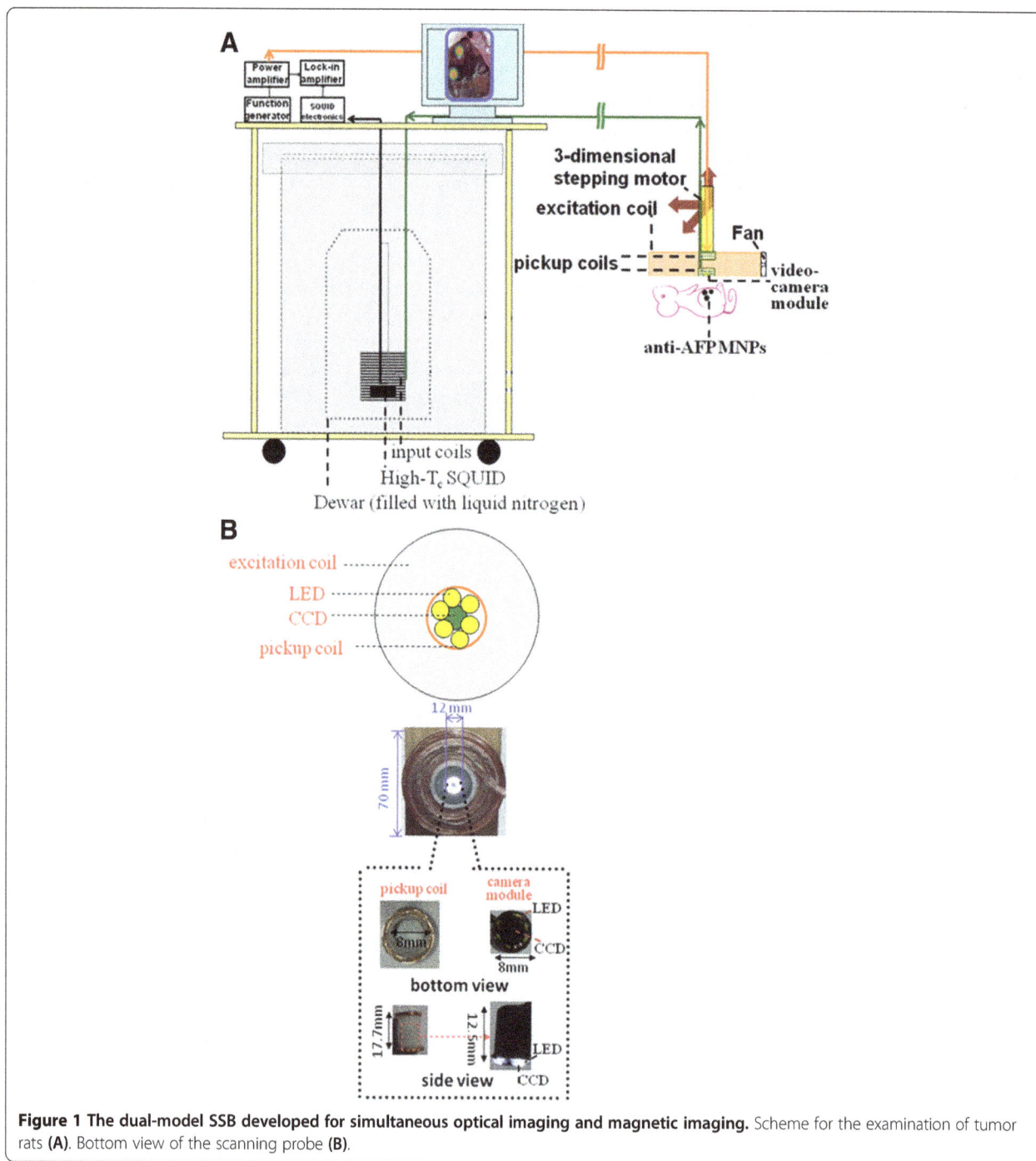

**Figure 1 The dual-model SSB developed for simultaneous optical imaging and magnetic imaging.** Scheme for the examination of tumor rats (**A**). Bottom view of the scanning probe (**B**).

MNPs were biodegraded by organs in the mononuclear phagocyte system, which is also called the reticuloendothelial system or macrophage system, and then excreted through other organs [18]. Therefore, at 24 h, the red spot was distributed in the back tumors only. Furthermore, the I of one tumor rat (Figure 3A) and the sum of the I of 2 tumor rats (Figure 3B) were apparently larger at 24 h than at 0 h (ie, before injection). However, the repeatability errors at 24 h and at 0 h were relatively small.

In the optical and fused images in Figure 3A, the blue dotted line and the red spot represents the contour of the implanted tumors and the distribution of anti-AFP MNPs, respectively. The blue dotted line and red spot exhibit adequate consistency, with a spatial error of 5 mm at both 0 h and 24 h. Thus, the SSB can be employed to locate MNP-targeted tumors. Furthermore, these results verify that the integral of I is a suitable indicator for detecting anti-AFP MNPs in tumors when

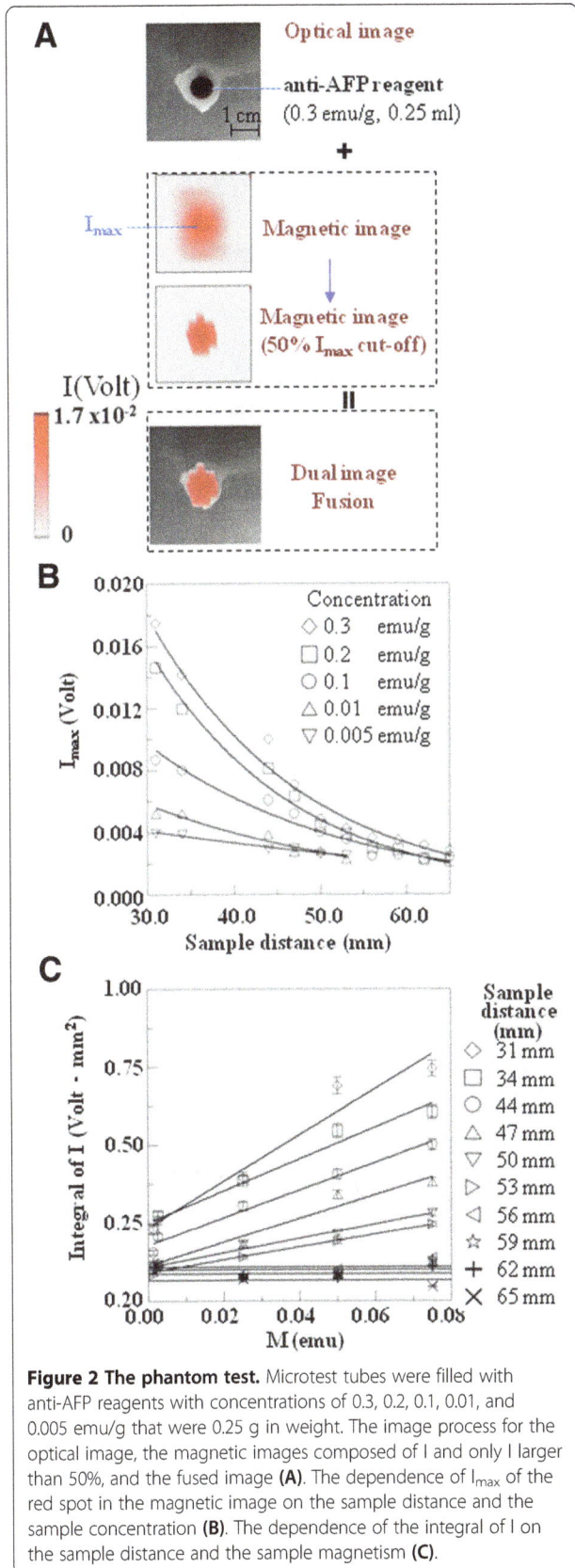

**Figure 2 The phantom test.** Microtest tubes were filled with anti-AFP reagents with concentrations of 0.3, 0.2, 0.1, 0.01, and 0.005 emu/g that were 0.25 g in weight. The image process for the optical image, the magnetic images composed of I and only I larger than 50%, and the fused image **(A)**. The dependence of $I_{max}$ of the red spot in the magnetic image on the sample distance and the sample concentration **(B)**. The dependence of the integral of I on the sample distance and the sample magnetism **(C)**.

the dual-imaging model SSB is used for in vivo imaging. Hence, the fused images revealed the spatial and functional results of the MNP-targeted tumors, and this targeting phenomenon is in agreement with a similar study that used an identical dose of the same anti-AFP reagent [23].

**Animal test of interior liver tumors**

The results of the animal tests for the surgical navigation of the liver tumors within the liver lobes are depicted in Figure 4. In the fused images of Rat B1's unexposed abdomen (Figure 4A), few red spots were observed at 0 h; however, the red spots were clearly observable in the liver region at 24 h. Consequently, exposing the abdomen for in vivo imaging at 24.5 h revealed nearly identical red spots, indicating that the skin did not interfere with the magnetic measurement.

Furthermore, after immersing the livers in formalin for 1 week (wk), the red spot on the preseparation liver lobes in the ex vivo image at 24.5 h was similar to that of the livers in the in vivo image of the exposed livers at 24.5 h, except in the lower left region (Figure 4A). This difference was probably because the short sample distance yielded a strong I in the in vivo test, whereas the lower-left part of the stacked livers was highly sustained by the other organs in the body. Conversely, the long distance yielded a weak I in the ex vivo test, and the lower-left part of the stacked livers was fixed without support from other organs. Similarly, the I of the ex vivo test was weaker because of the long sample distances for some regions of the stacked livers without the support of other organs. In other words, the distance between the scanning probe unit and each liver lobe was shorter in the in vivo test than in the ex vivo test. The result of the in vivo test was because of the support of other organs; the result of the ex vivo test was because of the formalin fixation without support from other organs.

In addition to the whole liver in the original preseparation (Figure 4A), Rat B1's discrete liver lobes were imaged (Figure 4B). The fused images of each liver lobe show dark spots in Lobes 1–4, and the red spot with the lowest intensity covered most of Lobe 5. Moreover, by using the same color scale, Figure 4B shows that the red on each separated liver lobe was more intense than that of all of the stacked liver lobes in Figure 4A. This occurred because each separated liver lobe on the same plane was at an identical distance from the scanning probe, whereas all of the liver lobes that were stacked together were at various distances from the probe. The lower lobes were the furthest from the scanning probe.

Moreover, a piece of the red spot region of the ex vivo images (Figure 4B) was stained using a hematoxylin and eosin (HE) stain and AFP stain. The morphology results of the HE staining revealed that most of the tissues in Lobes 1–4 exhibited abundant pink cytoplasms, whereas

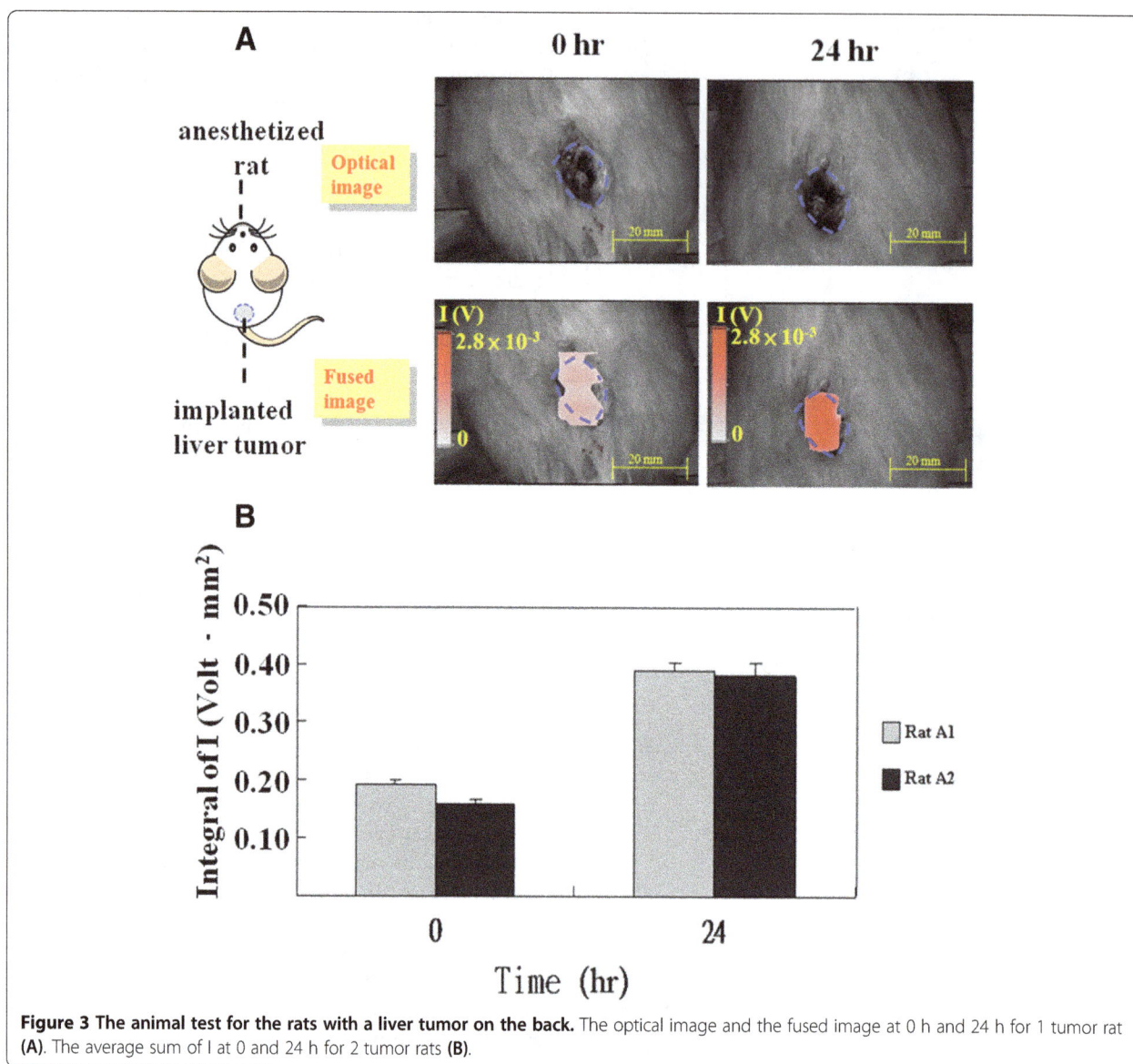

**Figure 3 The animal test for the rats with a liver tumor on the back.** The optical image and the fused image at 0 h and 24 h for 1 tumor rat (**A**). The average sum of I at 0 and 24 h for 2 tumor rats (**B**).

the entire region of Lobe 5 and a small portion of Lobes 3 and 4 exhibited purple because of normal amounts of cytoplasm. The 2 regions with light pink and dark purple in the HE stain corresponded to those with the dark brown and light brown in the AFP staining, respectively. Hence, these 2 regions were identified as tumor and normal tissues, respectively. Although small portions of normal tissue were present, the tissues were positive for tumors because of the presence of large tumor tissues. In other words, Lobes 1–4 were positive, but Lobe 5 was negative. Moreover, because the no-spot region of Lobes 1–4 in the ex vivo images yielded similar staining results to that of Lobe 5, this region was also negative. In summary, both the red-spot and no-spot regions in the ex vivo fused images of each lobe according to the dual-imaging model SSB correspond reasonably to the tissue

staining results. The intensity of the red spot in the ex vivo images depended on the darkness of the AFP stain in the tumor tissue recognized by the HE stain.

Analytically, for each liver lobe of the 3 rats (Rats B1–3), its integral of I can be divided into levels higher and lower than 0.10 Volt.mm$^2$ (Figure 4C). Similarly, its expression of the 2 tissue stains can determine positive and negative results. For example, for Rat B1 as shown in Figure 4B, positive results were confirmed by the expression of abundant pink cytoplasms in the HE stain and at least one brown region in the AFP stain in Lobes 1–4. The solid and dot pattern of the bar in Figure 4C represent the positive and negative results based on the 2 tissue stains. By comparing the integral of I and the judgment of positivity or negativity, a criterion was determined that the positive or negative judgment

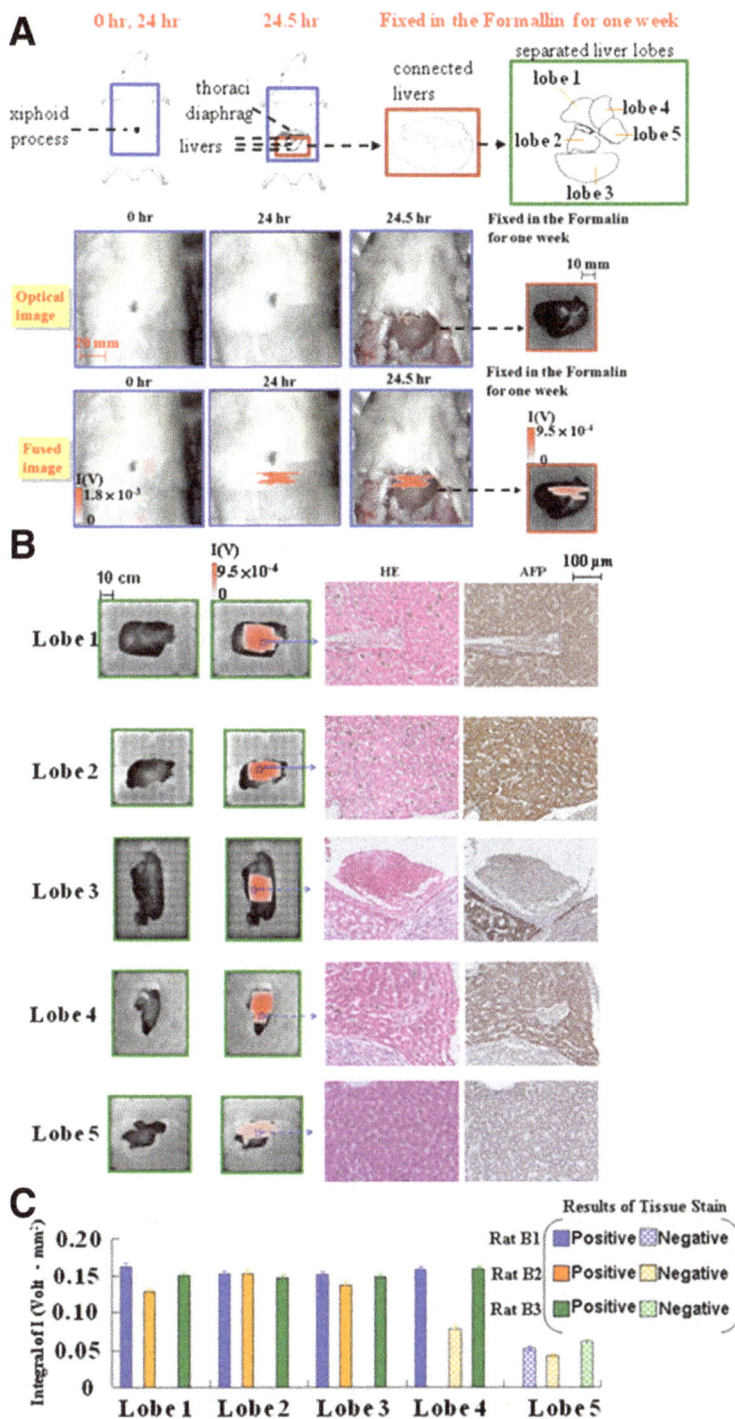

**Figure 4 The animal test for 3 rats with a liver tumor in the liver. Rat B1** was imaged in a supine position at 0 h and 24 h, and with its belly opened at 24.5 h. Its liver was immersed in diluted formalin with 10% concentration for 1 wk. Both the stacked block and separated lobe livers were magnetically examined ex vivo **(A)**. After identifying the red-spot and no-spot regions in the separated lobe livers by using the dual-model SSB for **Rat B1**, one small piece of liver tissue in the red-spot region was confirmed by HE and AFP staining **(B)**. The comparison between the integral of I according to the dual-model SSB and the positive and negative judgment according to the tissue staining for separated liver lobes (Lobes 1–5) of 3 tumor rats **(Rats B1–3) (C)**.

corresponds to the integral of I higher or lower than 0.10 Volt.mm$^2$, respectively.

## Conclusion

This study developed a novel dual-imaging model SSB by integrating an optical camera and magnetic SSB to fuse low-field magnetic images of MNP distributions and optical images for simultaneous functional and structural imaging. The feasibility of this novel dual-imaging model SSB was verified by the favorable spatial agreement in phantom and animal tests, as well as confirmation from tissue staining. Hence, the application of imaging technologies of simple $Fe_3O_4$ MNPs were expanded from preoperative diagnosis by MRI to intraoperative positioning of tumors and preoperative imaging in clinics by using this novel dual-imaging model SSB, demonstrating the high potential of this method in the surgical navigation of MNP-targeted tumors in future clinical applications.

## Methods

### Synthesis and characteristics of anti-AFP reagent

The anti-AFP reagent used in this study was anti-AFP-meditated MNPs in a phosphate buffered saline solution. The magnetic core, surfactant, and bioprobe coating of anti-AFP-meditated MNPs were $Fe_3O_4$, dextran, and AFP antibody (EA502-Q1053, EastCoast Bio, USA), respectively. The basic materials of $Fe_3O_4$ MNPs solved in a water solution were obtained from MagQu Co., Taiwan, and the details of the synthesis process were described in a previous study [24].

The average hydrodynamic diameter of the anti-AFP reagent was 57.3 ± 15.2 nm, as measured using a nanoparticle size analyzer (Microtrac, Montgomeryville, PA, USA) [19]. The superparamagnetic property was observed in a magnetism-field curve obtained using a vibrating sample magnetometer (EG&G PARC, Newnan, GA).

### Development of a dual-imaging model of SSB

A dual-imaging model of SSB (Figure 1) composed of a scanning probe and a SQUID sensor unit was developed for optical and magnetic imaging, respectively. The proposed model differs from traditional SSB systems that measure magnetic signals alone. The unique design features of this scanning probe unit include a dual-imaging model mechanism, charge-coupled-device (CCD) module (Singapsy Enterprise Corp., Taiwan), and first-order vertical pickup coils surrounding the CCD module. The dual-imaging model mechanisms were inserted into the center of the circular excitation coil to construct the scanning probe unit. To measure the actual AC susceptibility of the MNPs, the excitation field strength and frequency of the excitation coil were set at 120 Oe and 400 Hz, respectively. The reasons for selecting this frequency included the low power loading at low frequencies for the same excitation coil, the interval between 360 and 420 Hz of low background noises [25], and the superior characteristics of AC-susceptibility technology. The field strength was selected to achieve sufficient sensitivity for few MNPs targeted in rats; this is discussed in the section describing the phantom test. Moreover, because the product of these 2 excitation parameters was substantially smaller than that required for animal biosafety [26], the excitation exhibited low risk.

The CCD module with a focus of 1 cm was not influenced by the magnetic fields, and it yielded an optical video with a resolution of 0.2 in per pixel and a wide angle of 40°. In general, the recorded video of each scanning line was automatically converted to a panoramic photograph. Subsequently, only the approximately central 2/3 region of the panoramic photograph was retained as a single line image, which was then combined with the other line images to construct a 2-dimensional optical image. Moreover, light-emitting diodes were arranged surrounding the CCD to provide adequate lighting during the scanning processes, which involved close distances between the scanning probe and sample. In addition, the 7-cm-diameter scanning probe unit can be operated similarly to an ultrasound probe with the assistance of a 3-dimensional step motor similar to that used in robotic scanners.

The dual-imaging model signals were acquired as follows. The optical video from the CCD module was recorded using a personal computer, although the magnetic signal was too low to be directly sensed by any current or voltage meter. The SQUID sensor unit was composed of a high critical-temperature $T_c$ SQUID magnetometer (JSQ GmbH, Germany) in a dewar with a liquid nitrogen refrigerant and a set of shielding cans. Based on a typical conducting transfer coil [27] (as depicted in Figure 1), the weak magnetic flux was transferred from the pickup coils near the sample in an unshielded environment to the input coil surrounding the SQUID sensor, where it was amplified approximately 29-fold. The sensitivity of the entire dual-imaging model SSB was approximately 3 pT/√Hz. The white noise of the system is limited by the thermal noise of the normal-conducting flux transformer [27]. The environmental noise originated primarily from the concentric excitation coil and slightly from the CCD and cooling fan attached to the scanning probe unit.

The specificity of this dual-imaging model SSB in the measurement of anti-AFP reagents was characterized by conducting phantom and animal tests (Table 1).

### Phantom test

In the phantom test, microtest tubes (Eppendorf Corp., NY, USA) were filled with anti-AFP reagents at

**Table 1 Phantom and animal tests in this study**

| Test type | Test context |
|---|---|
| Phantom test | • **Anti-AFP reagent:**<br>0.25 g in volume and 0.3, 0.2, 0.1, 0.01, 0.005 emu/g in concentration.<br><br>• **Phantoms:**<br>Micro test tubes were filled with anti-AFP reagent.<br><br>• **Imaging:**<br>The fused images composed of the magnetic image for the spatial distribution of anti-AFP MNPs and the optic image of micro test tubes. |
| Animal tests | • **Dose of Anti-AFP reagent:**<br>0.9 g in volume and 0.3 emu/g in concentration.<br><br>• **Tumor rats:**<br>Liver tumors were implanted on backs for 2 rats and in livers for 3 rats, separately.<br><br>Anti-AFP reagents were intravenously injected through tail veins.<br><br>• **Imaging:**<br>The 2 tumor rats with back tumors were imaged in a prone position by using the dual-model SSB at 0 h.<br><br>The 3 tumor rats implanted with liver tumors were imaged in a supine position at 0 h, 24 h, and with their bellies opened at 24.5 h.<br><br>Both the stacked block and separated lobe livers of the 3 tumor rats implanted with liver tumors were magnetically examined ex vivo.<br><br>• **Tissue stain:**<br>After identifying the red-spot and no-spot regions in separated lobe livers by this dual-model SSB, small pieces of liver tissue in both regions for HE stain and AFP stain were performed. |

concentrations of 0.3, 0.2, 0.1, 0.01, and 0.005 emu/g. The samples weighed 0.25 g. Microtest tubes with a diameter of less than 8 mm were selected to imitate the size of early-stage tumors, and various concentrations of AFP reagent were used to simulate the dynamics of anti-AFP-meditated MNP-targeted tumors. In this test, the anti-AFP reagents of 0.01 and 0.005 emu/g were lower than the maximal MNP concentrations of approximately 0.045 emu/g in the livers of rats, as reported in the in vitro results of previous studies [22,23].

The anti-AFP reagents were scanned at a distance of 2–36 mm between the scanning probe and the top of the microtest tubes; this was approximately 31–65 mm between the scanning probe and the surface of anti-AFP reagents because the distance between the reagent surface and the top of the microtest tube was 29 mm. To calibrate the distance, 2 pieces of aluminum tape were attached to the upper surface of the samples and to the bottom surface of the scanning probe. Linking a copper wire from each aluminum tape to a resistance meter enabled the zero distance to be determined on the basis of the sound produced by the meter when the surface of aluminum tape contacted the wire. The relative position was controlled using the precision controller of a z-axis step motor. Each scanning path was commenced and terminated in free space, at least 1 cm from the animal body. The signal baseline of each line was determined according to the signal level in free space. Furthermore, the constant scanning speed and step size were 5 mm/s (for each line) and 5 mm, respectively. The pixel size of each line in the magnetic image was 5 mm, which was

determined on the basis of the scanning path over the sampling points, and the line interval was 5 mm (Figure 2A). In other words, each pixel in the magnetic image was constructed according to the signal of a scanning step. The preliminary test showed that the measurement results of this scanning process were identical to those obtained using a static process. The remanence of the MNPs were omitted from the AC-susceptibility measurement.

**Animal test**

Tumor masses of the GP7TB rat hepatoma cell line were implanted into 5 male F344/NNarl rats (age = 5 wk), which were divided into 2 groups. In one group, tumors were grafted onto the backs of 2 rats to enable easy identification of the tumors by using optical imaging; in the other group, the tumors were implanted in the livers of 3 rats to simulate real disease conditions. The tumors were confirmed using tissue stains. After 3 wk of incubation, anti-AFP reagents (dose = 0.9 g, concentration = 0.3 emu/g) were injected into the tail vein of these tumor rats. After administering a mixture of oxygen gas and isoflurane to anesthetize the rats, the tumor rats were imaged using the proposed dual-imaging model SSB. The imaging conditions were identical to those used in the phantom test. All experiments were conducted according to the animal care guidelines of National Taiwan University.

To verify the feasibility of tumor positioning by using the dual-model SSB, the tumor rats with back tumors were imaged in a prone position immediately before being injected with anti-AFP reagents (0 h), and again at 24 h after the injection (the tumor rat as shown in Figure 3). Each scanning time was approximately 2.5 minutes.

Similarly, to investigate the navigation of the interior liver tumors within the liver lobes, the 3 tumor rats with the implanted liver tumors were imaged in a supine position at 0 h, 24 h, and with their abdomens exposed at 24.5 h (Rat B1 as shown in Figure 4A). Each scanning time was approximately 8 minutes. The tumor rats were sacrificed and their livers were immersed in diluted formalin (concentration = 10%) for 1 wk. Both the stacked block and separated liver lobes were magnetically examined ex vivo (Rat B1 as shown in Figure 4B). Each scanning time was approximately 2 minutes. Opposite to the stacked livers, each liver lobe was observed at the same sample distance. After identifying the red-spot and no-spot regions in the separated liver lobes, small pieces of liver tissue in both regions were subjected to HE and AFP staining in the National Laboratory Animal Center, College of Medicine, at National Taiwan University.

## Abbreviations
MNPs: Magnetic nanoparticles; AFP: Antialpha-fetoprotein; SQUID: Superconducting-quantum-interference device; SSB: Scanning superconducting-quantum-interference-device biosusceptometry; CT: Computed tomography; MRI: Magnetic resonance imaging; PET: Positron emission tomography; AC: Alternate-current; CCD: Charge-coupled-device; LED: Light-emitting diode; $T_c$: Critical-temperature; ACUC: Animal Care and Use Committee; HE: Hematoxylin-and-Eosin.

## Competing interests
The authors declare that they have no competing interests.

## Authors' contributions
JJC designed and conducted this experiment and also wrote this manuscript; KWH carefully observed all stages in both the experimental and manuscript writing; YYL and WCW made the experiment in measurement and data process. All authors read and approved the final manuscript.

## Acknowledgments
This study was supported by the National Science Council of Taiwan (NSC101-2221-E-003-005, NSC 102-2221-E-003-008-MY2), the Ministry of Health and Welfare (MOHW103-TDU-N-211-133002), the Aim for the Top University Plan of National Taiwan Normal University, and the Ministry of Education, Taiwan, R.O.C. (103J1A27).

## Author details
[1]Institute of Electro-Optical Science and Technology, National Taiwan Normal University, Taipei 116, Taiwan. [2]Department of Surgery and Hepatitis Research Center, National Taiwan University Hospital, Taipei 100, Taiwan. [3]Graduate Institute of Clinical Medicine, National Taiwan University, Taipei 100, Taiwan.

## References
1. Ibraheem AA, Buck AK, Benz MR, Rudert M, Beer AJ, Mansour A, et al. 18F-Fluorodeoxyglucose positron emission tomography/computed tomography for the detection of recurrent bone and soft tissue sarcoma. Cancer. 2013;119:1227–34.
2. Yi CA, Lee KS, Lee HY, Kim S, Kwon OJ, Kim H, et al. Coregistered whole body magnetic resonance imaging-positron emission tomography (MRI-PET) versus PET-computed tomography plus brain MRI in staging resectable lung cancer. Cancer. 2013;119:1784–91.
3. Markides H, Rotherham M, Haj AJE. Biocompatibility and toxicity of magnetic nanoparticles in regenerative medicine. J Nanomater. 2012;2012:614094.
4. Maringhini A, Cottone M, Sciarrino E, Marceno MP, Seta F, Rinaldi F, et al. Ultrasonographic and radionuclide detection of hepatocellular carcinoma in cirrhotics with low alpha-fetoprotein levels. Cancer. 1984;54:2924–6.
5. Ni X, Yang J, Li M. Imaging-guided curative surgical resection of pancreatic cancer in a xenograft mouse model. Cancer Lett. 2012;324:179–85.
6. Buckle T, Chin PT, Leeuwen FW. (Non-targeted) radioactive/fluorescent nanoparticles and their potential in combined pre-and intraoperative imaging during sentinel lymph node resection. Nanotechnology. 2010;21:482001.
7. Jarzyna PA, Gianella A, Skajaa T, Knudsen G, Deddens LH, Cormode DP, et al. Multifunctional imaging nanoprobes. Wiley Interdisciplinary Rev Nanomed Nanobiotechnol. 2010;2:138–50.
8. Riegler J, Liewc A, Hynes SO, Ortega D, Brien TO, Day RM, et al. Superparamagnetic iron oxide nanoparticle targeting of MSCs in vascular injury. Biomaterials. 2013;34:1987–94.
9. U. S. Food and Drug Administration: Gadolinium-containing Contrast Agents for Magnetic Resonance Imaging (MRI): Omniscan, OptiMARK, Magnevist, ProHance, and MultiHance. Publ Health Advisory. 2006.
10. Riley K. New warnings required on use of gadolinium-based contrast agents- Enhanced screening recommended to detect kidney dysfunction. FDA News Release. 2010.
11. Song G, Xiangyang S, James RBJ, Mark BH, Bradford GO. Development of a remanence measurement-based SQUID system with in-depth resolution for nanoparticle imaging. Phys Med Biol. 2009;54:N177–88.
12. Tsukamoto A, Saitoh K, Suzuki D, Kandori A, Tsukada K, Sugiura Y, et al. Development of Multisample biological immunoassay system using HTS SQUID and magnetic nanoparticles. IEEE Transactions Appl Superconductivity. 2005;15:656–9.
13. Frank W, Uwe S, Dietmar E, Lutz T. Magnetorelaxometry assisting biomedical applications of magnetic nanoparticles. Pharm Res. 2012;29:1189–202.
14. Adolphi NL, Butler KS, Lovato DM, Tessier TE, Trujillo JE, Hathaway HJ, et al. Imaging of Her2-targeted magnetic nanoparticles for breast cancer detection: comparison of SQUID-detected magnetic relaxometry and MRI. Contrast Media Mol Imaging. 2012;7:308–19.
15. Chemla YR, Grossman HL, Poon Y, McDermott R, Stevens R, Alper MD, et al. Ultrasensitive magnetic biosensor for homogeneous immunoassay. PNAS. 2000;97:14268–72.
16. Weizenecker J, Gleich B, Rahmer J, Dahnke H, Borgert J. Three-dimensional real-time in vivo magnetic particle imaging. Phys Med Biol. 2009;54:L1–L10.
17. Chieh JJ, Tseng WK, Horng HE, Wu CC, Hong CY. In-vivo and real-time measurement of magnetic-nanoparticles distribution in animals by scanning SQUID Biosusceptometry for biomedicine study. IEEE Trans Biomed Eng. 2011;58:2719–24.
18. Tseng WK, Chieh JJ, Yang YF, Chiang CK, Chen YL, Yang SY, et al. A noninvasive method to determine the fate of $Fe_3O_4$ nanoparticles following intravenous injection using scanning SQUID biosusceptometry. PLoS One. 2012;7:e48510.
19. Huang KW, Chieh JJ, Horng HE, Hong CY, Yang HC. Characteristics of magnetic labeling on liver tumors with anti-alpha-fetoprotein-mediated $Fe_3O_4$ magnetic nanoparticles. Int J Nanomedicine. 2012;7:2987–96.
20. Huang KW, Yang SY, Hong YW, Chieh JJ, Yang CC, Horng HE, et al. Feasibility studies for assaying alpha-fetoprotein using antibody- activated magnetic nanoparticles. Int J Nanomedicine. 2012;7(1991):1996.
21. Hong CY, Chen WH, Chien CF, Yang SY, Horng HE, Yang LC, et al. Wash-free immunomagnetic detection for serum through magnetic susceptibility reduction. Appl Phys Lett. 2007;90:74105.
22. Tseng WK, Chieh JJ, Horng HE, Wu CC, Hong CY. In-vivo and fast examination of iron concentration of magnetic nano-particles in an animal torso via scanning SQUID Biosusceptometry. IEEE Trans Appl Supercond. 2011;21:2250.
23. Chieh JJ, Huang KW, Lee YD, Horng HE, Yang HC. In vivo screening of Hepatocellular Carcinoma Using the AC Susceptibility of Antialphafetoprotein-Activated Magnetic Nanoparticles. PLoS One. 2012;7:e46756.
24. Yang JW, Yang HC, Horng HE, Yang SY, Horng HE, Hung JC, Chen YC, et al. Preparation and properties of superparamagnetic nanoparticles with narrow size distribution and biocompatible. J Magn Mater. 2004;283:210–4.
25. Chieh JJ, Horng HE, Tseng WK, Yang SY, Hong CY, Yang HC, et al. Imaging the distribution of magnetic nanoparticles on animal bodies using scanning

SQUID biosusceptometry attached with a video camera. IEEE Trans Appl Supercond. 2013;23:1601503.

26. Atkinson WJ, Brezovich IA, Chakraborty DP. Usable frequencies in hyperthermia with thermal seeds. IEEE Trans Biomed Eng. 1984;BME-31:70–3175.

27. Kondo T, Itozaki H. Normal conducting transfer coil for SQUID NDE. Supercond Sci Technol. 2004;17:459–62.

# 13

# Novel pH-sensitive nanoformulated docetaxel as a potential therapeutic strategy for the treatment of cholangiocarcinoma

Nan Du[1†], Lin-Ping Song[1†], Xiao-Song Li[1], Lei Wang[2*], Ling Wan[1], Hong-Ying Ma[1] and Hui Zhao[1]

## Abstract

**Background:** Cholangiocarcinoma (CC) is one of the fatal malignant neoplasms with poor prognosis. The traditional chemotherapy has been resistant to CC and does not improve the quality of life. The aim of the present study is to investigate the potential of chondroitin sulphate (CS)-histamine (HS) block copolymer micelles to improve the chemotherapeutic efficacy of docetaxel (DTX).

**Results:** pH-responsive property of CS-HS micelles was utilized to achieve maximum therapeutic efficacy in CC. In the present study, docetaxel-loaded CS-HS micelles (CSH-DTX) controlled the release of drug in the basic pH while rapidly released its cargo in the tumor pH (pH 5 and 6.8) possibly due to the breakdown of polymeric micelles. A nanosize of <150 nm will allow its accumulation in the tumor interstitial spaces via EPR effect. CSH-DTX effectively killed the cancer kills in a time- and concentration-dependent manner and showed pronounced therapeutic action than that of free drug at all-time points. CSH-DTX resulted in higher apoptosis of cancer cells with ~30% and ~50 of cells in early apoptosis quadrant when treated with 100 and 1000 ng/ml of equivalent drug. The micellar formulations showed remarkable effect in controlling the tumor growth and reduced the overall tumor volume to 1/5$^{th}$ to that of control and half to that of free drug treated group with no sign of drug-related adverse effects. Immunohistochemical analysis of tumor sections showed that fewer number of Ki-67 cells were present in CSH-DTX treated group comparing to that of free DTX treated group.

**Conclusion:** Our data suggests that nanoformulation of DTX could potentially improve the chemotherapy treatment in cholangiocarcinoma as well as in other malignancies.

**Keywords:** Cholangiocarcinoma, Polymeric micelles, Docetaxel, Apoptosis, Cancer chemotherapy

## Introduction

Cholangiocarcinoma (CC) is one of the fatal malignant neoplasms which arise from epithelium of biliary tract with high rate of mortality and morbidity [1,2]. The CC constitutes the 3% of gastrointestinal cancers with ~15% of overall hepatic cancers [3]. The incidence of CC among Western countries is 1–2 cases per 100000 persons however East Asia has higher incidence of CC with ~8 cases per 1000 individuals [4]. The CC has poor prognosis rate with 5-year survival rate of less than 10% and has a steady increase in the incidence rate. Approximately, 50% of CC cases are diagnosed at unresectable stage, as the symptoms are largely unknown at initial stages [5,6]. At present, surgical resection of CC tumor is the main treatment option for advanced stage tumor. However, surgical biliary bypass often causes serious postoperative complications and increases the morbidity rate. Additionally, palliative therapies such as endoscopic stent, radiation therapy, photodynamic therapy, and chemotherapy are employed to treat the CC [7]. Among all, chemotherapy is regarded as the adjuvant or main alternative treatment to CC, however traditional chemotherapy is reported to be resistant to CC and does not improve the quality of life [8,9]. Therefore, we need an effective therapeutic strategy that can overcome the limitation of conventional

* Correspondence: wanglei5667@gmail.com
†Equal contributors
2Department of Medical, The First Affiliated Hospital of the General Hospital of the PLA, No. 51 Fucheng Road, Haidian District, Beijing 100048, China
Full list of author information is available at the end of the article

treatment modality and improve the chemotherapeutic effect in CC.

Nanotechnology-based drug delivery system has been reported to improve the pharmacological and anticancer property of chemotherapeutic drugs [10]. Specifically, fenestrated endothelium and heavy blood flow will allow the nanoparticles to be taken by the liver. This process can be accelerated by enhanced permeability and retention effect (EPR) that will allow the preferential accumulation or passive targeting of nanocarriers to the leaky vasculature of tumor tissues [11]. Importantly, the delivery carrier can be made responsive to the local microenvironment of tumor. The physiological pH of blood is ~7.2 while the pH of extracellular spaces around tumor is 6.8 and endolysosomes of cancer cells was very acidic (pH < 6) [12].

In this regard, block copolymer-based nanosized micelles have attracted significant attention as a promising delivery system towards cancer therapy [13]. Importantly, pH-responsive anticancer drug delivery has many benefits including high accumulation in tumor tissues, long blood circulation, limited release in physiological conditions, and utilizing EPR effect [14]. In the present study, we have conjugated chondroitin sulphate (CS) with histamine (HS) to form pH-responsive nanomicelles that can enhance the cancer cell killing effect. CS is a hydrophilic compound with excellent biocompatibility and biodegradability that made it an excellent choice for in vivo applications. CS is a vital structural component of cartilage and connective tissues. CS has been reported to target cancer cells by binding to the hyaluronic acid receptors expressed on the malignant cells and internalized actively. HS on the other hand was selected due to its imidazole ring characteristics [15]. The imidazole ring has a lone pair of electron on nitrogen that gives it amphoteric nature to protonate and deprotonate [16].

Docetaxel (DTX), is regarded as one of most effective chemotherapeutic agent for the cancer treatment. DTX is a typical microtubule inhibitor that binds with the microtubule assembly of cancer cells and prohibits its cell proliferation [17]. DTX is effective against wide range of cancers including ovarian, breast, head/neck, lung cancers, and liver cancers. Despite its promising clinical potential, severe side effects such as bone marrow suppression, hypersensitivity reactions, and peripheral neuropathy became a major obstacle. Additionally, poor water solubility and poor bioavailability limited its clinical application to a great extent [18].

Therefore, main aim of the present study was to load DTX in CS-HS-based nanomicelles and to utilize the pH-responsive property to achieve maximum therapeutic efficacy in Cholangiocarcinoma. The physicochemical characteristics of DTX-loaded CS-HS micelles (CSH-DTX) were studied in terms of size and release

kinetics. In vitro cytotoxicity assay and apoptosis assay of free drug and CSH-DTX was studied in QBC939 adenocarcinoma cells. Antitumor efficacy of CSH-DTX was studied in xenograft nude mice and immunohistochemical studies were performed to evaluate its systemic performance.

## Results and discussion

Cholangiocarcinoma (CC) which arises from epithelium of bialy tract is one of the fatal malignant neoplasms with high rate of mortality and morbidity. At present, conventional chemotherapy is the main treatment option; however it does not improve the quality of patient life [2,4]. In this regard, nanotechnological solutions have been reported to improve the therapeutic performance of anticancer drugs. Importantly, a pH-responsive strategy would increase the accumulation in tumor tissues, extend blood circulation, and effectively improve the overall chemotherapeutic efficacy. In the present study therefore, we have conjugated chondroitin sulphate (CS) with histamine (HS) to form pH-responsive nanomicelles that can enhance the cancer cell killing effect. DTX, a typical microtubule inhibitor has been selected in this study as an anticancer drug to improve its therapeutic efficacy against CC [18]. Since the therapeutic application of DTX is hindered by its limited solubility and systemic toxicity, in the present study, DTX was loaded into CS-HS conjugate based polymeric micelles. DTX and CS-HS block copolymer when dissolved in water, hydrophobic and hydrophilic part self-assemble to form a drug loaded micelles (Figure 1). The so formed micelle (CSH-DTX) has numerous advantages including pH-sensitive drug via protonation of histidine residue, high loading efficiency, and potential clinical translational ability.

### Preparation and characterization of DTX-loaded micelles

Physicochemical characterization of polymeric micelles was carried out in terms of particle size and polydispersity index. The particle size and PDI of CSH-DTX was measured by dynamic light scattering technique. The average size of CSH-DTX was observed to be around 110 nm with a fairly uniform dispersion of NP (PDI ~ 0.15) (Figure 2a). It has been previously reported that micelles size less than <200 nm could be preferentially accumulated in the tumor interstitial spaces via enhanced permeability and retention (EPR) effect [19].

The morphology of CSH-DTX was investigated using TEM and SEM. The TEM showed a spherical particle with uniform distribution in the copper grid (Figure 2b). The size measured by TEM was smaller than observed via DLS experiment. The discrepancy in size might be attributed to the hydrodynamic state and dried state measurement. The morphology was further confirmed

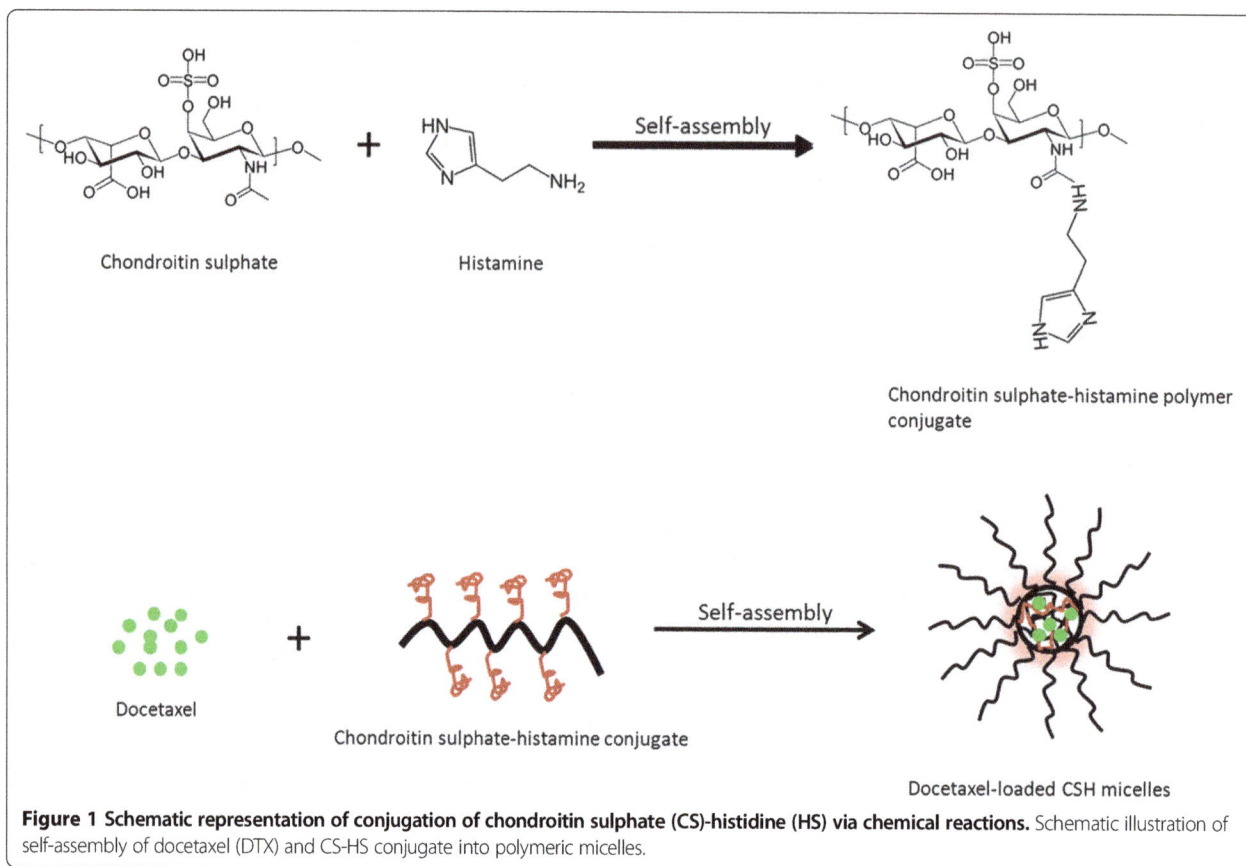

**Figure 1 Schematic representation of conjugation of chondroitin sulphate (CS)-histidine (HS) via chemical reactions.** Schematic illustration of self-assembly of docetaxel (DTX) and CS-HS conjugate into polymeric micelles.

by SEM which showed a smooth regular surface, spherical shaped particles (Figure 2c). The size was consistent with the TEM observation. The drug loading capacity of DTX was observed to be more than 20% with a high entrapment of >95%.

### In vitro drug release

The release study was carried out in phosphate buffered saline (PBS, pH 7.4) and acetate buffered saline (ABS, pH 6.8 and pH 5.0). As shown in Figure 3, release rate of DTX from CSH-DTX micelles markedly differed with the change in pH conditions. As expected, accelerated

release of DTX was observed at lower pH, while slow release profile was seen at basic pH conditions. At pH 7.4, nearly 30% of drug released while 70% of drug released when the pH of release media was decreased to pH 6.8. Importantly, release rate was further increased when micelles were incubated in pH 5.0 containing media. Nearly 95% of drug released in pH 5.0 at the end of 72 h of study period. In all the pH conditions, although slightly faster release was observed during the initial time points however no burst release pattern was observed. The micelles exhibited a sustained release profile for DTX. It could be expected that at physiological pH conditions,

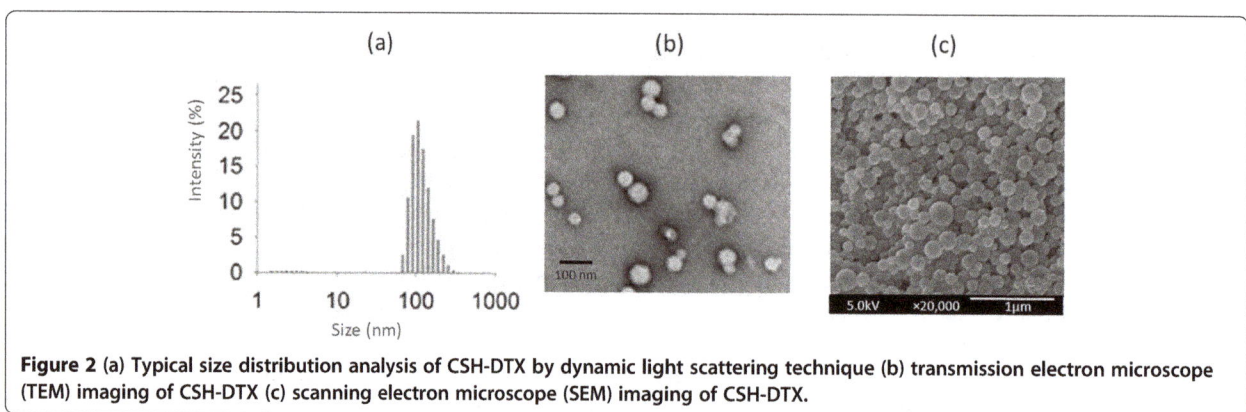

**Figure 2 (a) Typical size distribution analysis of CSH-DTX by dynamic light scattering technique (b) transmission electron microscope (TEM) imaging of CSH-DTX (c) scanning electron microscope (SEM) imaging of CSH-DTX.**

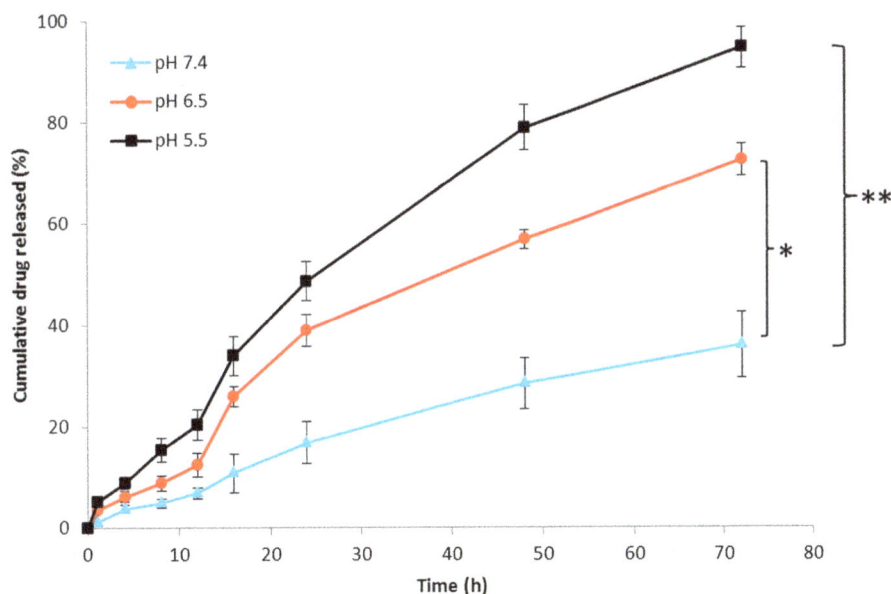

**Figure 3 Release profile of DTX from CSH-DTX micelles incubated at phosphate buffered saline (pH 7.4) and acetate buffered saline (pH 6.8 and 5.0).** The samples were incubated at 37°C in a rotary shaker (100 rpm). The data are presented as mean ± SD (n = 3). *p < 0.05, *p < 0.01 is the statistical difference between drug release at pH 5.0, pH 6.5, and pH 7.4.

core will be intact and DTX would be blocked in the highly hydrophobic core leading to low release rate. However when the pH decreased, accelerated release was observed due to the protonation of histidine residue. At lower pH, when the histidine was protonated, imbalance of hydrophilic and hydrophobic force destabilizes the micelles structure and the drug diffuses in higher rate [16]. Therefore, CSH micelles could effectively prevent the drug release or drug leakage in physiological (avoids toxicity) conditions while releases rapidly in acidic conditions in response to endosomal and lysosomal pH.

### In vitro cytotoxicity assay

The in vitro cytotoxicity of blank copolymer was studied in different concentrations against QBC939 CC cells to evaluate its safety profile. The cells were treated with concentrations between 0.1 µg/ml to 500 µg/ml. As seen (Figure 4a), blank polymeric micelles did not exhibit any significant toxicity in the tested concentration range after 24 h incubation. Especially, cell viabilities remained more than >94% at all the concentrations indicating its excellent safety profile. The least or negligible cytotoxicity of blank polymer makes it ideal for in vivo cancer targeting. Followed by which cytotoxicity of free DTX and CSH-DTX was evaluated in the same cell lines in a concentration and time dependent manner. As shown in Figure 4b-d, both free drug as well as drug loaded micellar formulations exhibited a greater cytotoxicity in a time- and concentration dependent manner. It has to be

noted that cytotoxicity of CSH-DTX was more pronounced than that of free drug in all the time points. IC50 value of individual formulation was calculated to quantify the cytotoxic effect. The IC50 value of free DTX remained at 6.45 µg/ml, 2.86 µg/ml, and 0.89 µg/ml after 24, 48, and 72 h incubation, respectively. On the other hand, IC50 value of CSH-DTX stood at 2.58 µg/ml, 0.98 µg/ml, and 0.49 µg/ml for the same time period, respectively. The superior cytotoxicity of CSH-DTX might be attributed to the pH-driven release of active therapeutic molecule in the cell cytoplasm. It could be expected that micelles were internalized into the cells via endocytosis mechanism where in the drug released at acidic compartments and travel to site of action [20]. The cytotoxicity was further confirmed by cellular morphology. As seen Figure 5a, control cells were densely packed on the cover slip and of regular shape, however, DTX treated cells showed signs of apoptosis and cells were round and circular. Importantly, CSH-DTX treated cells were fewer in number (viable cells were decreased) and scattered with a clear sign of membrane blebbing and apoptosis.

### Apoptosis measurements

Changes in cell morphology resulting in the rounding of cells are one of the prominent hallmarks of apoptosis. The apoptosis measurement was carried out by Hoechst 33258 staining. As shown in Figure 5b, untreated cells did not show any changes in morphology and remained same after 24 h. Additionally, cells were densely packed

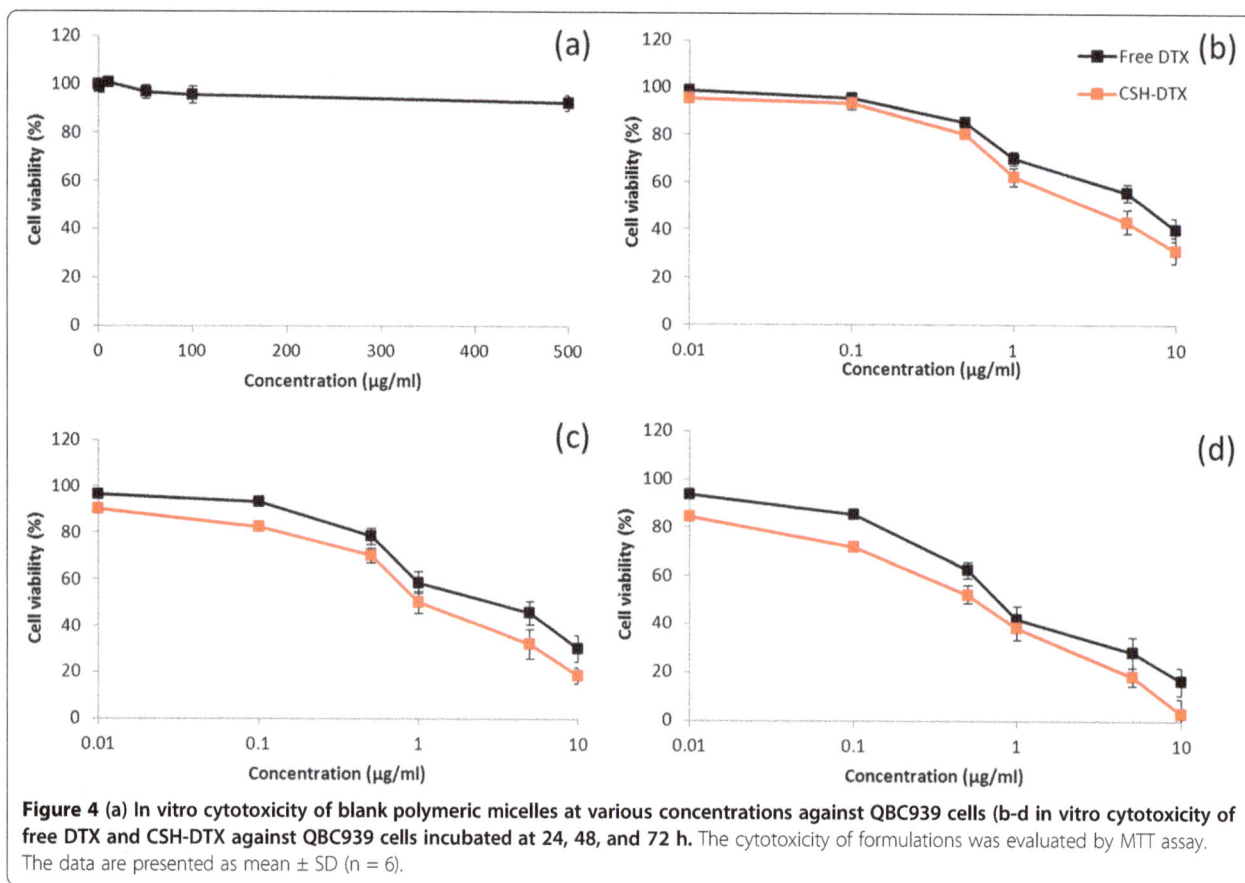

**Figure 4 (a) In vitro cytotoxicity of blank polymeric micelles at various concentrations against QBC939 cells (b-d in vitro cytotoxicity of free DTX and CSH-DTX against QBC939 cells incubated at 24, 48, and 72 h.** The cytotoxicity of formulations was evaluated by MTT assay. The data are presented as mean ± SD (n = 6).

and present large numbers covering the entire cover slip. The free DTX however reduced the number of viable cells and exhibited typical features of apoptosis. Notably, CSH-DTX remarkably induced the apoptosis in cancer cells with typical features of cell death such as chromatic condensation, membrane blebbing and apoptotic bodies were visible. Results indicate that the drug loaded micelles could cause marked condensation and fragmentation of nuclear bodies.

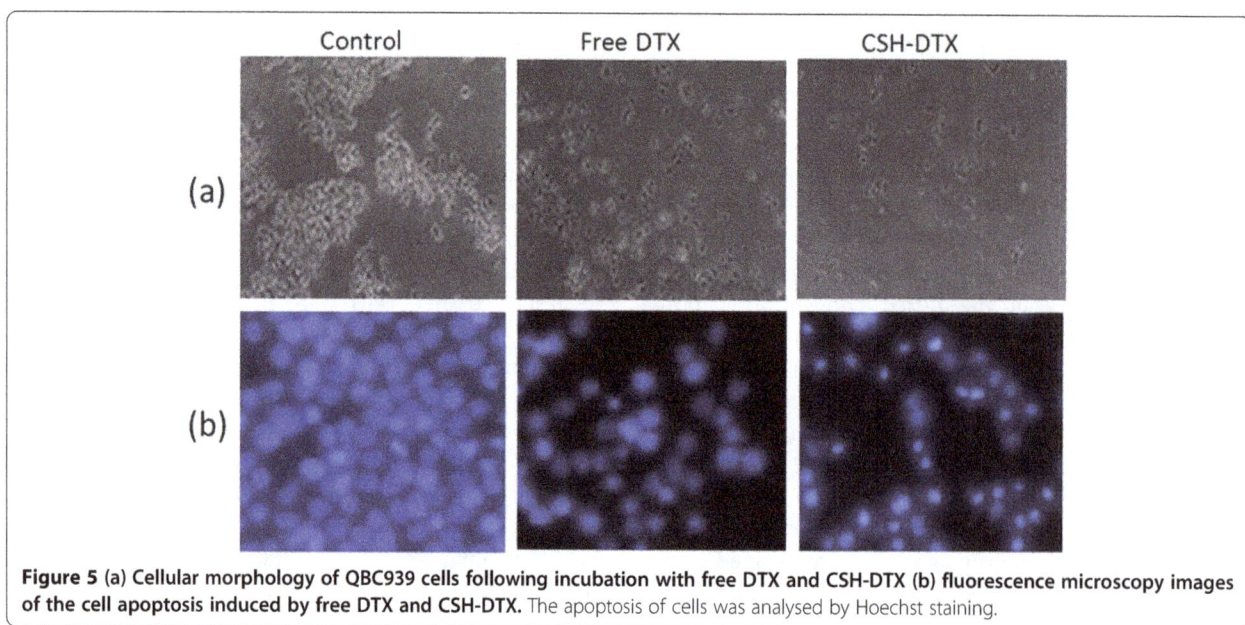

**Figure 5 (a) Cellular morphology of QBC939 cells following incubation with free DTX and CSH-DTX (b) fluorescence microscopy images of the cell apoptosis induced by free DTX and CSH-DTX.** The apoptosis of cells was analysed by Hoechst staining.

## Apoptosis assay by flow cytometry

Figure 6 shows the apoptosis analysis (early and late apoptosis) of QBC939 cells using Annexin V FITC and PI staining by flow cytometer. In the present study, cells were treated with 100 ng/ml and 1000 ng/ml of free DTX and equivalent CSH-DTX formulations and incubated for 24 h. Results indicate that the proportion of early and late apoptosis cells markedly increased with the increase in the concentration of chemotherapeutic drugs. For example, ~10% of cells were in early apoptosis quadrant when exposed with 100 ng/ml of free DTX, while it increased to ~32% for exposure to 1000 ng/ml of drug. As expected, CSH-DTX resulted in higher apoptosis of cancer cells with ~30% and ~50 of cells in early apoptosis quadrant for the same concentrations, respectively. Similarly, late apoptosis cells increased as well in a concentration-dependent manner. The result was consistent with the cytotoxicity that micellar formulation could remarkably induce the cell apoptosis.

## In vivo antitumor efficacy

The antitumor efficacy of free DTX and CSH-DTX was investigated in QBC939 cells bearing xenograft tumor model. The mice were intravenously injected with respective

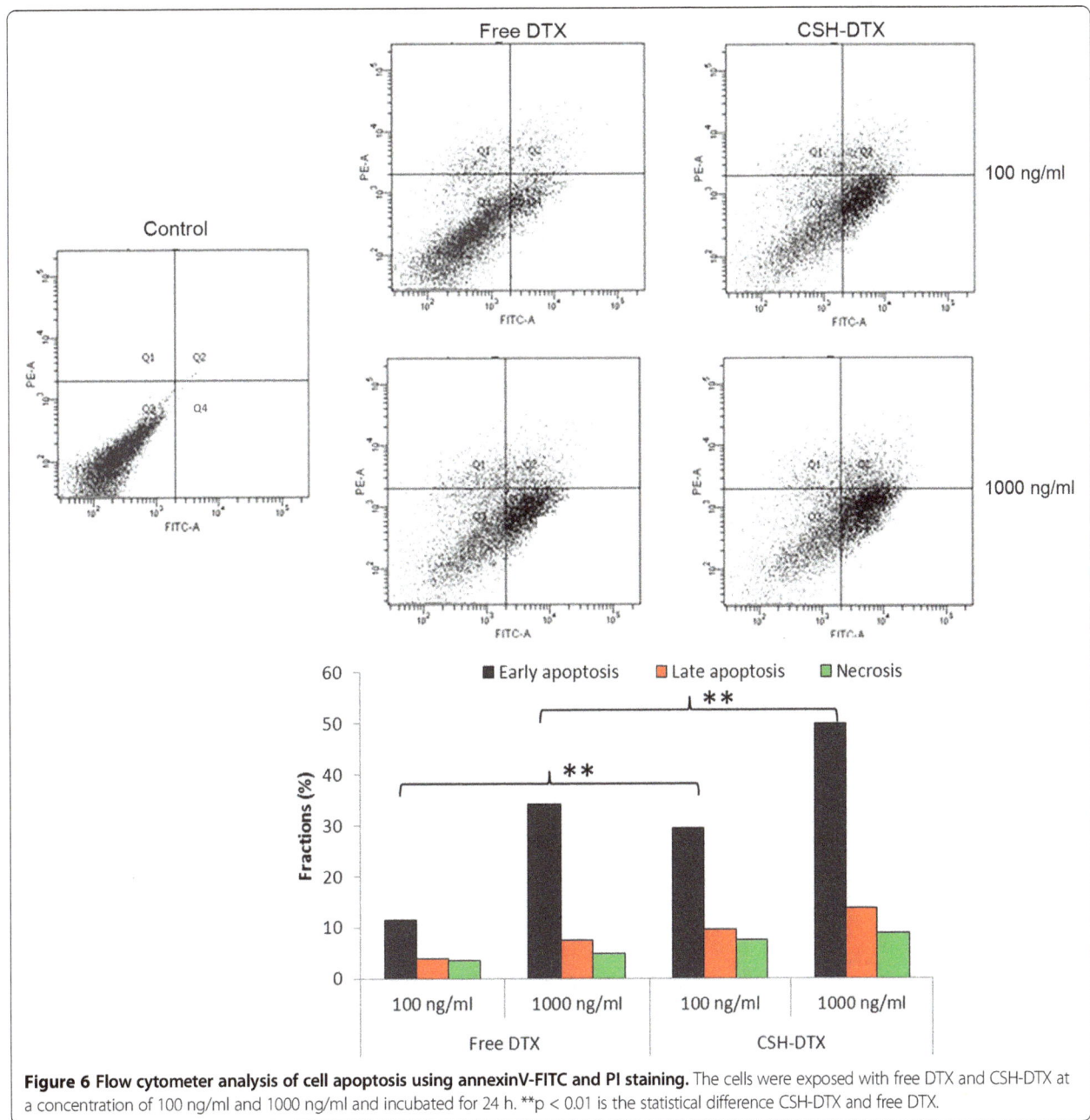

**Figure 6 Flow cytometer analysis of cell apoptosis using annexinV-FITC and PI staining.** The cells were exposed with free DTX and CSH-DTX at a concentration of 100 ng/ml and 1000 ng/ml and incubated for 24 h. **p < 0.01 is the statistical difference CSH-DTX and free DTX.

formulations every 3rd day for three times. The tumor volume and body weight was noted every alternative day up to day 20. As shown in Figure 7a, CSH-DTX significantly slowed down the growth of tumor in mice models comparing to that of free DTX and saline treated mice groups. As expected, blank micelles did not have any effect on the tumor volume of mice and grew along with control group. Administration of free DTX although showed some therapeutic effect however could not inhibit it's growth completely. The micellar formulations remarkably suppressed the tumor proliferation by comparison to that of control and free drug treated animal group. The final tumor volume of control, blank micelles, free DTX and CSH-DTX treated groups were ~2500, ~2500, ~1300, and ~600 mm³, respectively. The main reason behind the superior antitumor efficacy of CSH-DTX was attributed to increased accumulation of micelles in tumor regions due to EPR effect and enhanced sensitization of MDR cancer to DTX. The other reasons might be due to the sustained release of drug and prolonged blood circulation [21].

Along with therapeutic efficacy of anticancer drug loaded delivery system, minimization of side effects remains a big challenge for the successful cancer chemotherapy. The change in body weight has been considered to be an index to evaluate the systemic toxic effects. As shown in Figure 7b, mice group treated with free DTX significantly reduced its body weight. Approximately, 20% of body weight was reduced in this group indicating its systemic toxicity. On the other hand, when the same dose of drug was loaded in polymeric micelles, no body weight-loss was observed and throughout the study period the body weight was stable. It should be noted that the body weight of DTX treated group started recovering approximately after 8 days (after final injections). The body weight recovery might be due to the slow removal of free drug from the vital organs and clearance from the systemic circulation. The result therefore indicates that CS-HS based micelles effectively reduced the drug related side effects while at the same time improved its therapeutic efficacy as shown by reduced tumor volume [22].

### Histopathological and immunohistochemical analysis

H & E staining was performed to stain the tumor sections wherein nucleus was stained with hematoxylin (blue) and extracellular matrix was stained with eosin (pink). As shown in Figure 8a, control group exhibited clear cell morphology with excess chromatin and binucleolates. Whereas, free DTX treated group showed range of necrosis with irregular cellular morphology. The tissue necrosis further increased for CSH-DTX treated group with distinct damage to cancer cells. Lack

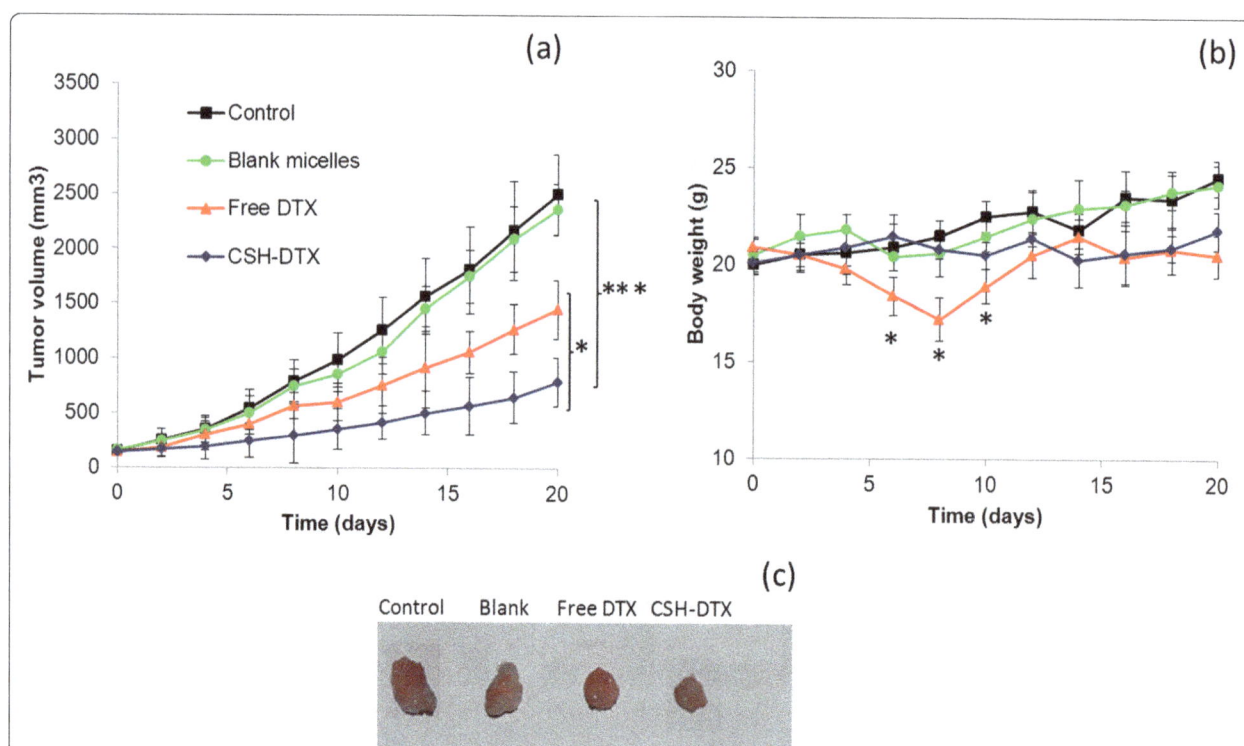

**Figure 7** In vivo antitumor efficacy study (a) changes in tumor volume (b) changes in mice body weight (c) images of tumor sections. The antitumor study was carried out in QBC939 cells -bearing xenograft model and administered thrice at a fixed dose of 5 mg/kg. *p < 0.05, ***p < 0.001 is the statistical difference in the tumor volume between CSH-DTX and free DTX or CSH-DTX and control group.

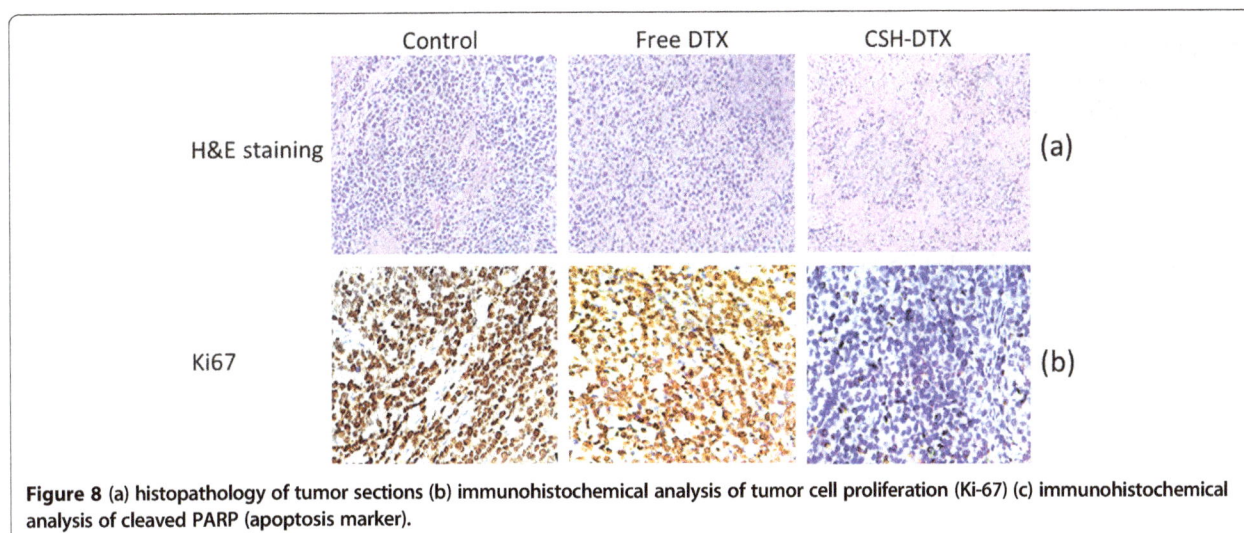

**Figure 8** (a) histopathology of tumor sections (b) immunohistochemical analysis of tumor cell proliferation (Ki-67) (c) immunohistochemical analysis of cleaved PARP (apoptosis marker).

of nuclei and lack of boundary regions were observed in this group.

Immunohistochemical staining of Ki-67 was performed to evaluate the tumor proliferation ability of individual formulations. As seen (Figure 8b), fewer number of Ki-67 cells were present in CSH-DTX treated cells comparing to that of free DTX treated group. This further confirms the enhanced accumulation of drug in the tumor tissues from micellar formulations and enhanced sensitization of MDR cancer to DTX.

PARP, a DNA binding enzyme is cleaved by caspase-3 and caspase-7. PARP is an important indicator of apoptosis in cancer cells. In this study, level of PARP was considered as a marker for level of cell apoptosis. As shown in Figure 8c, cleaved PARP was detected in DTX treated group, while it was more significant in CSH-DTX treated group. The enhanced apoptosis in CSH-DTX treated group was consistent with its excellent antitumor efficacy.

## Conclusions

An amphiphilic block copolymer CS-HS-based polymeric micelles was prepared and loaded with DTX to target cholangiocarcinoma. The pH-sensitive behaviour of histamine in the block copolymer will accelerate the release of DTX in the tumor region while protects the therapeutic load in the physiological conditions. In the present study, CSH-DTX controlled the release of drug in the basic pH while rapidly released its cargo in the tumor pH (pH 5 and 6.8) possibly due to the breakdown of polymeric micelles. A nanosize of <150 nm will allow its accumulation in the tumor interstitial spaces via EPR effect. CSH-DTX effectively killed the cancer kills in a time- and concentration-dependent manner and showed pronounced therapeutic action than that of free drug at all-time points. The superior cytotoxicity of CSH-DTX might be attributed to the pH-driven release of active

therapeutic molecule in the cell cytoplasm. CSH-DTX resulted in higher apoptosis of cancer cells with ~30% and ~50 of cells in early apoptosis quadrant when treated with 100 and 1000 ng/ml of equivalent drug. The micellar formulations showed remarkable effect in controlling the tumor growth and reduced the overall tumor volume to $1/5^{th}$ to that of control and half to that of free drug treated group with no sign of drug-related adverse effects. Immunohistochemical analysis of tumor sections showed that fewer number of Ki-67 cells were present in CSH-DTX treated cells comparing to that of free DTX treated group. Our data suggests that nanoformulation of DTX could potentially improve the chemotherapy treatment in cholangiocarcinoma as well as in other malignancies.

## Materials and methods
### Materials

Docetaxel was procured from Sigma-Aldrich (China). Chondroitin sulphate (CC) was procured from Shanghai Sangon Biological Engineering Technology & Services Co. Ltd. (Shanghai, China). Histamine dihydrochloride (HS) was purchased LSB Biotechnology Inc. (Xi'an, China). 1-(3-(Dimethylamino)propyl)-3-ethylcarbodiimide hydrochloride (EDC), N hydroxysuccinimide (NHS) was obtained from Sigma-Aldrich (China). All other chemicals were of reagent grade and used without further purification.

### Synthesis of chondroitin sulphate (CS)-histamine (HS) conjugate

Chondroitin sulphate was conjugated with histamine as reported previously [23]. Briefly, CS was dissolved in 120 ml of phosphate buffered saline (PBS, pH 6.0) maintained in a magnetic stirrer for 5 h. Carboxyl group of CS was activated by the addition of EDC and NHS in specific quantity one by one. After 30 min, HS was added and allowed the reaction mixture to proceed for 24 h. The resultant reaction mixture was dialyzed against phosphate buffer and then the process was repeated with distilled water. Finally, the product was lyophilized and stored in dark place.

### Preparation of docetaxel-loaded polymeric micelles

DTX-loaded CS-*b*-HS micelles (CSH-DTX) were prepared by a solvent extraction and evaporation method. Briefly, specific quantity of DTX and CS was dissolved in 10 ml of dichloromethane. This organic solution was poured in distilled water and immediately sonicated for 5 min to form an O/W emulsion system. The reaction was allowed to proceed for 24 h in the dark conditions.

### Particle size and zeta potential analysis

The mean diameter and surface charge was analyzed using dynamic light scattering technique by Zetasizer (Nano-ZS 90, Malvern, Worcestershire, UK). The samples were measured at 25°C at a fixed angle of 90°C. Each sample was measure in triplicate.

### Morphology analysis

The morphological examination of nanoparticles was carried out using transmission electron microscope (TEM) (JEM-2010; JEOL, Japan). Nanoparticle dispersion was placed on the carbon-coated copper grid and negatively stained with 2% (w/v) phosphotungstic acids and air dried. The morphology and surface texture was further confirmed by scanning electron microscopy (SEM; FEI Nova NanoSEM 230). The samples were freeze dried and coated with platinum before the SEM analysis.

### Drug-loading and encapsulation efficiency

UV–vis Spectrophotometer was used to calculate loading capacity and entrapment efficiency of DOX in CSH micelles was estimated by HPLC technique (LC 1200; Agilent Technologies, Santa Clara, CA, USA). The mobile phase consists of acetonitrile and 0.2% trimethylamine (pH adjusted to 6.4 with phosphoric acid) (48:52, v/v) at flow rate of 1 mL/min.

The dried solid samples were dissolved in 1 ml of dichloromethane and sonicated vigorously for 10 min. This solution was centrifuged (20000 rpm) and supernatant was collected and injected into HPLC column. A reverse-phase C18 column (250 mm × 4.6 mm; GL Science, Tokyo, Japan) was used. The mobile phase was run at 1 ml/min and detected at 254 nm.

$$DL\% = \frac{\text{Total Drug added}}{\text{Wt. of Polymer } + \text{ Wt. of drug in NP}} \times 100\%$$

$$EE\% = \frac{\text{Actual drug loading}}{\text{Theoretical drug loading}} \times 100\%$$

### Drug release study

The drug release study was carried out in various pH medium. For the release study, freeze dried micelles were reconstituted in distilled water and 1 ml of it was placed in dialysis tube and clipped at both the end. The dialysis tube was placed in a falcon tube with 30 ml of release media (different pH level). The whole assembly was placed in a shaking bath at 37°C. At predetermined time intervals, 1 ml of release sample was collected and replaced with equal amount of fresh release media. The amount of drug released in the release media was calculated from the HPLC technique.

### Cell culture

QBC939 cholangiocarcinoma cells were cultured in RPMI 1640 medium supplemented with 10% fetal bovine serum (FBS) and 1% penicillin streptomycin mixture. The cells were maintained in ambient conditions of 37°C and 5% $CO_2$.

### Cytotoxicity assay

The cytotoxicity assay was measured by 3-(4,5-dimethythiazol-2-yl)-2,5-diphenyl tetrazolium bromide (MTT) assay. It is based on the reduction of yellow MTT by mitochondrial succinate dehydrogenase. MTT enters the live cells and reduced into insoluble formazan complex. For this, QBC939 cells were seeded at a density of $1 \times 10^4$ in a 96-well plate. After 24 h, cells were exposed to blank polymer, free DTX and CSH-DTX at different dosing level. The cells were incubated for 24, 48 and 72 h accordingly. At each time point, plate was removed and treated with 100 μl of MTT solution (5 mg/ml) to each 96-well plate and incubated for 4 h. The formed formazan crystals were extracted by adding DMSO and incubated for additional 30 min. The absorbance of each plate was read at 570 nm using a microplate reader (Thermo-Fisher, USA). All experiments were repeated 6 times.

The morphology of cells was observed using a fluorescent microscope (Leica DM IRBE microscope) and representative images were selected.

### Apoptosis measurement

Hoechst 33258 was used to observe the cell apoptosis. During cell apoptosis, condensation of chromatin takes place and DNA gets cleaved into small fragments.

Generally, it enters the live cells and binds with adenosine-thymidine (AT) part of DNA while in apoptotic cells, it binds to condensed chromosome. Normal cells and apoptotic cells were different in their size and distinct morphology. The drug treated cells were washed with PBS and stained with Hoechst 33258 for 10 min. The cells were washed and fixed with 4% paraformaldehyde and observed under fluorescence microscope.

## Apoptosis analysis by flow cytometry

Apoptosis assay was carried out by flow cytometer. For this, cells were seeded, incubated for 24 h and treated with respective formulations (Free DTX and CSH-DTX). The treated cells were further incubated for 24 h. The cells were harvested and washed with PBS. The pellets were resuspended with 100 μl of binding buffer (10 mM HEPES pH 7.4, 150 mM NaCl, 5 mM KCl, 1 mM MgCl$_2$, and 1.8 mM CaCl$_2$). The cells were then treated with FITC-Annexin V and incubated for 20 min and then PI was added and incubated for additional 10 min. The cells were analysed for apoptotic cells using FACS (Becton Dickenson Biosciences, San Jose, CA, USA).

## In vivo antitumor efficacy study

In vivo antitumor efficacy study was performed in 7-week old xenograft nude mice. Briefly, $1 \times 10^6$ QBC939 cells (100 μl PBS) were subcutaneously injected into the right flank of nude mice to establish cholangiocarcinoma tumor models. The tumours were allowed to grow for two weeks until it reaches ~150 mm$^3$ size. The mice were equally divided into 4 groups with 8 mice in each group; untreated controls, blank micelles, free DTX, and CSH-DTX at a fixed dose of 5 mg/kg. The samples were injected thrice via tail vein injection during first two weeks. The tumor size was measured using Vernier calliper for every other alternative day. Tumor volume was calculated using the formula: volume = $1/2 \times D_{max} \times (D_{min})^2$. The body weight was measured simultaneously as an indicator of the systemic toxicity. At the end of the study period, tumors were surgically removed and fixed in 10% neutral formalin and embedded in paraffin.

## Histopathological and immunohistochemical evaluations

The histopathology of tumor sections was evaluated by hematoxylin and eosin (H & E) method. The embedded paraffin tumor sections were cut into 5 μm slices and stained with H & E staining agent and viewed by microscope (Nikon TE2000U). For immunohistochemical analysis, rabbit monoclonal primary antibody for cleaved poly-ADP-ribose polymerase (PARP) (Abcam, Cambridge, MA, USA) and rat anti-mouse Ki-67 monoclonal antibody (Maixin Biotechnology Co., Ltd) to quantify Ki-67 expression was used in the study.

## Statistical analysis

The experimental data are presented as the mean (standard deviation (SD). All statistical analyses were performed using ANOVA or a two-tailed Student's t-test (GraphPad Prism 5).

### Abbreviations
HS: Histidine; CS: Chondroitin sulphate; NP: Nanoparticles; DTX: Docetaxel.

### Competing interests
The authors declare that they have no competing interests.

### Authors' contributions
LW has guided and written the whole manuscript. ND and LPS prepared the formulations and performed in vitro experiments. XSL and LW performed all the biological and pharmacological experiments. HYM and HZ have carried out the in vivo anticancer efficacy study. All authors read and approved the final manuscript.

### Acknowledgments
This work supported by Grants from National Natural Science foundation of China (no.81000994), Beijing municipal Science and technology Commission (no Z121107001012080), and Beijing Nova program (no.Z131107000413104).

### Author details
[1]The Second Department of Oncology, The First Affiliated Hospital of the General Hospital of the PLA, Beijing 100048, China. [2]Department of Medical, The First Affiliated Hospital of the General Hospital of the PLA, No. 51 Fucheng Road, Haidian District, Beijing 100048, China.

### References
1. Khan SA, Davidson BR, Goldin RD, Heaton N, Karani J, Pereira SP, et al. Guidelines for the diagnosis and treatment of cholangiocarcinoma: an update. Gut. 2012;61:1657–69.
2. Patel T. Cholangiocarcinoma-controversies and challenges. Nat Rev Gastroenterol Hepatol. 2011;8:189–200.
3. Vauthey JN, Blumgart LH. Recent advances in the management of cholangiocarcinomas. Semin Liver Dis. 1994;14:109–14.
4. Patel T. Increasing incidence and mortality of primary intrahepatic cholangiocarcinoma in the United States. Hepatology. 2001;33:1353–7.
5. Matull WR, Khan SA, Pereira SP. Impact of classification of hilar cholangiocarcinomas (Klatskin tumors) on incidence of intra- and extrahepatic cholangiocarcinoma in the United States. J Natl Cancer Inst. 2006;21:873–5.
6. Parkin DM, Srivatanakul P, Khlat M, Chenvidhya D, Chotiwan P, Insiripong S, et al. Liver cancer in Thailand. I. A case–control study of cholangiocarcinoma. Int J Cancer. 1991;48:323–8.
7. Seehofer D, Kamphues C, Neuhaus P. Management of bile duct tumors. Expert Opin Pharmacother. 2008;9:2843–56.
8. Khan SA, Thomas HC, Davidson BR, Robinson SDT. Cholangiocarcinoma. Lancet. 2005;366:1303–10.
9. Tong R, Cheng J. Anticancer polymeric nanomedicines. Polym Rev. 2007;3:345–81.
10. Mura S, Nicolas J, Couvreur P. Stimuli-responsive nanocarriers for drug delivery. Nat Mater. 2013;12:991–1003.
11. Murakami M, Cabral H, Matsumoto Y, Wu S, Kano MR, Yamori T, et al. Improving drug potency and efficacy by nanocarrier-mediated subcellular targeting. Sci Transl Med. 2011;3:64ra2.
12. Owens III DE, Peppas NA. Opsonization, biodistribution, and pharmacokinetics of polymeric nanoparticles. Int J Pharm. 2006;307:93–102.
13. Wu XL, Kim JH, Koo H, Bae SM, Shin H, Kim MS, et al. Tumor-targeting peptide conjugated pH-responsive micelles as a potential drug carrier for cancer therapy. Bioconjug Chem. 2010;21:208–13.
14. Lv Y, Ding G, Zhai J, Guo Y, Nie G, Xu L. A superparamagnetic Fe3O4-loaded polymeric nanocarrier for targeted delivery of evodiamine with enhanced antitumor efficacy. Colloids Surf B Biointerfaces. 2013;110:411–8.
15. Li F, Na K. Self-assembled chlorin e6 conjugated chondroitin sulfate nanodrug for photodynamic therapy. Biomacromolecules. 2011;12:1724–30.

16. Lundberg P, Lynd NA, Zhang Y, Zeng X, Krogstad DV, Paffen T, et al. pH-triggered self-assembly of biocompatible histamine-functionalized triblock copolymers. Soft Matter. 2013;9:82–9.

17. Huang ZJ, Yang N, Xu TW, Lin JQ. Antitumor efficacy of docetaxel-loaded nanocarrier against esophageal cancer cell bearing mice model. Drug Res (Stuttg). 2014. [Epub ahead of print].

18. Noori Koopaei M, Khoshayand MR, Mostafavi SH, Amini M, Khorramizadeh MR, Jeddi Tehrani M, et al. Docetaxel loaded PEG-PLGA nanoparticles: optimized drug loading, in-vitro cytotoxicity and in-vivo antitumor effect. Iran J Pharm Res. 2014;13:819–33.

19. Matsumura Y. Preclinical and clinical studies of NK012, an SN-38-incorporating polymeric micelles, which is designed based on EPR effect. Adv Drug Deliv Rev. 2011;63:184–92.

20. Yu S, Wu G, Gu X, Wang J, Wang Y, Gao H, et al. Magnetic and pH-sensitive nanoparticles for antitumor drug delivery. Colloids Surf B Biointerfaces. 2013;103:1522.

21. Ramasamy T, Kim JH, Choi JY, Tran TH, Choi HG, Yong CS, et al. pH sensitive polyelectrolyte complex micelles for highly effective combination chemotherapy. J Mater Chem B. 2014;2:6324.

22. Danhier F, Feron O, Preat V. To exploit the tumor microenvironment: passive and active tumor targeting of nanocarriers for anti-cancer drug delivery. J Controlled Release. 2010;148:135–46.

23. Knight V, Koshkina NV, Waldrep JC, Giovanella BC, Gilbert BE. Anticancer exffect of 9-nitrocamptothecin liposome aerosol on human cancer xenografts in nude mice. Cancer Chemother Pharmacol. 1999;44:177–86.

# 14

# Micro CT visualization of silver nanoparticles in the middle and inner ear of rat and transportation pathway after transtympanic injection

Jing Zou[1,5*], Markus Hannula[2†], Superb Misra[3,7†], Hao Feng[1†], Roberto Hanoi Labrador[4], Antti S Aula[2,6], Jari Hyttinen[2] and Ilmari Pyykkö[1]

## Abstract

**Background:** Silver nanoparticles (Ag NPs) displayed strong activities in anti-bacterial, anti-viral, and anti-fungal studies and were reportedly efficient in treating otitis media. Information on distribution of AgNPs in different compartments of the ear is lacking.

**Objective:** To detect distribution of Ag NPs in the middle and inner ear and transportation pathways after transtympanic injection.

**Methods:** Contrast effect of Ag NPs in the micro CT imaging was assessed in a phantom. AgNPs at various concentrations (1.85 mM, 37.1 mM, and 370.7 mM) were administered to rat middle ear using transtympanic injection and cadaver heads were imaged using micro CT at several time points.

**Results:** The lowest concentration of Ag NPs that could be visualized using micro CT was 37.1 mM. No difference was observed between the solvents, deionized $H_2O$ and saline. Ag NPs at 37.1 mM were visible in the middle ear on 7 d post-administration. Ag NPs at 370.7 mM generated signals in the middle ear, ossicular chain, round window membrane, oval window, scala tympani, and Eustachian tube for both 4 h and 24 h time points. A gradient distribution of Ag NPs from the middle ear to the inner ear was detected. The pathways for Ag NPs to be transported from the middle ear into the inner ear are round and oval windows.

**Conclusion:** This study provided the imaging evidence that Ag NPs are able to access the inner ear in a dose-dependent manner after intratympanic administration, which is relevant to design the delivery concentration in the future clinic application in order to avoid adverse inner ear effect.

**Keywords:** Silver nanoparticles, Micro CT, Ear, Animal, Pathway

## Introduction

Silver nanoparticles (Ag NPs) displayed strong activities in anti-bacterial, anti-viral, and anti-fungal studies attributed to the mechanisms of inhibiting the formation of biofilm and destroying viral structures and boosting innate immune response among others [1-5]. Study performed by Radzig et al. supports the hypothesis that Ag NPs exert the antibacterial action through inducing generation of reactive oxygen species and causing DNA damage by oxidative stress, which can be also involved in the mechanisms of antiviral and antifungal activities [6]. Ag NPs also showed excellent behavior in surface-enhanced Raman scattering for the advanced Raman spectroscopy, which has potential for broad range of applications in clinical molecular imaging [7].

Potentially, Ag NPs will be used to treat otitis media and the consequential sensorineural hearing loss through intratympanic administration. Chronic otitis media, characterized by recurrent infections causing pain and purulent otorrhea, is still a significant public health problem affecting 0.5–30% of any given population in developing

\* Correspondence: Jing.Zou@uta.fi
†Equal contributors
[1]Hearing and Balance Research Unit, Field of Oto-laryngology, School of Medicine, University of Tampere, Medisiinarinkatu 3, 33520 Tampere, Finland
[5]Department of Otolaryngology-Head and Neck Surgery, Center for Otolaryngology-Head & Neck Surgery of Chinese PLA, Changhai Hospital, Second Military Medical University, Shanghai, China
Full list of author information is available at the end of the article

and developed countries. Complications with sensori-neural hearing loss and vestibular impairment were repeatedly reported in the literatures [8-12]. Endolymphatic hydrops secondary to the middle ear infection was demonstrated in both animal model and patient with Meniere's disease using gadolinium enhancement magnetic resonance imaging (MRI) [13,14]. However, antibiotic is not always efficient because of the appearance of multidrug resistant strains of bacteria. Formation of biofilm was recently reported in the middle ear of patients with chronic otitis media all over the world [15-18]. Through a completely different mechanism, Ag NPs may overcome all the disadvantages of any antibiotics and eliminate the microorganisms with high efficacy in the ear therapy. This therapeutic strategy was encouraged by a clinical study on treatment of relapses of chronic suppurative otitis media using a preparation containing Ag NPs. The study showed that Ag NPs eliminated clinical symptoms and positive dynamics of the objective signs of the disease, such as reduction or termination of pathological exudation and stimulation of the epidermization processes, which was stable during the observation time of 6 months [19]. In order to persuade this novel therapy with sophisticated design, detailed information on distribution and pathway of Ag NPs

in the middle and inner ear is necessary but currently lacking in the literature.

Micro computed tomography (CT) has been engaged in middle and inner ear imaging of animals and implicated to be a useful tool to trace kinetics of drugs in the inner ear [20,21]. The gray levels in a CT slice image correspond to X-ray attenuation, which reflects the proportion of X-rays scattered or absorbed as they pass through each voxel, and is affected by the density and composition of the material being imaged. Hence, Ag NPs are speculated to attenuate the X-rays and be visible in micro CT images. In the present work, first a phantom study was performed to check the dose response of the imaging system. Next, an *in vivo* experiment was carried out in rats by injecting Ag NP suspensions with different concentrations into the middle ear cavity and following the kinetics of Ag NPs in the middle and inner ear up to 7 d.

## Results

### Characterization of Ag NPs and potential interaction with artificial perilymph

The Ag NPs used in this study were highly faceted with a mean size of $21 \pm 8$ nm. The particles were polydispersed in size and shape, as shown in Figure 1. The transmission electron microscope (TEM) images and

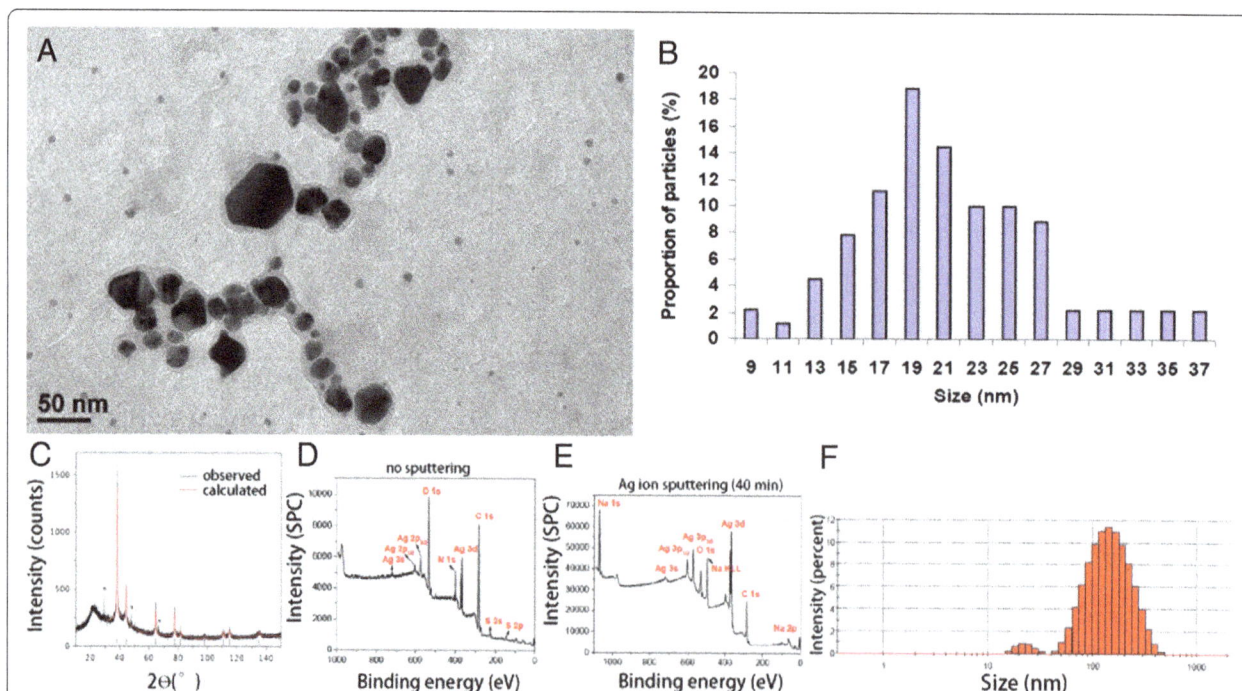

Figure 1 Characterization result of PVP coated Ag NPs using various analytical techniques. A) Transmission electron microscopy (TEM) image of NPs showing the polydispersity in size and shape of the PVP coated AgNPs. B) TEM particle size distribution of NPs (n = 200, mean = 21 ± 8 nm), C) X-ray diffraction pattern for Ag NPs indicating the presence of metallic silver (ICDD 004–0783). D-E) XPS analysis on Ag NPs without any sputtering indicating the presence of high amount of organic impurities (PVP used as a surfactant). Sputtered spectrum (E) confirms the presence of the organic components only on the surface. F) Hydrodynamic size of the NPs when suspended in deionized water, measured using dynamic light scattering.

Micro CT visualization of silver nanoparticles in the middle and inner ear of rat and transportation...

129

size distribution of the particles are shown in Figure 1a. X-ray diffraction (XRD) analysis confirmed the crystalline nature of the particles (ICDD: 004–0783). The mean hydrodynamic size of the particles when suspended in deionized water was $117 \pm 24$ nm, and the zeta potential was measured to be $-20 \pm 9$ mV. Inductively coupled plasma measurements on the particles showed a very low level of species other than silver, which were mostly cations (Figure 2). Because the nanoparticles were stabilized in the suspension using polyvinylpyrrolidone (PVP), XPS analysis was performed to characterize the surface of the particles. The un-sputtered spectrum of the particles showed a high presence of organic carbon, which was evidently due to the presence of PVP used as the capping agent/surfactant. However, after increasing the sputtering time, the Ag 3 d peak started to appear stronger, suggesting a core shell structure wherein the core was metallic silver and the shell was composed of an organic coating with PVP. Incubation with artificial perilymph for 4 h did not significantly affect the size distribution of the Ag NPs (Table 1).

### Sensitivity of micro CT imaging of Ag NPs

The current setup of micro CT showed a detection limit for Ag NPs at a concentration of 37 mM. Good linearity between the signal intensity and Ag NPs concentration was obtained in the range of 37–370.7 mM that were dissolved in $H_2O$ (Figure 3). Significant correlation was observed between signal intensities of Ag NPs generated in $H_2O$ and NaCl solutions, but the $H_2O$ provided significantly higher signal intensities than the NaCl with normalized value of 1.04 (p < 0.001, paired samples t-test).

### Distribution of AgNPs in the middle and inner ear and pathways

The heterogeneous fine structures of rat cochlea were demonstrated by iodine-contrast micro CT in Figure 4.

The optimized protocol for rat ear micro CT imaging had a resolution of 21.9 µm, which can utilize both the middle ear and inner ear for detecting the distribution of the Ag NPs in both compartments. At 4 h after transtympanic injection of 370.7 mM Ag NPs, the nanoparticles distributed along the middle ear mucosa, diffused to the Eustachian tube, and the extra Ag NPs flowed out into the external ear canal. Abundant Ag NP accumulation on the surface of ossicular chain and stapes artery was detected. The Ag NPs significantly distributed in the round window membrane and continuously moved to the mesothelium of the scala tympani and the annular ligament across the stapediovestibular joint, which is the junctional site between the middle ear and vestibule (Figure 5). At 24 h, Ag NPs showed abundant distribution on in the round window membrane and oval window, and became more visible within the cochlea (Figure 5). Ag NPs was detected in the middle ear mucosa at 4 h post-transtympanic injection at 37 mM in one rat. Aggregated Ag NPs were visualized in both middle ear and cochlea on 7 d after injection at 37 mM (Figure 5). Higher estimated concentrations of Ag NPs in various locations of the ear than the applied concentrations supported the aggregation or accumulation of Ag NPs in the corresponding area (Table 2). However, transtympanic injection of Ag NPs at 1.85 mM did not produce any signal of Ag NP at the time points of 4 h, 24 h, and 7 d post-administration. There was not any fluid detected in the middle ear cavity at these time points indicating that there was no infiltration.

### Discussion

The present work demonstrated that the PVP-coated Ag NPs were visible in the ear by micro CT after transtympanic injection and entered in the inner ear through the round and oval windows. The detected bright signals in the ear by micro CT could be either aggregated Ag NPs or silver compound formed upon contacting the

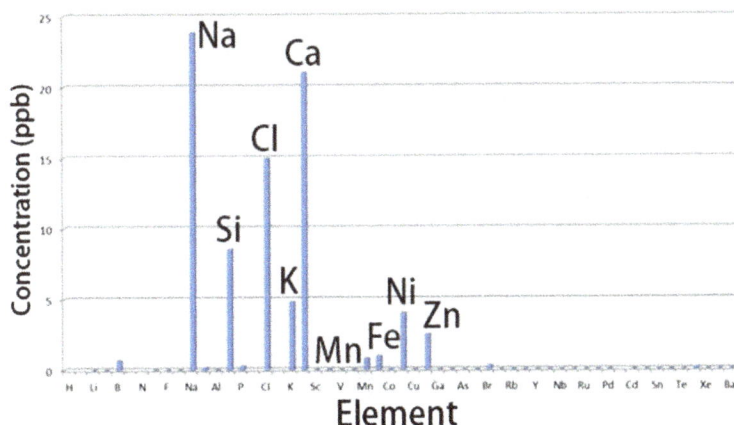

**Figure 2** Level of impurities found in the Ag NPs shown by inductively couple plasma-mass spectrometry.

**Table 1 Size distribution of AgNPs in artificial perilymph for 4 h at different dilutions**

| Concentration (dilution) | $Z_{mean}$ (nm) |
|---|---|
| x10 | 106.9 ± 0.3 |
| X100 | 102.9 ± 0.7 |
| X1000 | 100.2 ± 1.0 |
| X10000 | 100.7 ± 1.2 |

extracellular or cellular fluids. Ag NPs encounter different extracellular environments in the external ear canal, middle ear, and inner ear. The plentiful perilymph in the inner ear may interact with Ag NPs and form a compound immediately after the entry. However, the incubation of Ag NPs with artificial perilymph did not change the size distribution over a period of 25 h, suggesting that the bright signals in the ear represent the Ag NPs. It was reported that silver might be developed as a radiographic contrast agent in dual-energy breast X-ray imaging [22]. However, the detection sensitivity of Ag NPs by micro CT is rather low and the detection limit is 37 mM, a concentration that demonstrated toxicity in the rat ear [23]. These results did not support that the current form of Ag NPs will be used as a contrast agent for CT imaging. Clinical feasibility, however, warrants further studies.

The oval window pathway was recently proved to be more efficient than the round window to transport chelated-gadolinium from the middle ear to the inner ear in animals and human shown by MRI [24,25]. The pathways for the Ag NPs to enter the inner ear were clearly shown to be the round and oval windows. This indicates that the oval window potentially has a broad spectrum of substance transportation in addition to chelated-gadolinium. At 24 h post-administration to the middle ear at a concentration of 370.7 mM, Ag NPs accumulated in the round window membrane and oval

window, and concentrated in the scala tympani, which indicates that the entry of Ag NPs into the inner ear is a dynamic process. This conclusion was further supported by the quantification of Ag NPs in various regions of the ear (Table 2). Obvious Ag NP signal was detected in the middle ear after administration at a concentration of 37.1 mM that was the lowest detection limit of the present setup, which may result from accumulation or aggregation of Ag NPs in the middle ear as supported by the quantification result (Table 2). No signal was detected in the inner ear when Ag NPs were administered at a concentration of 37 mM. This might be caused by the low sensitivity of micro CT visualization. Our explanation is that the layer of Ag NPs formed on tissue surfaces of the inner ear is too thin to raise the value of the voxel as a result of the partial volume effect (the grayscale value of a voxel is the volume fraction weighted sum of all the materials present in the voxel). A previous study demonstrated that hearing loss occurred in rats after middle ear administration of 37.1 mM Ag NPs, which suggests that certain amount of Ag NPs (below the detection threshold of the micro CT) should have entered the inner ear [23].

The long term remaining of Ag NPs in the middle ear cavity for 7 d post-transtympanic injection supports that Ag NP is a potential candidate to combat otitis media. Although no signal was detected in the inner ear on 7 d post-administration of 37.1 mM Ag NP, it did not rule out the penetration of Ag NPs into the inner ear because hearing loss and pathological changes were detected in rats exposed to Ag NPs at this concentration [23]. 1.85 mM Ag NPs did not generate either micro CT signal of AgNPs or infiltration in the middle ear cavity. No infiltration indicates that 1.85 mM of Ag NPs is a safe level for the ear, which is in accordance with our observation that neither hearing loss nor cytokine up-regulation in the inner ear was induced by Ag NPs at this concentration (unpublished data). Importantly, 1.85 mM of Ag NPs

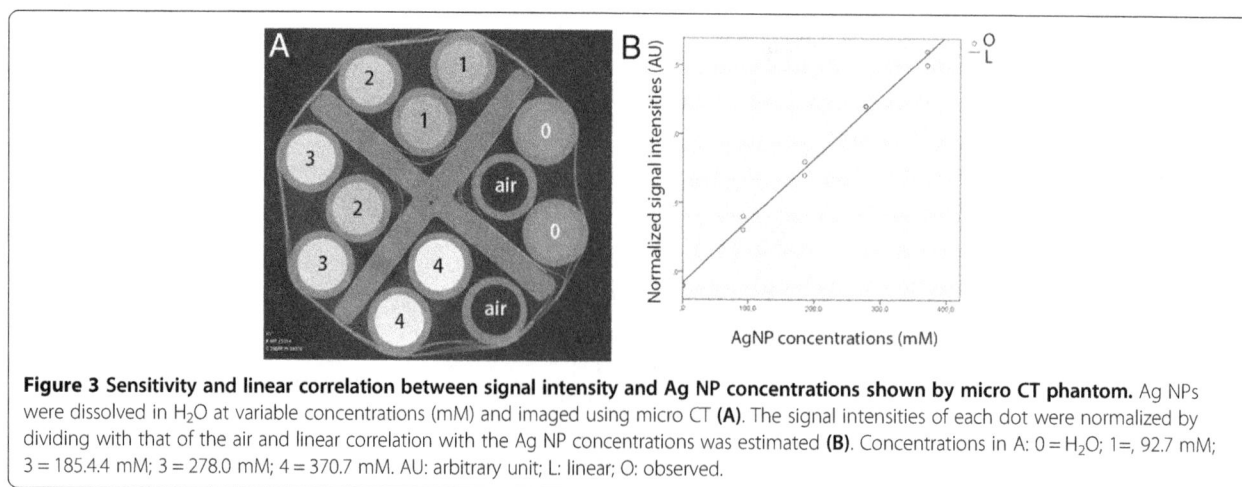

**Figure 3 Sensitivity and linear correlation between signal intensity and Ag NP concentrations shown by micro CT phantom.** Ag NPs were dissolved in $H_2O$ at variable concentrations (mM) and imaged using micro CT (**A**). The signal intensities of each dot were normalized by dividing with that of the air and linear correlation with the Ag NP concentrations was estimated (**B**). Concentrations in A: 0 = $H_2O$; 1=, 92.7 mM; 3 = 185.4.4 mM; 3 = 278.0 mM; 4 = 370.7 mM. AU: arbitrary unit; L: linear; O: observed.

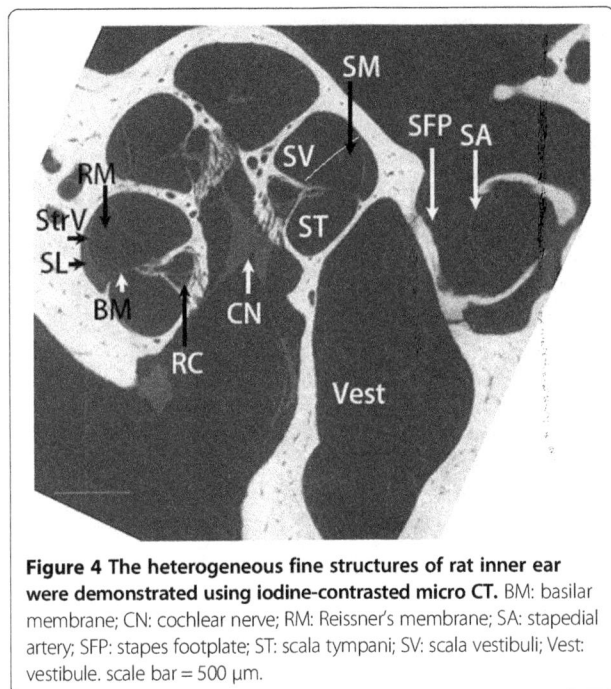

**Figure 4 The heterogeneous fine structures of rat inner ear were demonstrated using iodine-contrasted micro CT.** BM: basilar membrane; CN: cochlear nerve; RM: Reissner's membrane; SA: stapedial artery; SFP: stapes footplate; ST: scala tympani; SV: scala vestibuli; Vest: vestibule. scale bar = 500 μm.

is sufficient to inhibit biofilm formation during bacterial infection which only demands 0.1-2 mM Ag NPs [26].

In addition, the extra Ag NPs were secreted to the nasal pharynx through the Eustachian tube and flowed to the external ear canal through the tympanic membrane penetration. Dysfunction of the Eustachian tube is a common complication of otitis media. The distribution of Ag NPs in the Eustachian tube suggest that Ag NPs may have direct effect on the extension of otitis media. The dendrimer-stabilized silver nanoparticles, that have similar sizes as the Ag NPs utilized in the present study, were reportedly effective in X-ray computed tomography (CT) imaging and stable in water, PBS buffer, fetal bovine serum, and resistant to changes in pH and temperature [27]. There is a possibility that the dendrimer-stabilized silver nanoparticles may be used as a contrast agent in the CT imaging of the external, middle, and inner ears and the Eustachian tube in the future based on the present results.

## Conclusions

The distribution of Ag NPs in the middle and inner ear is visible by micro CT and a gradient concentration from the middle ear to the inner ear was detected. The pathways for Ag NPs to be transported from the middle ear into the inner ear are round and oval windows. This study provided the imaging evidence that Ag NPs are able to access various regions of the ear after intratympanic administration in a dosage-dependent manner, which is relevant to design the delivery concentration in

the future clinic application in order to avoid adverse inner ear effect.

## Materials and methods
### Materials

The Ag NPs was supplied by Colorobbia (Firenze, Italy). Ten male Sprague Dawley rats, weighing between 330 g and 410 g, were maintained in the Experimental Animal Unit, School of Medicine, University of Tampere, Finland. All animal experiments were approved by the Ethical Committee of University of Tampere (permission: ESAVI/3033/04.10.03/2011). Animal care and experimental procedures were conducted in accordance with European legislation. Two rats were assigned into each group with respect to concentrations of AgNPs and imaging time (Table 3). Animal care and experimental procedures were conducted in accordance with European legislation. All experiments were performed under general anesthesia with intraperitoneal injection of a mixture of 0.8 mg/kg of medetomidine hydrochloride (Domitor, Orion, Espoo, Finland) and 80 mg/kg of ketamine hydrochloride (Ketalar; Pfizer, Helsinki, Finland) followed by intramuscular injection of Enrofloxacin (Baytril®vet, Orion, Turku, Finland) at a dose of 10 mg/kg to prevent potential infection. During experiments, the animal's eyes were protected by Viscotears® (Novartis Healthcare A/S, Denmark).

### Characterization of Ag NPs

The Ag NPs were dispersed in water (370.7 mM) and characterized using a range of analytical techniques, to assess various physicochemical properties (eg. size, shape, zeta potential, surface properties etc.). For TEM measurements, a diluted suspension of Ag NPs was deposited on a copper grid for TEM imaging (Hitachi 7100, 100 kV). XRD was performed on the NPs using an Enraf-Nonius diffractometer coupled to INEL CPS 120 position-sensitive detector with Co-$K_\alpha$ radiation, and the phase identification was performed using STOE software. The hydrodynamic size and zeta potential of the nanoparticles were measured using a Malvern Zetasizer (Malvern Instruments, Malvern, UK). ICP-AES (Varian Instruments) analysis was performed to determine the initial concentration of silver in the aqueous nanoparticulate suspension and to measure the level of any impurities present in the matrix. X-ray photoelectron spectroscopy (XPS, Omicron Nanotechnology) was used to study the chemical composition and chemical state of the Ag NPs. The XPS analyses were performed in an ultra-high vacuum medium (pressure of $10^{-10}$ mbar) using an Al, K$\alpha$ (hv = 1486.7 eV) X-ray source, with power given by the emission of 16 mA at a voltage of 12.5 kV. For the silver element, the high-resolution spectra were obtained with analyzer pass energy of 50 eV and a step size of 0.01 eV. The argon ion flux was employed to sputter the

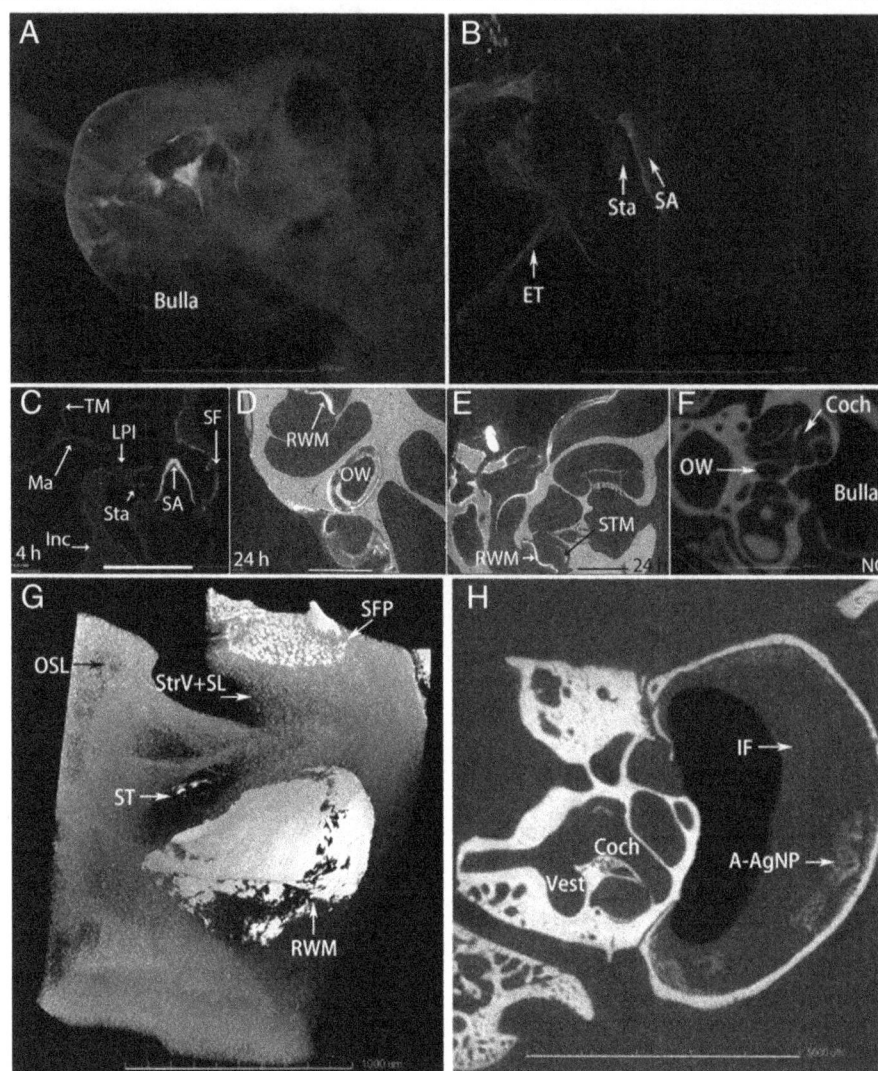

**Figure 5 Distribution of Ag NPs in the ear after transtympanic injection shown by micro CT.** Either 370.7 mM **(A-E, G)** or 37.1 mM (H) of Ag NPs were injected at a volume of 50 μl. At 4 h post-administration (370.7 mM), AgNPs generated bright signal that appeared in the bulla, tympanic membrane (TM) Eustachian tube (ET), and the ossicular chain including malleus (Ma), incus (Inc) and stapes (Sta) **(A-C)**. Abundant Ag NPs were found in the stapedial artery (SA) **(C)**. At 24 h (370.7 mM), abundant distribution of AgNPs was detected in the round window membrane (RWM), oval window (OW), and scala tympani medial wall (STM) of the cochlea **(D, E, G)**. On 7 d (37 mM), middle ear infiltration (IF) and AgNP aggregation (A-AgNPs) were observed **(H)**. No Ag NPs were detected in the ear of non-treatment control (NC) **(F)**. Coch: cochlea; LPI: lenticular process of incus; SF: stapes footplate; ST: scala tympani. Scale bars = 5 mm **(A)**, 2 mm **(B, F)**, 1 mm **(C-E)**. A-F, **H**: 4x, Pixel size 21.8498; G: 10x, pixel size 1.7 um.

surface and remove the adsorbed species, with an energy of 3.5 kV, emission of 20 mA, and incidence angle of 45° over a period of 20 and 40 min. The binding energies were referred to the carbon 1 s level, which was set as 284.6 eV.

### Potential impact of perilymph on Ag NPs

Since the Ag NPs will interact with perilymph once enter the inner ear, the potential impact of perilymph on Ag NPs was evaluated. The artificial perilymph containing 145.5 mM NaCl, 2.7 mM KCl, 2.0 mM MgSO$_4$, 1.2 mM CaCl$_2$, and 5.0 mM HEPES, with the pH adjusted to 7.4,

was prepared as previously reported [28]. Ag NPs were diluted with artificial perilymph at 10, 100, 1000 and 10000-fold and stored at room temperature for 4 h before the size distribution was measured using DLS (Malvern Zeta Sizer Nano ZS, UK). For the change in the DLS over 25 h, the dilutions were 10-fold.

### Micro CT studies
#### Phantom study

The first round experiment was designed to check the sensitivity of the imaging system using solutions of Ag

**Table 2 Concentrations (mM) of AgNPs distributes in various locations of rat ear after transtympanic injection measured by μCT**

| AgNP con delivered | Time | ME | ME-flu | Mall | Inc | Stap | StapArt | StapFoot | OW | RWM | Coc | EEC |
|---|---|---|---|---|---|---|---|---|---|---|---|---|
| 371 | 5 h | 1270 | | 547 | 677 | 500 | 769 | | 1038 | | 639 | 1177 |
| 371 | 4 h | 1084 | | 232 | 269 | 408 | 677 | | 232 | | | |
| 371 | 24 h | | | 816 | 639 | 769 | | 639 | 1177 | | | |
| 371 | 24 h | | | 677 | 593 | 723 | 1084 | 769 | 955 | 1177 | 593 | |
| 37 | 4 h | 139 | | | | | | | | | | |
| 37 | 1 w | 232 | 93 | | | | | | | | | |
| 37 | 1 w | 185 | | | | | | | | | | |

Intensities in various locations of rat ear after transtympanic injection of AgNPs were normalized by the intensities of the cochlear perilymph imaged by μCT. The concentrations of AgNPs were estimated using the formula of y = 4.88x-4.86 obtained in a phantom study, where "y" is the concentration and "x" is the normalized intensity. AgNP con: AgNP concentration; Coc: cochlea; EEC: external ear canal; Inc: incus; ME: middle ear mocusa; ME-flu: middle ear fluid; Mall: malleus; OW: oval window; RWM: round window membrane; Stap: stapes; StapArt: stapedial artery.

NPs with broad concentration range (370.7 mM, 37.1 mM, 3.7 mM, 0.37 mM, and 0.037 mM) that were prepared with either deionized $H_2O$ or saline and placed into plastic phantom tubes arranged concentrically on the modified piston rod of a 50 ml syringe. Negative controls were prepared using saline. Each sample was prepared in duplicate. The phantom was firmly installed on the specimen stage of the MicroXCT-400 (Carl Zeiss X-ray Microscopy, Inc, Jena, Germany) and imaged using the following parameters: Voltage 120 kV, current 83 μA, pixel size 33.95 μm, exposure time 0.5 s. The detection limit of the imaging system with the defined parameters was shown to be 37.1 mM based on the first round experiment. The second round experiment was performed using solutions of Ag NPs with smaller concentration range (370.7 mM, 278.0 mM, 185.4 mM, 92.7 mM) suspended in $H_2O$ according to the above protocol to determine the accurate correlation between the concentration and signal intensity.

### Animal study

Under general anesthesia, 50 μl of Ag NPs at defined concentrations were injected into the left middle ear cavity through the tympanic membrane penetration under an operating microscope according to a previously reported procedure [29]. After injection, the animals were kept in the lateral position with the injected ear oriented upward for 15 min to ensure the sufficient amount of Ag NPs to remain in the middle ear cavity

before intraperitoneal injection of Antisendan (atipamezole hydrochloride, Orion Pharma, Finland) (2 mg/kg) to accelerate recovery from anesthesia. At certain observation time points post-administration (Table 3), animals were injected intraperitoneally with pentobarbital sodium at a dosage of 100 mg/kg. The temporal bones were fixed through cardiac perfusion with 0.01 M PBS containing 0.6% (v/v) heparin (pH 7.4) and then 4% paraformaldehyde (Merck, Espoo, Finland).After decapitation, the animal head was further fixed with 4% paraformaldehyde for 2 h, covered with parafilm, and placed on the specimen stage of the micro CT. During imaging, three objectives were used, 1X for the large field of view images, 4X for the images that were focused onto the cochlea, 10x for imaging the oval and round windows. The voltage varied from 60 to 120 kV, the source distance was adjusted to 60–100 mm, and the detector distance was 38–40 mm. The pixel size ranged from 1.7 to 35.4 μm according to different setup parameters. Afterwards, one bulla was processed for iodine-contrast micro CT imaging in order to demonstrate the soft tissue in the inner ear. The stapes was displaced and about 5 μl iodixanol (VisipaqueTM, 320 g I/ml, GE Healthcare, Helsinki, Finland) was infused into the inner ear using a high-performance polyimide tubing (MicroLumen, Tampa, FL, USA) that was connected to polyethylene tubing (PE10, Becton, Dickinson and Company, Franklin Lakes, NJ, USA) [28].The images were acquired with a 4x-objective, source voltage of 40 kV and current 200 μA, pixel size of 5.6 μm. Images were

**Table 3 Assignments of rats in micro CT measurements and distribution of AgNPs in the ear post-intratympanic administration**

| AgNPs conc | 370.7 mM | 37.1 mM | 1.85 mM | | |
|---|---|---|---|---|---|
| Time points | 4 h* | 24 h* | 4 h* | 7 d2* | 7 d* |
| Locations of AgNPs in the ear | ME, OC, SA, RWM, OW, ET, ST | ME, OC, SA, RWM, OW, ET, ST | ND | ME | ND |

*Two rats were assigned into each group. conc: concentration; ET: Eustachian tube; ME: middle ear; ND: not detected; OC: ossicular chain; OW: oval window; RWM: round window membrane; SA: stapes artery; ST: scala tympani.

collected using the Xradia TXMController software and reconstructed using the Xradia TXMR econstructor software.

## Image analysis and statistics

Signal intensities in the region of interest were evaluated using Image J 1.46r software (National Institutes of Health, Bethesda, MD). Linear equation was used for the curve estimation between Ag NP concentration and signal intensity obtained using micro CT in phantom. Paired samples T-test (IBM SPSS statistics 20) was used to compare the signal intensity generated by Ag NPs in deionized $H_2O$ and NaCl solutions. Intensities in various locations of rat ear after transtympanic injection of Ag NPs were normalized by the intensities of the cochlear perilymph imaged by $\mu$CT. The concentrations of Ag NPs were estimated according to the linear curve obtained in the phantom study.

### Abbreviations
AgNPs: Silver nanoparticles; CT: Computed tomography; MRI: Magnetic resonance imaging; PVP: Polyvinylpyrrolidone; TEM: Transmission electron microscope; XRD: X-ray diffraction.

### Competing interests
The authors declare that they have no competing interests.

### Authors' contributions
Conceived and designed the experiments: JZ. Performed the experiments: JZ, MH, SM, HF, RHL, ASA. Analyzed the data: JZ, SM, MH. Wrote the paper: JZ, SM. Edited the paper: JH, IP. All authors read and approved the final manuscript.

### Acknowledgements
This study was supported by the EU FP7 large-scale integrating project NanoValid (contract: 263147). The authors acknowledge the support of Dr. Joyce Rodrigues de Araujo (Inmetro, Brazil) for performing the XPS analysis on the Ag NPs.

### Author details
[1]Hearing and Balance Research Unit, Field of Oto-laryngology, School of Medicine, University of Tampere, Medisiinarinkatu 3, 33520 Tampere, Finland. [2]BioMediTech and Department of Electronics and Communications Engineering, Tampere University of Technology, Tampere, Finland. [3]School of Geography, Earth and Environmental Sciences, University of Birmingham, Birmingham, UK. [4]Nanologica AB, Stockholm, Sweden. [5]Department of Otolaryngology-Head and Neck Surgery, Center for Otolaryngology-Head & Neck Surgery of Chinese PLA, Changhai Hospital, Second Military Medical University, Shanghai, China. [6]Department of Medical Physics, Imaging Centre, Tampere University Hospital, Tampere, Finland. [7]Materials Science and Engineering, Indian Institute of Technology-Gandhinagar, Ahmedabad, India.

### References
1. Martinez-Gutierrez F, Boegli L, Agostinho A, Sanchez EM, Bach H, Ruiz F, et al. Anti-biofilm activity of silver nanoparticles against different microorganisms. Biofouling. 2013;29(6):651–60.
2. Doudi M, Naghsh N, Setorki M. Comparison of the effects of silver nanoparticles on pathogenic bacteria resistant to beta-lactam antibiotics (ESBLs) as a prokaryote model and Wistar rats as a eukaryote model. Med Sci Monit Basic Res. 2013;19:103–10.
3. Lu Z, Rong K, Li J, Yang H, Chen R. Size-dependent antibacterial activities of silver nanoparticles against oral anaerobic pathogenic bacteria. J Mater Sci Mater Med. 2013;24(6):1465–71.
4. Pinto RJ, Almeida A, Fernandes SC, Freire CS, Silvestre AJ, Neto CP, et al. Antifungal activity of transparent nanocomposite thin films of pullulan and silver against Aspergillus niger. Colloids Surf B: Biointerfaces. 2013;103:143–8.
5. Xiang D, Zheng Y, Duan W, Li X, Yin J, Shigdar S, et al. Inhibition of A/Human/Hubei/3/2005 (H3N2) influenza virus infection by silver nanoparticles in vitro and in vivo. Int J Nanomedicine. 2013;8:4103–13.
6. Radzig MA, Nadtochenko VA, Koksharova OA, Kiwi J, Lipasova VA, Khmel IA. Antibacterial effects of silver nanoparticles on gram-negative bacteria: influence on the growth and biofilms formation, mechanisms of action. Colloids Surf B: Biointerfaces. 2013;102:300–6.
7. Zhang C, Wang K, Han D, Pang Q. Surface enhanced Raman scattering (SERS) spectra of trinitrotoluene in silver colloids prepared by microwave heating method. Spectrochim Acta A Mol Biomol Spectrosc. 2014;122:387–91.
8. Margolis RH, Hunter LL, Rykken JR, Giebink GS. Effects of otitis media on extended high-frequency hearing in children. Ann Otol Rhinol Laryngol. 1993;102(1 Pt 1):1–5.
9. Papp Z, Rezes S, Jokay I, Sziklai I. Sensorineural hearing loss in chronic otitis media. Otol Neurotol. 2003;24(2):141–4.
10. Luntz M, Yehudai N, Haifler M, Sigal G, Most T. Risk factors for sensorineural hearing loss in chronic otitis media. Acta Otolaryngol. 2013;133(11):1173–80.
11. Mostafa BE, Shafik AG, El Makhzangy AM, Taha H, Abdel Mageed HM. Evaluation of vestibular function in patients with chronic suppurative otitis media. ORL J Otorhinolaryngol Relat Spec. 2013;75(6):357–60.
12. Chang CW, Cheng PW, Young YH. Inner ear deficits after chronic otitis media. Eur Arch Otorhinolaryngol. 2014;271(8):2165–70.
13. Zou J, Pyykkö I, Börje B, Toppila E. In vivo MRI visualization of endolymphatic hydrops induced by keyhole limpet hemocyanin round window immunization. Audiol Med. 2007;5:182–7.
14. Zou J, Pyykkö I. Endolymphatic hydrops in Meniere's disease secondary to otitis media and visualized by gadolinium-enhanced magnetic resonance imaging. World J Otorhinolaryngol. 2013;3(1):22–5.
15. Hall-Stoodley L, Hu FZ, Gieseke A, Nistico L, Nguyen D, Hayes J, et al. Direct detection of bacterial biofilms on the middle-ear mucosa of children with chronic otitis media. Jama. 2006;296(2):202–11.
16. Wessman M, Bjarnsholt T, Eickhardt-Sorensen SR, Johansen HK, Homoe P. Mucosal biofilm detection in chronic otitis media: a study of middle ear biopsies from Greenlandic patients. Eur Arch Otorhinolaryngol. 2014; Jan 30. [Epub ahead of print].
17. Gu X, Keyoumu Y, Long L, Zhang H. Detection of bacterial biofilms in different types of chronic otitis media. Eur Arch Otorhinolaryngol. 2014;271(11):2877–83.
18. Nguyen CT, Robinson SR, Jung W, Novak MA, Boppart SA, Allen JB. Investigation of bacterial biofilm in the human middle ear using optical coherence tomography and acoustic measurements. Hear Res. 2013;301:193–200.
19. Semenov FV, Fidarova KM. The treatment of the patients presenting with chronic inflammation of the trepanation cavity with a preparation containing silver nanoparticles following sanitation surgery of the open type. Vestn Otorinolaringol. 2012;6:117–9.
20. Seifert H, Roher U, Staszyk C, Angrisani N, Dziuba D, Meyer-Lindenberg A. Optimising muCT imaging of the middle and inner cat ear. Anat Histol Embryol. 2012;41(2):113–21.
21. Haghpanahi M, Gladstone MB, Zhu X, Frisina RD, Borkholder DA. Noninvasive technique for monitoring drug transport through the murine cochlea using micro-computed tomography. Ann Biomed Eng. 2013;41(10):2130–42.
22. Karunamuni R, Tsourkas A, Maidment AD. Exploring silver as a contrast agent for contrast-enhanced dual-energy X-ray breast imaging. British J Radiol. 2014;87(1041):20140081.
23. Zou J, Feng H, Mannerström M, Heinonen T, Pyykkö I. Toxicity of silver nanoparticle in rat ear and BALB/c 3T3 cell line. J Nanobiotechnol. 2014;12 (1):52 [Epub ahead of print].
24. Zou J, Poe D, Ramadan UA, Pyykko I. Oval window transport of Gd-dOTA from rat middle ear to vestibulum and scala vestibuli visualized by in vivo magnetic resonance imaging. Ann Otol Rhinol Laryngol. 2012;121(2):119–28.
25. Shi H, Li Y, Yin S, Zou J. The predominant vestibular uptake of gadolinium through the oval window pathway is compromised by endolymphatic hydrops in Meniere's disease. Otol Neurotol. 2014;35(2):315–22.
26. Markowska K, Grudniak AM, Wolska KI. Silver nanoparticles as an alternative strategy against bacterial biofilms. Acta Biochim Pol. 2013;60(4):523–30.

27. Liu H, Wang H, Guo R, Cao X, Zhao J, Luo Y, et al. Size-controlled synthesis of dendrimer-stabilized silver nanoparticles for X-ray computed tomography imaging applications. Polym Chem. 2010;1(10):1677–83.

28. Takemura K, Komeda M, Yagi M, Himeno C, Izumikawa M, Doi T, et al. Direct inner ear infusion of dexamethasone attenuates noise-induced trauma in guinea pig. Hear Res. 2004;196(1-2):58–68.

29. Zou J, Ramadan UA, Pyykko I. Gadolinium uptake in the rat inner ear perilymph evaluated with 4.7 T MRI: a comparison between transtympanic injection and gelatin sponge-based diffusion through the round window membrane. Otol Neurotol. 2010;31(4):637–41.

# 15

# Lactosaminated mesoporous silica nanoparticles for asialoglycoprotein receptor targeted anticancer drug delivery

Guilan Quan[1], Xin Pan[1], Zhouhua Wang[1], Qiaoli Wu[1], Ge Li[2], Linghui Dian[3], Bao Chen[1*] and Chuanbin Wu[1*]

## Abstract

**Background:** Mesoporous silica nanoparticles (MSNs) have several attractive properties as a drug delivery system, such as ordered porous structure, large surface area, controllable particle size as well as interior and exterior dual-functional surfaces. The purpose of this study was to develop novel lactosaminated mesoporous silica nanoparticles (Lac-MSNs) for asialoglycoprotein receptor (ASGPR) targeted anticancer drug delivery.

**Results:** Lac-MSNs with an average diameter of approximately 100 nm were prepared by conjugation of lactose with 3-aminopropyl triethoxysilane modified MSNs. Characterization of Lac-MSNs indicated a huge Brunauer-Emmett-Teller (BET) surface area (1012 $m^2$/g), highly ordered 2D hexagonal symmetry, an unique mesoporous structure with average pore size of 3.7 nm. The confocal microscopy and flow cytometric analysis illustrated Lac-MSNs were effectively endocytosed by ASGPR-positive hepatoma cell lines, HepG2 and SMMC7721. In contrast, non-selective endocytosis of Lac-MSNs was found in ASGPR-negative NIH 3T3 cells. The cellular uptake study showed the internalization process was energy-consuming and predominated by clathrin-mediated pathway. Model drug docetaxel (DTX) was loaded in the mesopores of Lac-MSNs by wetness impregnation method. *In vitro* cytotoxicity assay showed that DTX transported by Lac-MSNs effectively inhibited the growth of HepG2 and SMMC7721 cells in a time- and concentration- dependent manner.

**Conclusions:** These results demonstrated that Lac-MSNs could be a promising inorganic carrier system for targeted intracellular anti-cancer drug delivery.

**Keywords:** Mesoporous silica nanoparticles, Lactose, Asialoglycoprotein receptor, Docetaxel

## Background

In recent years, more than ten million people per year worldwide have suffered from cancers, and cancer is one of the deadliest killers to human being [1]. Currently, systemic chemotherapy is the indispensable treatment for malignant tumors. However, many anticancer drugs have severe toxic side effects due to their unspecific actions on normal cells and tissues [2]. Therefore, development of an effective cancer targeting drug delivery system is extremely necessary for improving the drug efficacy to cancer cells, reducing toxic side effects systematically, and prolonging survivals of patients.

With recent advances in nanotechnology research, nanocarries have shown great potential to improve the therapeutic efficacy while minimize the side effects, especially for highly toxic anticancer drugs [3,4]. It is known that the vascular architecture and the lymphatic system in tumors are impaired and may allow the permeation of macromolecules. So, passive targeting of nanocarriers to these abnormal tumors may be partially achieved with the enhanced permeability and retention (EPR) effect [5,6], leaving the surrounding healthy tissues barely touched. It is expected that the application of nanotechnology would be beneficial to millions of cancer patients with more efficient, safe, and affordable treatment.

Though the common organic nanocarriers including polymeric micelles [7], nanocapsules [8], polymer nanoparticles [9], and liposomes [10] have been extensively studied, their physicochemical instability and undesirable drug

* Correspondence: lsscb@mail.sysu.edu.cn; chuanbin_wu@126.com
[1]School of Pharmaceutical Sciences, Sun Yat-Sen University, Guangzhou 510006, People's Republic of China
Full list of author information is available at the end of the article

leakage have severely impeded their further applications. In contrast, inorganic silicate ($SiO_2$) carriers possess many advantages, such as great physicochemical and biochemical stabilities, good biocompatibility, and excellent degradability [11]. Recently, silica nanoparticles in the form of Cornell dots (C dots) received FDA's approval for stage I human clinical trial [12-14], representing an important step towards clinical acceptance of silica-based nanoparticles.

Among silica-based nanomaterials, mesoporous silica nanoparticles (MSNs) have attracted great attention due to their unique properties, including highly regular mesoporous structure, tunable pore size (2–10 nm), huge surface area (>700 $m^2$/g), large pore volume (>1 $cm^3$/g), excellent endocytotic behavior, and good biocompatibility both *in vitro* and *in vivo* [15-17]. Several chemotherapeutic agents have been successfully delivered by using MSNs as cancer cell-specific delivery vehicles [18-20]. More importantly, the external surface of MSNs can be modified with tumor-recognition molecules to increase the active targetability through the receptor-mediated endocytosis. Several well-known targeting molecules, such as folate [21], mannose [22], hyaluronic acid [23], arginine-glycine-aspartate (RGD) [24], and lactobionic acid [25] have been conjugated to MSNs successfully, resulting in significantly enhanced antitumor efficiency.

Among various targeting ligands, lactose, a glucosyl-galactose disaccharide, shows great promise as a tumor-homing agent, because it has a specific interaction with the asialoglycoprotein receptor (ASGPR) which is a well-characterized molecular target expressed on the cell surface of hepatocytes and hepatomas. ASGPR can actively internalize the bound galactose or galactose-derived complexes via receptor-mediated endocytosis [26,27]. Moreover, due to its low cost, nonimmunogenicity, high stability, and ease for modification, lactose has been recognized as a promising candidate for hepatocellular carcinoma targeting agent. Many researchers have applied lactose to target drug delivery system [28-30]. However, to the best of our knowledge, there is no report on combining lactose with MSNs to construct a drug delivery system for hepatocellular carcinoma targeting.

So, in this study, the targeting property of lactose was integrated with the excellent drug delivery and endocytotic behaviors of MSNs to build a novel drug delivery system, which was expected to possess not only a passive targeting capability via EPR effect but also an active targeting character (Figure 1). Moreover, the internalization mechanism of MSNs by hepatoma cells was investigated to thoroughly understand the efficiency of the lactosaminated MSNs.

## Results and discussion

### Preparation and characterization of MSNs and Lac-MSNs

MSNs were synthesized by the sol–gel method using surfactant as the template. The as-synthesized MSNs prior to removing the template were firstly functionalized with $NH_2$-silane on the outer surface, while leaving the inner pores available for drug loading. After conjugation of MSNs with lactose, the template was removed by refluxing the product in acidic ethanol. In addition, fluorescein isothiocyanate (FITC) as a fluorescent probe was encapsulated in the Lac-MSNs through co-condensation in order to monitor the interaction between the nanoparticles and the cells [31].

The scanning electron microscopy (SEM) and transmission electron microscopy (TEM) images (Figure 2) showed that both MSNs and Lac-MSNs were roughly spherical in shape and uniform in diameter of approximately 100 nm. The mesoporous structure of MSNs was revealed in details by TEM, as the clearly observed bright and dark domains (Figure 2C and D), corresponding to the pores and the silica walls respectively, confirmed the hexagonal arrays of nanochannels. It is known the particle size of nanoparticles plays an important role on pharmacokinetics. Nanoparticles with particle size smaller than 200 nm can generally increase accumulation of anticancer drug in tumor via EPR effect [5]. Though the particle size of Lac-MSNs was measured as approximately 100 nm based on the TEM images, this only represented the size of inorganic silica core, while the organic $NH_2$-silane coating was transparent under TEM observation [32]. Therefore, dynamic light scattering (DLS) was employed to measure the overall size of Lac-MSNs as 170 nm approximately. The difference in particle size obtained from TEM and DLS measurements confirmed the successful deposition of a $NH_2$-silane layer on the nanoparticle surface. These silane-layer coated, well-dispersed, small nanoparticles should be favorable for passive tumor targeting and cellular uptake [32,33].

The mesostructure ordering of nanoparticles was analyzed by X-ray diffraction (XRD) patterns (Figure 3), where three distinct diffraction peaks indexed at (100), (110), and (200) revealed that both MSNs and Lac-MSNs had a highly ordered 2D hexagonal (*P*6mm) symmetry [34]. Nitrogen adsorption-desorption measurements are usually employed to obtain precise information about the structure of porous materials. As shown in Figure 4, both MSNs and Lac-MSNs exhibited the classical type-IV isotherms with H1-type hysteresis. According to the International Union of Pure and Applied Chemistry (IUPAC) classification [35], this suggests that both MSNs and Lac-MSNs have uniform mesoporous channels and relatively narrow pore size distribution (the insert of Figure 4), in consistence with the TEM images and the results of XRD. Moreover, the mean surface area, pore volume, and pore size of MSNs and Lac-MSNs were calculated as 1335 and 1012 $m^2$/g, 1.85 and 1.33 $cm^3$/g, 4.1 and 3.7 nm, respectively.

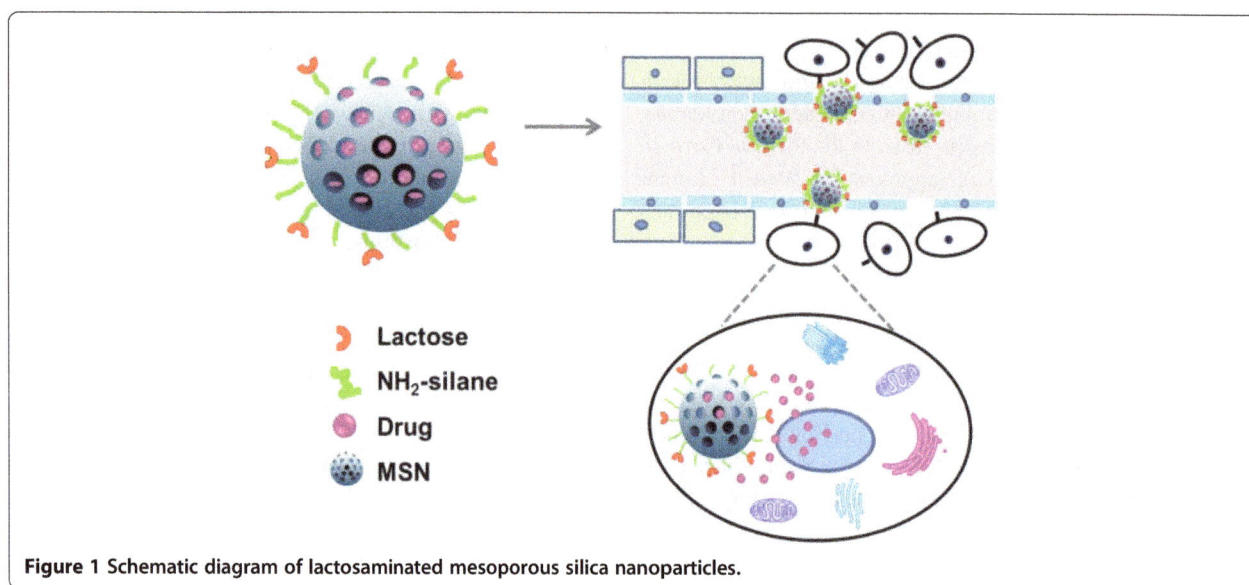

**Figure 1** Schematic diagram of lactosaminated mesoporous silica nanoparticles.

The cationic surfactant cetyltrimethyl ammonium bromide (CTAB) was used as a mesoporous template for synthesis of MSNs and removed through postsynthesis extraction with acidic ethanol. Because the marked cytotoxicity of CTAB was reported by other researchers [36], fourier-transform infrared spectra (FTIR) analysis was carried out to confirm the complete removal of CTAB. Typically,

CTAB shows two intense peaks at 2800–3200 cm$^{-1}$, which correspond to the symmetric (2849 cm$^{-1}$) and asymmetric (2918 cm$^{-1}$) stretching vibrations of the methylene chains (Figure 5). These peaks were observed in as-synthesized MSNs but absent in the extracted MSNs, indicating the complete removal of CTAB through extraction. Moreover, in FTIR spectra the standard silica, as-synthesized MSNs,

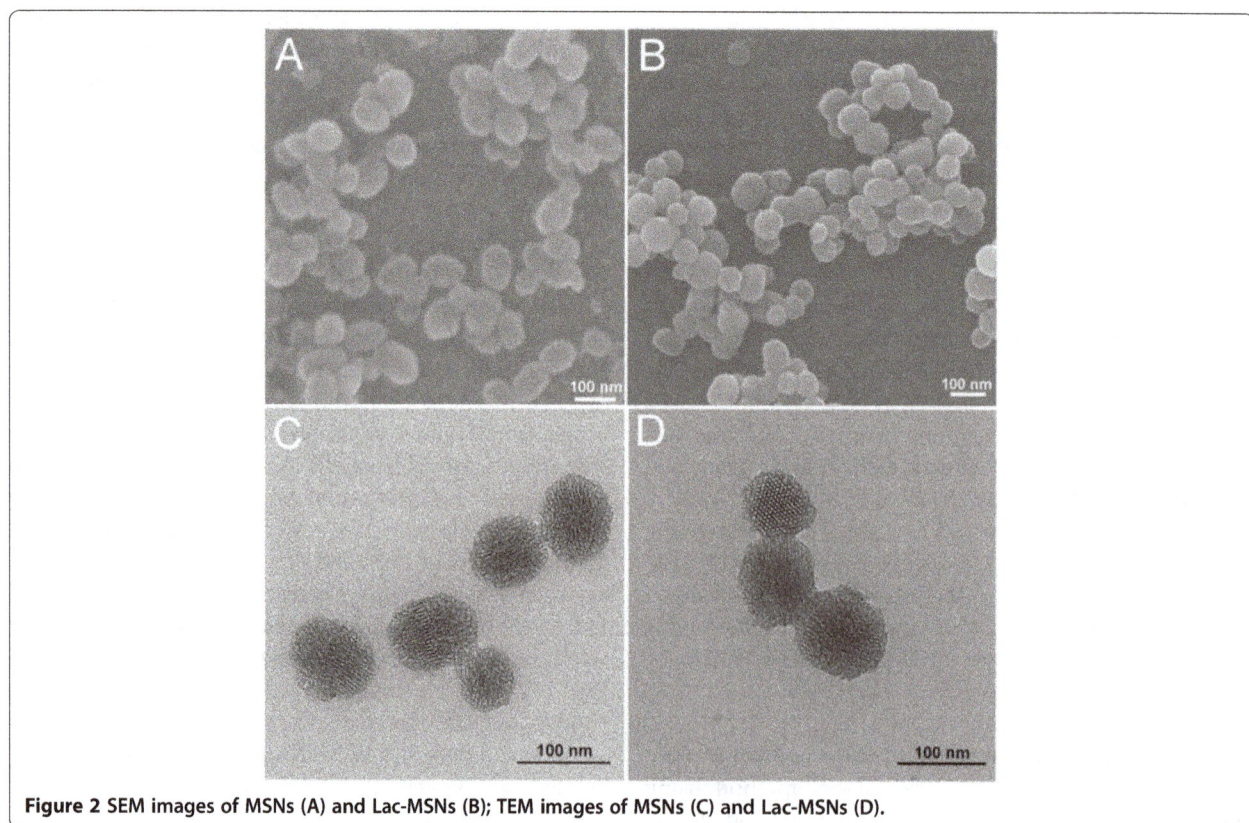

**Figure 2** SEM images of MSNs (A) and Lac-MSNs (B); TEM images of MSNs (C) and Lac-MSNs (D).

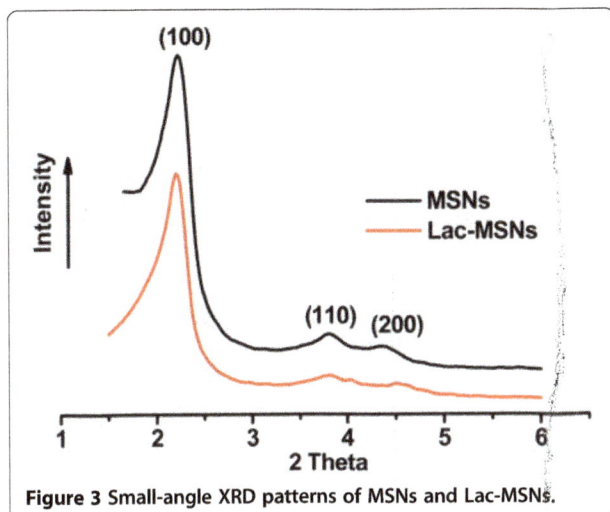

**Figure 3** Small-angle XRD patterns of MSNs and Lac-MSNs.

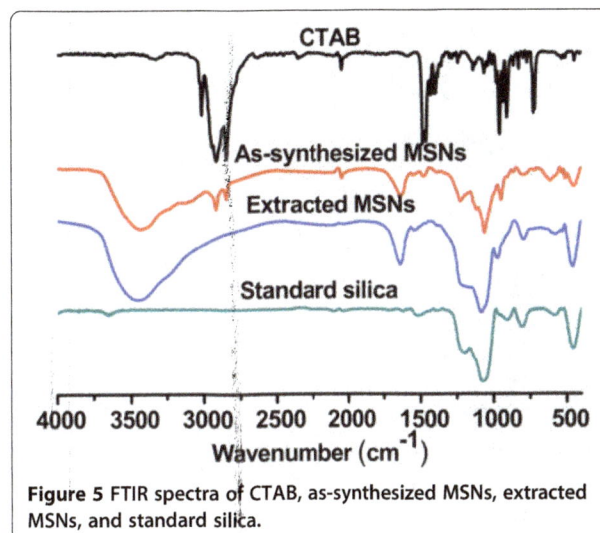

**Figure 5** FTIR spectra of CTAB, as-synthesized MSNs, extracted MSNs, and standard silica.

and extracted MSNs all showed the same characteristic peaks in the region of 400–1800 $cm^{-1}$, indicating the MSNs had the same chemical constituents as the pure silica.

Lactose was conjugated to MSNs through the formation of Schiff base between the aldehyde group on the ring-open form of glucose moiety in lactose and the amino-silane groups in MSNs [28]. Lactose content of 2.11 μg/mg in MSNs was measured by the phenol/sulfuric acid method, indicating an efficient lactose-binding on MSNs was achieved.

## Targeting efficiency of Lac-MSNs

The cellular uptake of FITC labeled nanoparticles was studied on two kinds of ASGPR-positive hepatoma cells HepG2 and SMMC7721, as well as ASGPR-negative fibroblast cells NIH 3T3 via laser scanning confocal microscope (Figure 6). The HepG2 and SMMC7721 cells incubated

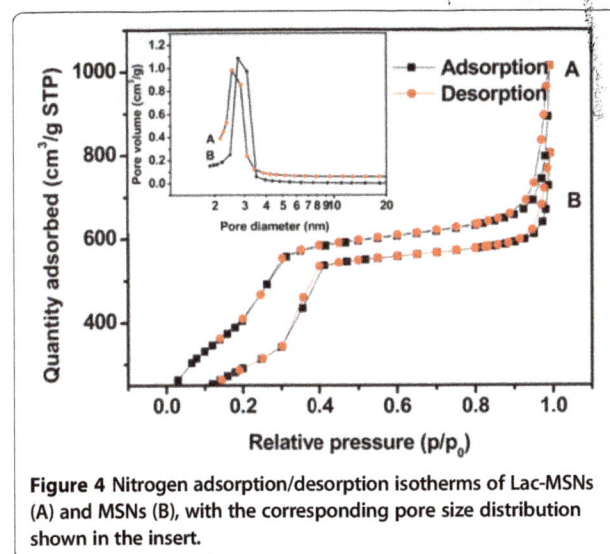

**Figure 4** Nitrogen adsorption/desorption isotherms of Lac-MSNs (A) and MSNs (B), with the corresponding pore size distribution shown in the insert.

with Lac-MSNs showed stronger green appearance than those with MSNs, indicating that lactose modification significantly enhanced the cell uptake by ASGPR-positive cells. However, low cellular uptake by NIH 3T3 cells was observed for both Lac-MSNs and MSNs, suggesting the low affinity between ASGPR-negative cells and nanoparticles. Moreover, the cellular internalization of Lac-MSNs by HepG2 and SMMC7721 cells markedly decreased in the presence of excess free lactose. This corroborates that ASGPR on the membrane of hepatoma cells facilitates the recognition of lactose on Lac-MSNs and increases the cellular uptake through ASGPR-mediated endocytosis.

Flow cytometry was employed to quantitatively evaluate the cellular internalization of nanoparticles. The logarithmic autofluorescence intensity of untreated cells was set between $10^0$ and $10^1$, and any higher fluorescence intensity might indicate the cellular internalization of FITC labeled nanoparticles [2], as the extracellular fluorescence was already quenched by trypan blue solution [36]. As shown in Figure 7, the uptake efficiency for Lac-MSNs was 2.1 and 1.8 times higher than that for MSNs in HepG2 and SMMC7721 cells respectively. Moreover, the presence of excess free lactose markedly decreased the cellular internalization of Lac-MSNs approximately by 30% and 40% in HepG2 and SMMC7721 cells, respectively. This further proved that Lac-MSNs were transported into ASGPR-positive cells via receptor-mediated endocytosis. Consistent with the confocal microscope images, both MSNs and Lac-MSNs showed similar lower cellular uptake efficiency in ASGPR-negative NIH 3T3 cells.

Therefore, our hypothesis that lactosaminated MSNs might have a greater ability to actively target the hepatoma cells through ASGPR expressed on the cell surface was proved, and the Lac-MSNs could serve as nanoreservoirs for targeted drug delivery.

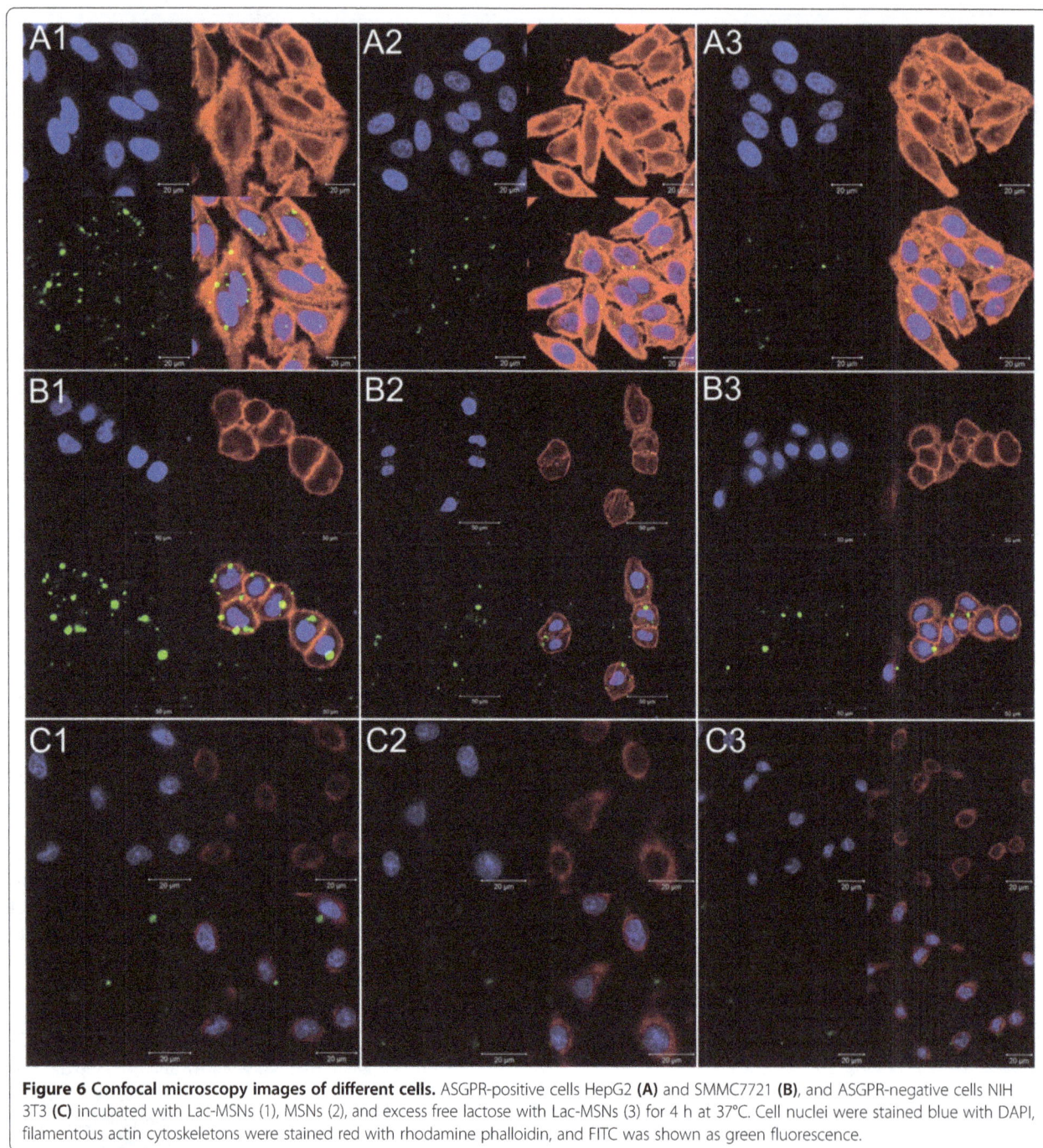

**Figure 6 Confocal microscopy images of different cells.** ASGPR-positive cells HepG2 **(A)** and SMMC7721 **(B)**, and ASGPR-negative cells NIH 3T3 **(C)** incubated with Lac-MSNs (1), MSNs (2), and excess free lactose with Lac-MSNs (3) for 4 h at 37°C. Cell nuclei were stained blue with DAPI, filamentous actin cytoskeletons were stained red with rhodamine phalloidin, and FITC was shown as green fluorescence.

## Mechanism for nanoparticle uptake

Bio-TEM observation on the ultrathin sections of HepG2 cells after being treated with Lac-MSNs for varying time was used to explore the process of cellular uptake and intracellular trafficking. Firstly, a part of Lac-MSNs were found near the cell membrane, interacting with the cell surface and inducing the cell membrane invagination after 10 min of treatment (Figure 8A). Then the cell membrane pinched off to form endocytic vesicles which carried the nanoparticles into the cytoplasm at 1 h (Figure 8B). After uptake by cancer cells via endocytosis at 4 h, the nanoparticles were processed in endosomes, as clearly marked by the circle in Figure 8C. The membrane of endosome surrounding the clumpy nanoparticles finally broke to release the nanoparticles at 24 h (Figure 8D) [37]. This step is very important, because the drug can only be released into cytoplasm after the delivery vesicle escapes from the endosome. Moreover, a large number of MSNs

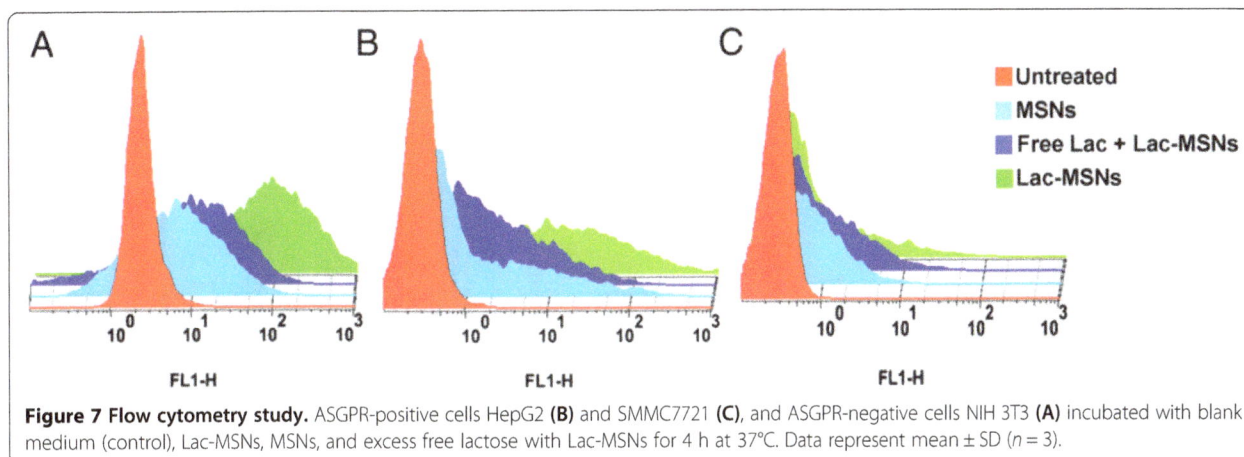

**Figure 7 Flow cytometry study.** ASGPR-positive cells HepG2 **(B)** and SMMC7721 **(C)**, and ASGPR-negative cells NIH 3T3 **(A)** incubated with blank medium (control), Lac-MSNs, MSNs, and excess free lactose with Lac-MSNs for 4 h at 37°C. Data represent mean ± SD ($n = 3$).

found in the cytoplasm maintained their spherical morphology, and no nanocarriers were found in the nucleus at 24 h, which is consistent with the literature [38,39].

The influence of incubation temperature on the cellular uptake of Lac-MSNs was also studied. As shown in Figure 9, incubation of cells with Lac-MSNs at 4°C significantly impeded the uptake, resulting in approximately 90% less uptake than that of control incubated at 37°C. This indicates that the cellular uptake of Lac-MSNs requires an appropriate temperature, and endocytosis is an energy-dependent process rather than a passive diffusion.

Furthermore, a series of inhibition experiments were conducted on HepG2 cells to explore the role of specific endocytotic pathways involving in the cellular internalization. The influence of various pharmacological inhibitors on the cellular uptake of Lac-MSNs was also investigated. Sodium azide, which is widely used as an inhibitor of cellular oxidative respiration, acts by inhibiting cytochrome C oxidase and thereby blocking the cellular adenosine triphosphate (ATP) synthesis [40]. Chlorpromazine is used to inhibit the clathrin-mediated endocytosis by inhibiting the formation of clathrin vesicles. Nystatin binds sterols and disrupts the formation of caveolae, leading to inhibition of caveolae-mediated endocytosisn [41]. Colchicine is an inhibitor of non-clathrin non-caveolae-dependent endocytosis. As shown in Figure 9, the presence of sodium

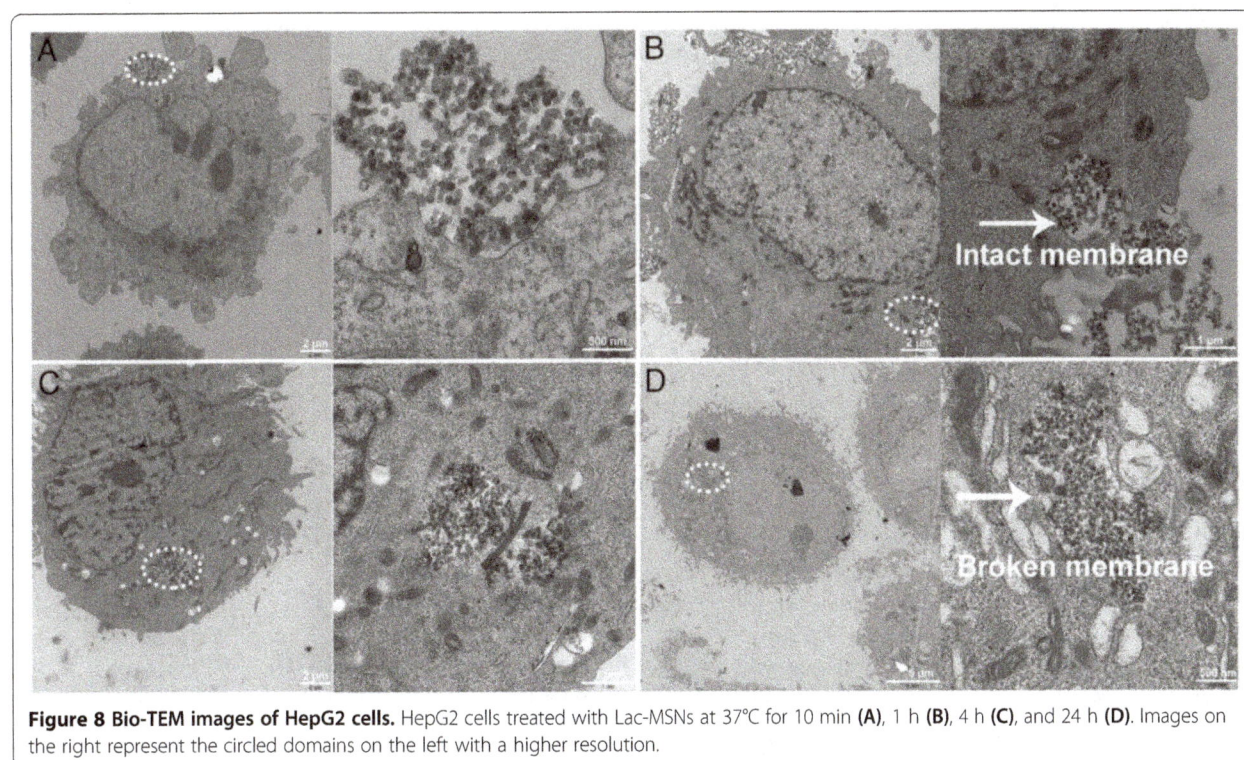

**Figure 8 Bio-TEM images of HepG2 cells.** HepG2 cells treated with Lac-MSNs at 37°C for 10 min **(A)**, 1 h **(B)**, 4 h **(C)**, and 24 h **(D)**. Images on the right represent the circled domains on the left with a higher resolution.

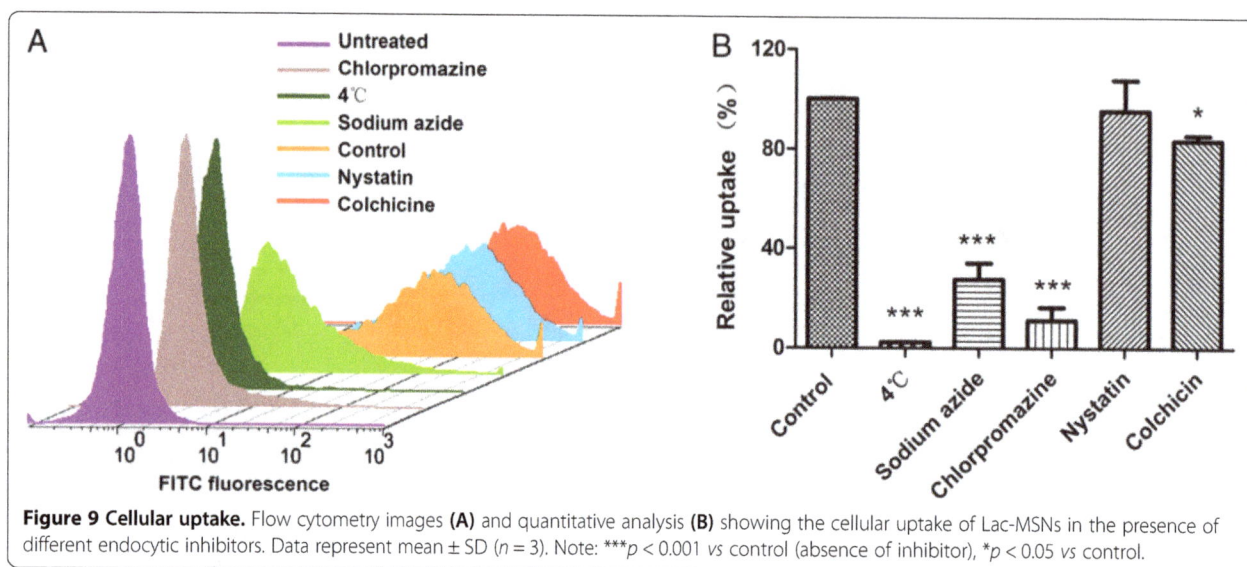

**Figure 9 Cellular uptake.** Flow cytometry images **(A)** and quantitative analysis **(B)** showing the cellular uptake of Lac-MSNs in the presence of different endocytic inhibitors. Data represent mean ± SD ($n = 3$). Note: ***$p < 0.001$ *vs* control (absence of inhibitor), *$p < 0.05$ *vs* control.

azide significantly decreased the cellular uptake of Lac-MSNs approximately by 70%, indicating that the uptake is energy-dependent. Compared with the uptake at 4°C, the cellular uptake with the presence of sodium azide was apparently higher, which is probably because of the presence of exogenous ATP and glucose in the media [42]. Similarly, the presence of chlorpromazine and colchicine decreased the cellular uptake of Lac-MSNs approximately by 80% and 20% respectively. In contrast, HepG2 cells pretreated with nystatin showed negligible reduction in uptake. Therefore, the results suggested that endocytosis of Lac-MSNs into HepG2 cells was an energy-dependent process predominated by clathrin-mediated endocytosis, and non-clathrin non-caveolae-dependent endocytosis may represent an additional endocytotic route. This is consistent with the reported literature [41-43], in which the endocytosis mechanism of MSNs by A549, KB, and 3T3 cells was investigated.

### Drug loading and *in vitro* release of DTX

One critical challenge for cancer therapy is the limited availability of effective carriers for most hydrophobic anticancer drugs. In this study, hydrophobic anticancer drug DTX was successfully loaded into the channels of MSNs, obtaining drug loading of 10.1 and 12.4 nmol in 1 mg of Lac-MSNs and MSNs respectively as determined by high performance liquid chromatography (HPLC). The cumulative DTX release profiles from DTX-MSNs and DTX-Lac-MSNs in phosphate buffered saline (PBS) at 37°C are shown in Figure 10. Only 20% of DTX was released from DTX-Lac-MSNs at 10 h, showing a slower release rate as compared with DTX-MSNs. Moreover, it took 96 h for DTX-Lac-MSNs to release 80% of drug, whereas DTX-MSNs only needed half of the time. It has been reported that modifying the

surface of mesoporous silica materials could restrict water diffusing into the matrix and subsequently slow down the release process [44]. So, the reduced drug release rate noted for DTX-Lac-MSNs can be explained by surface modification.

### *In vitro* cytotoxicity of DTX loaded nanoparticles

The biosafety of the drug carriers must be taken into consideration before application. Herein, MSNs and Lac-MSNs were incubated with HepG2, SMMC7721, and NIH 3T3 cells for 72 h at a broad concentration range of 10–200 μg/ml and their cytotoxicity was evaluated via MTT assay. As shown in Figure 11, both MSNs and Lac-MSNs showed negligible cytotoxicity in spite of sample concentration and cell species, as the cell viabilities all remained above 90%.

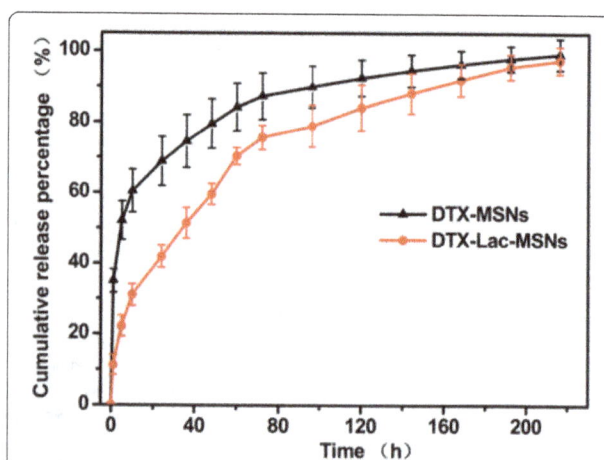

**Figure 10 *In vitro* Drug release.** Release profiles of DTX from DTX-MSNs and DTX-Lac-MSNs in PBS at 37°C. Data represent mean ± SD ($n = 3$).

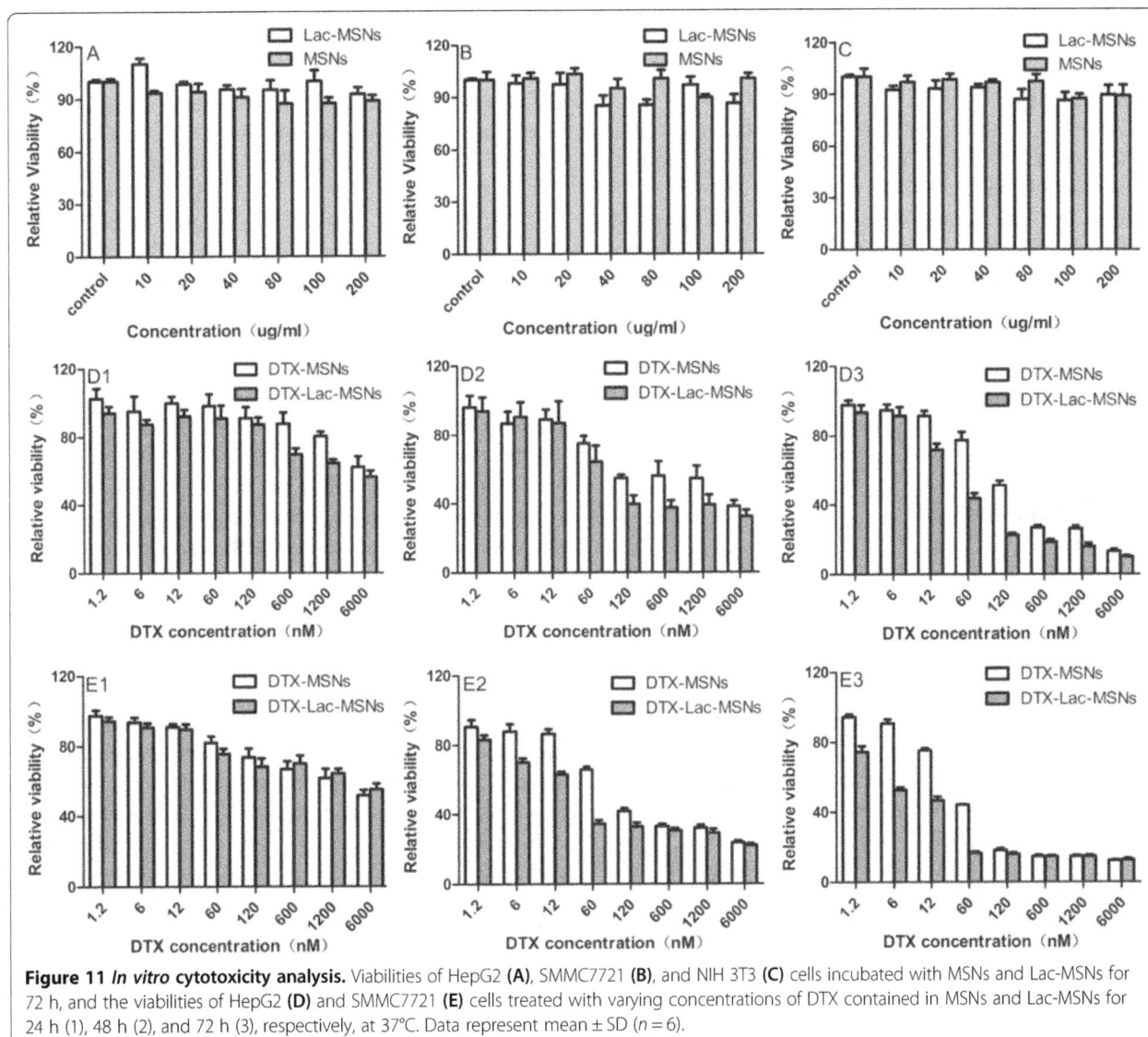

**Figure 11** *In vitro* **cytotoxicity analysis.** Viabilities of HepG2 **(A)**, SMMC7721 **(B)**, and NIH 3T3 **(C)** cells incubated with MSNs and Lac-MSNs for 72 h, and the viabilities of HepG2 **(D)** and SMMC7721 **(E)** cells treated with varying concentrations of DTX contained in MSNs and Lac-MSNs for 24 h (1), 48 h (2), and 72 h (3), respectively, at 37°C. Data represent mean ± SD (*n* = 6).

The *in vitro* cytotoxicity of DTX-Lac-MSNs and DTX-MSNs against both HepG2 and SMMC7721 cells was measured to assess their specific tumor targeting effect. It was found the cytotoxicity of DTX-Lac-MSNs and DTX-MSNs was strongly dependent on the drug concentration and treatment time. After 48 and 72 h treatment, both HepG2 and SMMC7721 cells exhibited appreciable level of cell death. Further calculation was performed to determine concentrations needed to cause 50% inhibition (IC50). As shown in Table 1, the IC50 values were much lower for DTX-Lac-MSNs than for DTX-MSNs against two kinds of human hepatoma cell lines (*p* < 0.05). These results suggested that Lac-MSNs transported DTX into hepatoma cells more effectively than MSNs, resulting in distinctly enhanced cytotoxicity, which was correlated to the aforementioned enhanced cellular uptake. Therefore,

**Table 1** *In vitro* **cytotoxicity of drug loaded nanoparticles**

| Cells | Treatment | IC50 (nM) | |
|---|---|---|---|
| | Time (h) | DTX-MSNs | DTX-Lac-MSNs |
| HepG2 | 24 | — | — |
| | 48 | 122.43 ± 8.02 | 51.6 ± 5.51* |
| | 72 | 117.04 ± 20.38 | 31.55 ± 6.35* |
| SMMC7721 | 24 | — | — |
| | 48 | 72.77 ± 11.14 | 16.65 ± 3.31* |
| | 72 | 32.61 ± 6.24 | 10.51 ± 1.01* |

IC50 values of DTX-MSNs and DTX-Lac-MSNs against HepG2 and SMMC7721 cells after 24, 48 and 72 h of treatment. Data represent mean ± SD (*n* = 6).
*Significantly different from DTX-MSNs according to a Student's *t*-test and Mann–Whitney *U* test (*p* < 0.05).

Lac-MSNs may potentially be used as vehicles for loading anticancer drugs and targeted cancer therapy.

## Conclusions

In summary, a hepatoma targeting drug delivery system was successfully constructed by conjugation of mesoporous silica nanoparticles with the active targeting agent lactose. The Lac-MSNs were demonstrated to specifically target ASGPR-positive HepG2 and SMMC7721 cells, and their internalization into hepatoma cells is an energy-consuming process and predominated by clathrin-mediated endocytosis. Water insoluble anticancer drug DTX was effectively loaded in the pores of Lac-MSNs, showing significantly enhanced cytotoxicity. Therefore, Lac-MSNs provide a promising approach for targeted intracellular anti-cancer drug delivery.

## Materials and methods

### Materials

Docetaxel (DTX, purity > 99%) was purchased from Yikangsida Med. Tech. Ltd. (Beijing, China). Lactose monohydrate and sodium cyanoborohydride were obtained from Aladdin (Shanghai, China). Cetyltrimethyl ammonium bromide (CTAB), tetraethoxysilane (TEOS), (3-aminopropyl) triethoxysilane (APTES), 3-(4,5-dimethylthiazol-2-yl)-2,5-diphenyltetrazolium bromide (MTT), 4',6-diamidino-2-phenylindole (DAPI), phalloidin-tetramethylrhodamine B isothiocyanate conjugate (rhodamine phalloidin), and fluorescein isothiocyanate (FITC) were purchased from Sigma-Aldrich (St Louis, MO, USA). Propidium iodide (PI) and Hoechst 33258 were obtained from MP Biomed. (Santa Ana, USA). Chlorpromazine, nystatin, colchicines, and sodium azide were obtained from Yuelai Med. Tech. Ltd. (Xi'an, China). Dulbecco's modified Eagle's medium (DMEM), trypsin-EDTA, fetal bovine serum (FBS), and penicillin-streptomycin were acquired from GIBCO (Gaithersburg, MD, USA). All other reagents used were of analytical grade.

Human hepatoma cell lines HepG2 and SMMC7721, and mouse embryonic fibroblast cell line NIH 3T3 were obtained from Shanghai Institute of Cell Biology (Chinese Academy of Sciences, Shanghai, China). The cells were cultured in Dulbecco's modified eagle's medium (DMEM) supplemented with 10% fetal bovine serum and 100 U/mL of penicillin-streptomycin, and maintained at 37°C in a humidified incubator containing 5% $CO_2$. The media were changed every 2 days prior to experimental operation.

### Methods

#### Synthesis of MSNs

Mesoporous silica nanoparticles were synthesized in alkaline media using CTAB as the template and TEOS as silicon source according to Zink's report with minor modification [45]. Briefly, 11 mg of FITC was dissolved in 6 mL of absolute ethanol and then 24 μL of 3-aminopropyl triethoxysilane (APTES) was added in. The solution reacted in the dark for 2 h and then 5 mL of TEOS was added. In another three-necked flask, 1.0 g of CTAB and 0.28 g of sodium hydroxide were dissolved in 480 mL of water, and the resulting mixture was constantly stirred at 80°C till CTAB was completely dissolved and the temperature became stable. Subsequently, the mixture of TEOS and FITC-APTES was added dropwise in the flask, and 2 h later, the particles were collected by centrifugation, washed with water till the filtrate was neutral, and rinsed twice with alcohol before dried at 60°C.

#### Synthesis of lactosaminated MSNs (Lac-MSNs)

Briefly, 1 g of MSNs were dispersed in 150 mL of toluene, followed by adding 2 mL of $NH_2$-silane (APTES) and reaction for 4 h at 120°C. Then the obtained particles were centrifuged, washed with absolute ethanol, and dried at 60°C. Subsequently, 500 mg of the dried nanoparticles were mixed with 6 mL of lactose solution (0.34 g/L) and 6 mL of sodium cyanoborohydride solution (0.31 g/L) sequentially. With gentle shaking several times daily, the mixture was allowed to react for 7 days. Finally, the Lac-MSNs were centrifuged, washed with water to remove the unconjugated lactose, and dried at 60°C. To further remove the template, 500 mg of dry nanoparticles were redispersed in 100 mL of absolute ethanol containing 2 mL of concentrated hydrochloric acid and refluxed for 24 h. Then the particles were collected and washed to remove the template.

### Characterization of MSNs

The morphology of MSNs was characterized by SEM (JSM-6330 F, JEOL, Japan). The samples were sputter-coated with gold for two cycles prior to imaging. Mesostructure of the nanoparticles was observed by TEM (JEM-1400, JEOL, Japan) with a drop of dispersed sample solution being deposited on a carbon-coated copper grid and dried at room temperature before examination. The particle size of MSNs was measured at 25°C by dynamic light scattering at a scattering angle of 90° using Zetasizer Nano ZS90 (Malvern Instruments, Worcestershire, UK). The mesostructure ordering was analyzed by small-angle X-ray diffraction (SAXRD, D/MAX 2200 VPC, Tokyo, Japan) using Cu Kα radiation with 2θ in the range of 0.6°-6° at a scanning rate of 0.5°/min. Brunauer-Emmett-Teller (BET) surface area, pore volume and diameter distribution of MSNs were measured at −196°C by using a surface area and pore size analyzer (ASAP 2020C, Micromeritics, USA). FTIR spectra of MSNs were obtained by using a FTIR spectrophotometer (Bruker, German) to scan over a region of 400–4000 $cm^{-1}$ on a thin KBr slice containing MSNs.

## Lactose content in Lac-MSNs

Lactose content was measured by the phenol/sulfuric acid method [46]. Since the secondary amine formed between amino-MSNs and glucosyl by reductive amination is acid-stable, only galactose is produced during the hydrolysis [47]. Briefly, 2 mL of standard galactose solution at various concentrations, 1 mL of phenol (5%), and 4 mL of concentrated sulfuric acid were added in a tube. The tube was sealed and allowed to react for 15 min, and the absorbance after reaction was measured at 490 nm to build a standard curve. Then, dispersion of Lac-MSNs (50 mg) in deionized water (2 mL) was treated similarly, the absorbance was measured and the lactose content was calculated according to the standard curve.

## Confocal microscopy study

The cellular uptake of nanoparticles was visualized by confocal microscopy [36]. HepG2, SMMC7721, and NIH 3T3 cells were seeded at $1 \times 10^5$ per dish in special glass dishes and allowed to attach for 24 h. Then, Lac-MSNs and MSNs suspensions in DMEM at a final concentration of 50 μg/mL were added in. After 4 h of incubation, the medium was removed and the cells were washed with cold PBS (pH 7.4) three times. Trypan blue PBS solution (0.4%) was added to quench any fluorescence outside the cells for 10 min. Afterwards, the cells were fixed with 4% paraformaldehyde at room temperature for 10 min and extracted with 0.1% Triton X-100 in PBS for 3 min. Subsequently, the filamentous actin cytoskeleton was stained with 200 ng/mL rhodamine phalloidin for 20 min, followed the nuclei staining with DAPI for 10 min. Finally, the samples were analyzed with the laser scanning confocal microscope (LSCM, Zessi LSM 710, Germany).

## Flow cytometry study

Cellular uptake was quantitatively analyzed by flow cytometry. HepG2, SMMC7721, and NIH 3T3 cells were seeded into 12-well plates at the density of $2 \times 10^5$ cells per well and allowed to attach for 24 h. Then, Lac-MSNs and MSNs suspensions in DMEM at a final concentration of 50 μg/mL were added in for cell incubation. After 4 h of incubation, the medium was removed and 0.4% trypan blue PBS solution was added to neutralize the extracellular fluorescence. Then the cells were harvested by trypsinization, collected by centrifugation, and resuspended in 4% paraformaldehyde PBS solution. Finally, the collected cells were analyzed by a Beckman Coulter EPICS XL flow cytometer (Beckman Coulter, Fullerton, CA, USA). The regular DMEM was applied as the blank control. All the tests were performed in triplicate.

In order to assess the competitive uptake efficacy, the cells were preincubated with 50 μg/mL of excessive free lactose for 30 min at 37°C. Then 50 μg/mL of Lac-MSNs were added for incubation at 37°C for another 4 h. Following the similar procedures above, the fluorescent images were taken with confocal microscopy and the quantitative results were measured by flow cytometer.

## Cell transmission electron microscopy (TEM)

Bio-TEM observation was performed on ultrathin sections of HepG2 cells after being treated with Lac-MSNs to reveal the endocytic process of the nanoparticles into cancer cells and their intracellular locations [48]. Cells were seeded into 12-well plates at the density of $2 \times 10^5$ cells per well and allowed to attach for 24 h. Then Lac-MSNs were added in for incubation at 37°C for 10 min, 1 h, 4 h, and 24 h. After that, the cells were harvested and centrifuged at 4000 rpm for 1 min, immediately fixed with 2.5% glutaraldehyde solution in PBS for at least 1 h, post-fixed with 1% aqueous osmium tetroxide for another hour, dehydrated by ethanol series, washed three times with acetone, and embedded in Spurr resin medium overnight. Ultrathin sections of the cells were obtained by 300 mesh copper grids and contrasted with 0.3% lead citrate and 50% uranyl acetate. Finally, the samples were visualized with TEM.

## Endocytosis-inhibition experiments

A series of endocytosis-inhibition experiments were performed on HepG2 cells to further investigate the endocytosis mechanism of Lac-MSNs as follows [41,42]. Cells were cultured in a 12-well plate at the density of $2 \times 10^5$ cells per well for 24 h. First, the cells were pretreated with various endocytosis inhibitors for 30 min, including chlorpromazine (20 μg/mL) for inhibition of clathrin-mediated endocytosis, nystatin (30 μg/mL) for inhibition of caveolae-mediated endocytosis, colchicine (20 μg/mL) for inhibition of non-clathrin non-caveolae-dependent endocytosis, and sodium azide (3 mg/mL) for ATP. Then the medium was replaced with 50 μg/mL Lac-MSNs suspension. After incubation at 37°C for 4 h, the cells were harvested and analyzed by flow cytometer. Another uptake study was performed similarly at 4°C for inhibition of cell respiration to further determine whether the uptake of Lac-MSNs into human hepatoma cells was energy-dependent. All the tests were performed in triplicate.

## Drug loading and release study

Model drug DTX was loaded in the pores of the nanoparticles by wetness impregnation method [21]. MSNs and Lac-MSNs (100 mg each) were added to 5 mL of ethanol solution containing 5 mg/mL of DTX, respectively. Magnetic stirring was applied at room temperature for 24 h to maximize drug loading in the pores. Then the drug-loaded nanoparticles (DTX-MSNs and DTX-Lac-MSNs) were collected by centrifugation, washed twice with PBS to remove the free drug on the particle surface, and dried under vacuum.

The drug-loaded nanoparticles (10 mg) were resuspended in methanol because of the high solubility of DTX in methanol to determine the amount of drug actually loaded in the nanoparticles. The suspension was sonicated to dissolve DTX from the pores, and then the supernatant was collected by centrifugation. This process was repeated twice to ensure the loaded drug was completely removed from the pores. The concentration of DTX in the supernatant was determined by HPLC (Daojing, Japan).

Pretreated dialysis bags with dialyzer molecular weight cutoff 14,000 Da were used in the drug release experiments. DTX-MSNs and DTX-Lac-MSNs samples (20 mg each) were dispersed in 2 mL of PBS, and the solutions were placed into the pretreated dialysis bags. The sealed bags were immersed in 10 mL of PBS and shaken at 100 rpm at 37°C. The release medium was taken and replaced with fresh medium at given time intervals. Each release study was performed in triplicate. The concentration of DTX in samples was measured by HPLC.

## Cytotoxicity study

The cytotoxicity of MSNs, Lac-MSNs, DTX, DTX-MSNs, and DTX-Lac-MSNs was evaluated against HepG2 and SMMC7721 cells by MTT viability assay. Cells were seeded in 96-well plates at a density of $5 \times 10^3$ cells per well. After incubation in 5% $CO_2$ at 37°C for 24 h, the medium was replaced with 200 µL of fresh medium containing different concentrations of samples. Cells treated with pure medium were used as the blank control. After incubation with the samples for 24, 48, and 72 h, the medium was replaced with 20 µL of MTT (5 mg/mL) and 180 µL of fresh medium for another 4 h of incubation at 37°C. Finally, 150 µL of DMSO was added in each cell to dissolve the purple formazan crystals and the absorbance was measured at 490 nm by an ELX 800 micro-plate reader. The cytotoxicity was calculated as the percentage of cell viability as compared with the blank control, and data were expressed as mean ± standard deviation (SD) of six independent wells. The IC50 values of different formulations were calculated via nonlinear regression of the log(dose)-response profiles using GraphPad Prism 5.

## Statistical analysis

IC50 values of DTX-MSNs and DTX-Lac-MSNs were compared using the Student's $t$-test and Mann–Whitney $U$ test following normality and equal variance tests (SPSS 13.0). Statistical analysis of the effects of various pharmacological inhibitors on the cellular uptake of Lac-MSNs was performed using a one-way ANOVA (SPSS 13.0). The post-hoc comparisons of the means of individual groups were performed using least significant difference test. Differences were considered significant if $P < 0.05$.

## Abbreviations

MSNs: Mesoporous silica nanoparticles; Lac: Lactose; Lac-MSNs: Lactosaminated mesoporous silica nanoparticles; ASGPR: Asialoglycoprotein receptor; DTX: Docetaxel; CTAB: Cetyltrimethyl ammonium bromide; TEOS: Tetraethoxysilane; APTES: 3-Aminopropyl triethoxysilane; DAPI: 4',6-diamidino-2-phenylindole; FITC: Fluorescein isothiocyanate; SEM: Scanning electron microscopy; TEM: Transmission electron microscopy; XRD: X-ray diffraction; MTT: 3-(4,5-dimethylthiazol-2-yl)-2,5-diphenyltetrazolium bromide; DLS: dynamic light scattering; FTIR: Fourier-transform infrared spectra.

## Competing interests

The authors declare that they have no competing interests.

## Authors' contributions

GQ performed the majority of the experiments and wrote the manuscript with XP and ZW. XP, ZW and QW assisted to prepare the formulations and evaluate the physical characteristics. LD helped to perform the confocal microscopy study. BC and CW designed the overall project, supervised the whole work, and finalized the manuscript. GL revised the whole manuscript critically. All authors read and approved the final manuscript.

## Acknowledgements

The authors appreciate financial support from the National Natural Science Foundation of China (81173002), the National Science and Technology Pillar Program (2012BAI35B02), and the International Cooperation and Exchanges Program of China (2008DFA31080).

## Author details

[1]School of Pharmaceutical Sciences, Sun Yat-Sen University, Guangzhou 510006, People's Republic of China. [2]Guangzhou Neworld Pharmaceutical Ltd. Co., Guangzhou 510006, People's Republic of China. [3]School of Pharmaceutical Sciences, Guangdong Medical College, Dongguan 523808, People's Republic of China.

## References

1. Jemal A, Center MM, DeSantis C, Ward EM. Global patterns of cancer incidence and mortality rates and trends. Cancer Epidem Biomar. 2010;19:1893–907.
2. Wu HX, Zhang SJ, Zhang JM, Liu G, Shi JL, Zhang LX, et al. A hollow-core, magnetic, and mesoporous double-shell nanostructure: in situ decomposition/reduction synthesis, bioimaging, and drug-delivery properties. Adv Funct Mater. 2011;21:1850–62.
3. Barreto JA, O'Malley W, Kubeil M, Graham B, Stephan H, Spiccia L. Nanomaterials: applications in cancer imaging and therapy. Adv Mater. 2011;23:H18–40.
4. Shi D, Bedford NM, Cho HS. Engineered multifunctional nanocarriers for cancer diagnosis and therapeutics. Small. 2011;7:2549–67.
5. Maeda H, Wu J, Sawa T, Matsumura Y, Hori K. Tumor vascular permeability and the EPR effect in macromolecular therapeutics: a review. J Control Release. 2000;65:271–84.
6. Xiao K, Luo J, Fowler WL, Li Y, Lee JS, Xing L, et al. A self-assembling nanoparticle for paclitaxel delivery in ovarian cancer. Biomaterials. 2009;30:6006–16.
7. Khosroushahi AY, Naderi-Manesh H, Yeganeh H, Barar J, Omidi Y. Novel water-soluble polyurethane nanomicelles for cancer chemotherapy: physicochemical characterization and cellular activities. J Nanobiotech. 2012;10:2.
8. Vonarbourg A, Passirani C, Desigaux L, Allard E, Saulnier P, Lambert O, et al. The encapsulation of DNA molecules within biomimetic lipid nanocapsules. Biomaterials. 2009;30:3197–204.
9. Zhou J, Pishko MV, Lutkenhaus JL. Thermoresponsive layer-by-layer assemblies for nanoparticle-based drug delivery. Langmuir. 2014;30:5903–10.
10. Muthu MS, Kulkarni SA, Raju A, Feng SS. Theranostic liposomes of TPGS coating for targeted co-delivery of docetaxel and quantum dots. Biomaterials. 2012;33:3494–501.

11. Wang X, Li X, Ito A, Sogo Y, Ohno T. Particle-size-dependent toxicity and immunogenic activity of mesoporous silica-based adjuvants for tumor immunotherapy. Acta Biomater. 2013;9:7480–9.

12. Mamaeva V, Sahlgren C, Linden M. Mesoporous silica nanoparticles in medicine-recent advances. Adv Drug Deliver Rev. 2013;65:689–702.

13. Benezra M, Penate-Medina O, Zanzonico PB, Schaer D, Ow H, Burns A, et al. Multimodal silica nanoparticles are effective cancer-targeted probes in a model of human melanoma. J Clin Invest. 2011;121:2768–80.

14. Ow H, Larson DR, Srivastava M, Baird BA, Webb WW, Wiesner U. Bright and stable core-shell fluorescent silica nanoparticles. Nano Lett. 2005;5:113–7.

15. He QJ, Shi JL, Zhu M, Chen Y, Chen F. The three-stage in vitro degradation behavior of mesoporous silica in simulated body fluid. Micropor Mesopor Mat. 2010;131:314–20.

16. Liu T, Li L, Teng X, Huang X, Liu H, Chen D, et al. Single and repeated dose toxicity of mesoporous hollow silica nanoparticles in intravenously exposed mice. Biomaterials. 2011;32:1657–68.

17. Zhang Q, Neoh KG, Xu LQ, Lu SJ, Kang ET, Mahendran R, et al. Functionalized mesoporous silica nanoparticles with mucoadhesive and sustained drug release properties for potential bladder cancer therapy. Langmuir. 2014;30:6151–61.

18. He Q, Gao Y, Zhang L, Zhang Z, Gao F, Ji X, et al. A pH-responsive mesoporous silica nanoparticles-based multi-drug delivery system for overcoming multi-drug resistance. Biomaterials. 2011;32:7711–20.

19. Lu J, Liong M, Zink JI, Tamanoi F. Mesoporous silica nanoparticles as a delivery system for hydrophobic anticancer drugs. Small. 2007;3:1341–6.

20. Li L, Tang F, Liu H, Liu T, Hao N, Chen D, et al. In vivo delivery of silica nanorattle encapsulated docetaxel for liver cancer therapy with low toxicity and high efficacy. ACS NANO. 2010;4:6874–82.

21. Liong M, Lu J, Kovochich M, Xia T, Ruehm SG, Nel AE, et al. Multifunctional inorganic nanoparticles for imaging, targeting, and drug delivery. ACS NANO. 2008;2:889–96.

22. Brevet D, Gary-Bobo M, Raehm L, Richeter S, Hocine O, Amro K, et al. Mannose-targeted mesoporous silica nanoparticles for photodynamic therapy. Chem Commun (Camb). 2009;12:1475–7.

23. Ma M, Chen HR, Chen Y, Zhang K, Wang X, Cui XZ, et al. Hyaluronic acid-conjugated mesoporous silica nanoparticles: excellent colloidal dispersity in physiological fluids and targeting efficacy. J Mater Chem. 2012;22:5615–21.

24. Fang IJ, Slowing II, Wu KC, Lin VS, Trewyn BG. Ligand conformation dictates membrane and endosomal trafficking of arginine-glycine-aspartate (RGD)-functionalized mesoporous silica nanoparticles. Chemistry. 2012;18:7787–92.

25. Luo Z, Cai K, Hu Y, Zhao L, Liu P, Duan L, et al. Mesoporous silica nanoparticles end-capped with collagen: redox-responsive nanoreservoirs for targeted drug delivery. Angew Chem Int Edit. 2011;50:640–3.

26. Kim KS, Lei Y, Stolz DB, Liu D. Bifunctional compounds for targeted hepatic gene delivery. Gene Ther. 2007;14:704–8.

27. Wu J, Nantz MH, Zern MA. Targeting hepatocytes for drug and gene delivery: emerging novel approaches and applications. Front Biosci. 2002;7:d717–25.

28. Huang G, Diakur J, Xu Z, Wiebe LI. Asialoglycoprotein receptor-targeted superparamagnetic iron oxide nanoparticles. Int J Pharm. 2008;360:197–203.

29. Ma P, Liu S, Huang Y, Chen X, Zhang L, Jing X. Lactose mediated liver-targeting effect observed by ex vivo imaging technology. Biomaterials. 2010;31:2646–54.

30. Jule E, Nagasaki Y, Kataoka K. Lactose-installed poly(ethylene glycol)-poly(d, l-lactide) block copolymer micelles exhibit fast-rate binding and high affinity toward a protein bed simulating a cell surface. A surface plasmon resonance study. Bioconjugate Chem. 2003;14:177–86.

31. Lin YS, Tsai CP, Huang HY, Kuo CT, Hung Y, Huang DM, et al. Well-ordered mesoporous silica nanoparticles as cell markers. Chem Mater. 2005;17:4570–3.

32. De Palma R, Peeters S, Van Bael MJ, Van den Rul H, Bonroy K, Laureyn W, et al. Silane ligand exchange to make hydrophobic superparamagnetic nanoparticles water-dispersible. Chem Mater. 2007;19:1821–31.

33. Kwon S, Singh RK, Kim TH, Patel KD, Kim JJ, Chrzanowski W, et al. Luminescent mesoporous nanoreservoirs for the effective loading and intracellular delivery of therapeutic drugs. Acta Biomater. 2014;10:1431–42.

34. He Q, Shi J, Chen F, Zhu M, Zhang L. An anticancer drug delivery system based on surfactant-templated mesoporous silica nanoparticles. Biomaterials. 2010;31:3335–46.

35. He Q, Zhang J, Chen F, Guo L, Zhu Z, Shi J. An anti-ROS/hepatic fibrosis drug delivery system based on salvianolic acid B loaded mesoporous silica nanoparticles. Biomaterials. 2010;31:7785–96.

36. Tsai CH, Vivero-Escoto JL, Slowing II, Fang IJ, Trewyn BG, Lin VSY. Surfactant-assisted controlled release of hydrophobic drugs using anionic surfactant templated mesoporous silica nanoparticles. Biomaterials. 2011;32:6234–44.

37. Tsai CP, Chen CY, Hung Y, Chang FH, Mou CY. Monoclonal antibody-functionalized mesoporous silica nanoparticles (MSN) for selective targeting breast cancer cells. J Mater Chem. 2009;19:5737–43.

38. Chen Y, Chen HR, Ma M, Chen F, Guo LM, Zhang LX, et al. Double mesoporous silica shelled spherical/ellipsoidal nanostructures: Synthesis and hydrophilic/hydrophobic anticancer drug delivery. J Mater Chem. 2011;21:5290–8.

39. Chen Y, Chen H, Zeng D, Tian Y, Chen F, Feng J, et al. Core/shell structured hollow mesoporous nanocapsules: a potential platform for simultaneous cell imaging and anticancer drug delivery. ACS NANO. 2010;4:6001–13.

40. Torchilin VP, Rammohan R, Weissig V, Levchenko TS. TAT peptide on the surface of liposomes affords their efficient intracellular delivery even at low temperature and in the presence of metabolic inhibitors. P Natl Acad Sci USA. 2001;98:8786–91.

41. Liu Q, Zhang J, Xia W, Gu H. Magnetic field enhanced cell uptake efficiency of magnetic silica mesoporous nanoparticles. Nanoscale. 2012;4:3415–21.

42. Yang H, Lou C, Xu M, Wu C, Miyoshi H, Liu Y. Investigation of folate-conjugated fluorescent silica nanoparticles for targeting delivery to folate receptor-positive tumors and their internalization mechanism. Int J Nanomed. 2011;6:2023–32.

43. Chung TH, Wu SH, Yao M, Lu CW, Lin YS, Hung Y, et al. The effect of surface charge on the uptake and biological function of mesoporous silica nanoparticles in 3T3-L1 cells and human mesenchymal stem cells. Biomaterials. 2007;28:2959–66.

44. Tang Q, Xu Y, Wu D, Sun Y, Wang J, Xu J, et al. Studies on a new carrier of trimethylsilyl-modified mesoporous material for controlled drug delivery. J Control Release. 2006;114:41–6.

45. Lu J, Li Z, Zink JI, Tamanoi F. In vivo tumor suppression efficacy of mesoporous silica nanoparticles-based drug-delivery system: enhanced efficacy by folate modification. Nanomedicine. 2012;8:212–20.

46. Dubois M, Gilles KA, Hamilton JK, Rebers P, Smith F. Colorimetric method for determination of sugars and related substances. Anal Chem. 1956;28:350–6.

47. Jeong JM, Hong MK, Lee J, Son M, So Y, Lee DS, et al. 99mTc-neolactosylated human serum albumin for imaging the hepatic asialoglycoprotein receptor. Bioconjugate Chem. 2004;15:850–5.

48. Morelli C, Maris P, Sisci D, Perrotta E, Brunelli E, Perrotta I, et al. PEG-templated mesoporous silica nanoparticles exclusively target cancer cells. Nanoscale. 2011;3:3198–207.

# 16

# Entrapment of an EGFR inhibitor into nanostructured lipid carriers (NLC) improves its antitumor activity against human hepatocarcinoma cells

Maria Luisa Bondì[1*], Antonina Azzolina[2], Emanuela Fabiola Craparo[3], Chiara Botto[3], Erika Amore[1], Gaetano Giammona[3] and Melchiorre Cervello[2]

## Abstract

**Background:** In hepatocellular carcinoma (HCC), different signaling pathways are de-regulated, and among them, the expression of the epidermal growth factor receptor (EGFR). Tyrphostin AG-1478 is a lipophilic low molecular weight inhibitor of EGFR, preferentially acting on liver tumor cells. In order to overcome its poor drug solubility and thus improving its anticancer activity, it was entrapped into nanostructured lipid carriers (NLC) by using safe ingredients for parenteral delivery.

**Results:** Nanostructured lipid carriers (NLC) carrying tyrphostin AG-1478 were prepared by using the nanoprecipitation method and different matrix compositions. The best system in terms of mean size, PDI, zeta potential, drug loading and release profile was chosen to evaluate the anti-proliferative effect of drug-loaded NLC versus free drug on human hepatocellular carcinoma HA22T/VGH cells.

**Conclusions:** Thanks to the entrapment into NLC systems, tyrphostin AG-1478 shows an enhanced *in vitro* anti-tumor activity compared to free drug. These finding raises hope of future drug delivery strategy of tyrphostin AG-1478 -loaded NLC targeted to the liver for the HCC treatment.

**Keywords:** Nanostructured lipid carriers, Tyrphostin AG-1478, Drug release, Hepatocellular carcinoma, EGFR inhibitor

## Background

Hepatocellular carcinoma (HCC) represents the fifth most common cancer worldwide and third leading cause of cancer-related mortality globally, maintaining a dismal prognosis since intermediate and advanced stages still account for a large percentage of cases [1]. Therapeutic options in advanced stage have been quite limited so far, until the discovery of new therapeutic agents that target the molecular pathways involved in hepatocarcinogenesis [1].

Epidermal growth factor receptor (EGFR) is expressed at high levels in a variety of solid tumors. In HCC, the overexpression of this receptor has been associated with late-stage disease, increased cell proliferation, and degree of tumor differentiation [2-4]. In addition, activation of EGFR pathway is a prognostic predictor of survival in patients with HCC [5]. Therefore, EGFR represents a good potential molecular target for biologic therapy of HCC.

Tyrphostins are protein tyrosine kinase inhibitors. Among them, the tyrphostin AG-1478, 4-(3-chloroanilino)-6,7-dimethoxyquinazoline, a competitive inhibitor of the ATP binding site in the kinase domain of EGFR, inhibits proliferation and induces death of liver tumor cells through EGF receptor-dependent and independent mechanisms [6,7]. Previous studies also revealed that tyrphostin AG-1478 has no cytotoxic effects per se against normal hepatocytes, while it prevents proliferation and induces apoptosis in human HCC cells [6]. Moreover, it enhances the sensitivity to cytotoxic drugs like cisplatin and doxorubicin. Therefore, tyrphostin AG-1478 could be a

* Correspondence: marialuisa.bondi@ismn.cnr.it
[1]Istituto per lo Studio dei Materiali Nanostrutturati, U.O.S. Palermo, Consiglio Nazionale delle Ricerche, Via Ugo la Malfa 153, Palermo 90146, Italy
Full list of author information is available at the end of the article

potential therapeutic drug for the treatment of HCC. However, it has not been proposed as a potential antineoplastic drug in HCC yet.

Recently we have successfully realized novel lipid-based drug delivery systems for several lipophilic anticancer compounds by selecting the proper lipid mixture to obtain nanostructured lipid carriers (NLC) and by using the nanoprecipitation method [8-11]. By *in vitro* studies, we have also demonstrated the increased antitumor efficacy of the drug when loaded into NLC compared with free drug.

Thus, in the present study, we describe the preparation of novel tyrphostin AG-1478 -loaded NLC by selecting the suitable matrix composition in order to achieve the chemical-physical characteristics and release profile suitable for parenteral administration of this drug. Moreover, on the best formulation, *in vitro* cell viability assays were carried out to compare the anti-proliferative activity of the drug entrapped into NLC versus free drug on HA22T/VGH cells.

## Results and discussion

In this paper, we describe the preparation of empty and tyrphostin AG-1478 -loaded Nanostructured Lipid Carriers (NLC) and their characterization from the chemical-physical, technological and biological point of view in order to realize a drug delivery system with suitable characteristics for the treatment by parenteral administration.

Tyrphostin AG-1478, a potent and specific inhibitor of EGFR tyrosine kinase, plays a key role in the control of normal cellular growth and abnormal cell proliferation [12]. This molecule is promising for the therapeutic treatment of highly malignant forms of tumors, but it is poorly soluble in aqueous media. Thus, the formulation of this molecule into colloidal nanoparticulate systems, such as NLC, could give many advantages being these particles already proposed for drug administration in cancer therapy [8,10].

In order to obtain a suitable carrier for tyrphostin AG-1478, four NLC formulations were successfully prepared by using the precipitation technique. In particular, a solid un-pegylated lipid (Compritol 888 ATO) or a solid pegylated lipid (Compritol HD5 ATO) were used to obtain the lipid nanoparticles, respectively named NLC-A or NLC-B; while a mixture between a solid lipid (Tripalmitin) with either un-pegylated (Captex 355EP/NF) or pegylated (Acconon CC-6) liquid lipid were used to obtain the lipid nanoparticles, respectively named NLC-C or NLC-D. The choice of different mixtures of solid and/or liquid lipids is based on the consideration that the use of a liquid lipid to prepare NLC systems could give a higher drug loading capacity and a longer term stability during storage than that obtained by using only solid lipids; while the use of a pegylated lipid could give a surface modification of the obtained

nanostructures which could improve their pharmacokinetic behaviour by increasing the mean residence time in the bloodstream [11].

In detail, in order to obtain drug-loaded NLC, each chosen lipid or lipid mixture was melted and tyrphostin AG-1478 was added; then to this solution a warm ethanolic solution of Epikuron 200 was added. Preliminary studies were performed in order to ensure the drug stability above the lipid melting points for a time period required to obtain the nanoparticles. No degradation process occurs on the drug at tested conditions (data not shown). To obtain empty NLC samples, the step involving the addition of the drug to the melted lipid was avoided.

Empty or drug-loaded NLC were produced by dispersing the obtained warm organic solution, containing or not the drug, in a cold aqueous solution containing taurocholate sodium salt under mechanical stirring, to allow the lipid solidification.

Finally, each colloidal aqueous NLC dispersion was purified by exhaustive dialysis and freeze-dried. NLC samples were stored at $4 \pm 1°C$ for successive characterization.

Since some physical-chemical and technological properties such as size, surface charge, polydispersity index (PDI) and loading capacity (LC%) are quite critical for biopharmaceutical behavior of NLC, all the obtained empty and drug-loaded samples, after preparation and purification, were characterized in terms of mean particle size and PDI in different aqueous media (bidistilled water, NaCl 0.9 wt% and PBS aqueous saline solutions). Obtained data are reported in Table 1.

Data indicate that the average diameter of either empty or drug-loaded NLC samples were in the order of nanometer scale in all aqueous media, ranging between 60 and 250 nm.

However, PDI values are too high for NLC-A and NLC-B samples, obtained by using only a solid lipid, especially in isotonic saline solutions. Otherwise, for those systems obtained by using a mixture between solid and liquid lipids, that is NLC-C and NLC-D samples, PDI values are acceptable in all investigated media.

The results indicate that these systems could be injected intravenously, being the mean size values suitable to minimize the uptake from macrophages of Mononuclear Phagocyte System (MPS) [13]. In this way, these particles could circulate in the bloodstream and potentially accumulate in tumor masses as a consequence of the well-known Enhanced Permeability and Retention (EPR) effect [14,15]. In fact, a critical advantage in treating tumors with nanoparticulate systems comes from the unique patho-physiological characteristics of solid tumors: extensive angiogenesis and hence hypervascularization, coupled with poor lymphatic drainage, which allow a facilitate extravasation into the tumor and EPR effect of colloidal systems [14,15].

**Table 1 Mean size, PDI in different aqueous media, Loading Capacity (LC%) and Entrapment Efficiency (EE%) values of empty and tyrphostin AG-1478 -loaded NLC**

| Sample | H$_2$O | | NaCl 0.9 wt% | | PBS pH 7.4 | | LC (wt%) | EE (wt%) |
|---|---|---|---|---|---|---|---|---|
| | Size (nm) | PDI | Size (nm) | PDI | Size (nm) | PDI | | |
| Empty NLC-A | 139.7 | 0.38 | 146.2 | 0.43 | 122.2 | 0.59 | —— | —— |
| Drug-loaded NLC-A | 176.2 | 0.41 | 207.2 | 0.90 | 145.6 | 0.79 | 2.8 | 28.0 |
| Empty NLC-B | 62.6 | 0.46 | 120.3 | 0.75 | 106.6 | 0.76 | —— | —— |
| Drug-loaded NLC-B | 80.1 | 0.49 | 108.4 | 0.49 | 180.1 | 0.58 | 1.7 | 17.0 |
| Empty NLC-C | 175.9 | 0.34 | 129.2 | 0.33 | 117.1 | 0.41 | —— | —— |
| Drug-loaded NLC-C | 209.7 | 0.46 | 203.7 | 0.22 | 248.1 | 0.29 | 24.0 | 70.0 |
| Empty NLC-D | 185.5 | 0.29 | 125.6 | 0.28 | 143.8 | 0.25 | —— | —— |
| Drug-loaded NLC-D | 189.3 | 0.42 | 248.1 | 0.65 | 181.5 | 0.52 | 24.0 | 70.0 |

In Table 1, the LC% (expressed as weight percent ratio between entrapped tyrphostin AG-1478 and the total dried sample weight) and the EE% (expressed as weight percent ratio between entrapped tyrphostin AG-1478 and total amount of tyrphostin AG-1478 used to prepare the nanoparticles) of drug-loaded NLC are also reported. Also in this case, the best values in terms of LC and EE, evaluated by HPLC analysis on each drug-loaded system (as reported in the Materials and Methods section), were obtained when a mixture of solid and liquid lipids was used as matrix composition. In fact, when tripalmitin mixed with either un-pegylated or pegylated liquid lipid are used as matrix composition (named respectively NLC-C and NLC-D samples), a LC of about 24 wt% was obtained (with a EE of 70 wt%); while when un-pegylated or pegylated solid lipid is used as lipid matrix composition (named respectively NLC-A and NLC-B samples), a LC of 1.7 and 2.8 were obtained (with a EE of 17 and 28 wt%, respectively).

These results can be explained considering an increasing effect of the liquid lipid on the drug solubility into the lipid matrix, as other authors have already reported [11].

The zeta potential values were also determined on the obtained samples, and reported in Table 2.

These values resulted to be high and negative especially in bidistilled water and decreased in isotonic media such as NaCl 0.9 wt% and PBS aqueous solutions probably for the charge shielding effect of solution ions. However, these values assured a potential stability of all the aqueous NLC dispersions. Moreover, a slight increase of NLC surface charge in the presence of tyrphostin AG-1478 compared to empty systems was evidenced, and this result could be explained considering the drug localization probably also onto the nanoparticle surface.

In order to evaluate the storage stability of the obtained systems, each sample (empty or drug-loaded) was lyophilised and stored at 0°C for 3 months in the dark;

after this time, mean size, PDI, zeta potential values and LC were evaluated in bidistilled water. Obtained data, reported in Table 3, showed that all empty and tyrphostin AG-1478 -loaded NLC were stable during storage in the tested conditions, being comparable to those of fresh samples.

Thanks to all their chemical–physical properties and their stability after storage, these systems could be proposed for the administration by all the routes, also intravenously.

All together these results in terms of LC, mean size and zeta potential values indicated that the best NLC to be proposed as drug delivery systems for tyrphostin AG-1478 seem to be those obtained by using the mixture between tripalmitin and the liquid lipid (pegylated or not), that is NLC-D and NLC-C. For this reason, these latter systems were chosen to perform successive characterization in terms of drug release studies and *in vitro* biological assay. In particular, release studies were carried out in different incubating media such as phosphate buffer solution (PBS) at pH 7.4/ethanol mixture (80:20 v/v) or human plasma. The use of this modified dissolution medium (containing ethanol) to test preparation

**Table 2 Zeta potential values in different aqueous media of empty and tyrphostin AG-1478 -loaded NLC**

| Sample | ζ-potential (mV) ± S.D. | | |
|---|---|---|---|
| | In H$_2$O | In NaCl 0.9 wt% | In PBS pH 7.4 |
| Empty NLC-A | −20.1 ± 5.5 | −12.3 ± 4.5 | −19.6 ± 3.3 |
| Drug-loaded NLC-A | −30.3 ± 7.7 | −13.6 ± 3.7 | −20.4 ± 7.7 |
| Empty NLC-B | −18.7 ± 4.6 | −10.4 ± 3.6 | −15.4 ± 4.2 |
| Drug-loaded NLC-B | −28.5 ± 10.3 | −13.2 ± 2.3 | −15.1 ± 6.3 |
| Empty NLC-C | −35.7 ± 5.2 | −15.9 ± 4.2 | −19.7 ± 5.1 |
| Drug-loaded NLC-C | −46.9 ± 8.4 | −13.1 ± 2.9 | −19.6 ± 5.4 |
| Empty NLC-D | −36.7 ± 5.9 | −09.4 ± 2.5 | −16.6 ± 3.9 |
| Drug-loaded NLC-D | −38.4 ± 6.5 | −11.4 ± 3.5 | −16.6 ± 3.7 |

**Table 3 Mean size, PDI and zeta potential in bidistilled water of lyophilised empty and tyrphostin AG-1478 -loaded NLC after storage at 0°C for 3 months in the dark**

| Sample | Size (nm) | | PDI | | ζ-potential (mV) | | L.C. (wt%) | |
|---|---|---|---|---|---|---|---|---|
| | Before storage | After storage | Before storage | After storage | Before storage | After storage | Before storage | After storage |
| Empty NLC-A | 139.7 | 134.9 | 0.38 | 0.39 | −20.1 ± 5.5 | −19.1 ± 4.5 | —— | —— |
| Drug-loaded NLC-A | 176.2 | 179.5 | 0.41 | 0.44 | −30.3 ± 7.7 | −29.4 ± 7.9 | 2.8 | 2.6 |
| Empty NLC-B | 62.6 | 64.4 | 0.46 | 0.49 | −18.7 ± 4.6 | −19.5 ± 4.9 | —— | —— |
| Drug-loaded NLC-B | 80.1 | 84.4 | 0.49 | 0.50 | −28.5 ± 10.3 | −29.9 ± 16.2 | 1.7 | 1.5 |
| Empty NLC-C | 175.9 | 175.9 | 0.34 | 0.34 | −35.7 ± 5.2 | −35.7 ± 5.2 | —— | —— |
| Drug-loaded NLC-C | 209.7 | 220.5 | 0.46 | 0.48 | −46.9 ± 8.4 | −42.7 ± 7.3 | 24.0 | 21.4 |
| Empty NLC-D | 185.5 | 192.5 | 0.29 | 0.32 | −36.7 ± 5.9 | −32.7 ± 4.4 | —— | —— |
| Drug-loaded NLC-D | 189.3 | 199.3 | 0.42 | 0.48 | −38.4 ± 6.5 | −36.3 ± 4.4 | 24.0 | 21.8 |

containing poorly aqueous-soluble active substances was in accordance to the European Pharmacopoea [16]. In Figures 1 and 2, the released drug, expressed as weight percent ratio between released drug and the total entrapped drug, is reported as a function of incubation time respectively in PBS/ethanol and in human plasma.

The release trend could be explained considering the high hydrophobic behaviour of the drug that shows a higher affinity for the system obtained by using the un-pegylated liquid lipid mixed with tripalmitin as for lipid matrix composition than for that obtained by using the pegylated lipid. On the other hand, the lower affinity for the pegylated lipid could give a preferential drug deposition in the outsides shell of the NLC during the preparation process, and consequently a burst effect in the release profile of the drug could be evidenced.

Therefore, a modified release of tyrphostin AG-1478 from the un-pegylated systems (NLC-C sample) can be seen in the graphic, being the amount of released tyrphostin AG-1478 about the 90 wt% of the total entrapped amount after 72 hrs incubation.

It was also evaluated that the amount of un-released tyrphostin AG-1478 was still inside NLC sample in the intact form at every incubation time (data not shown). This result supports the great potential of these nanostructures as drug delivery systems for systemic administration of drugs with low solubility and/or instability in aqueous media.

The release profile of tyrphostin AG-1478 was also investigated in human plasma, and obtained data are reported in Figure 2.

Compared to the drug release profiles obtained in PBS at pH 7.4, a faster drug release is evidenced from either

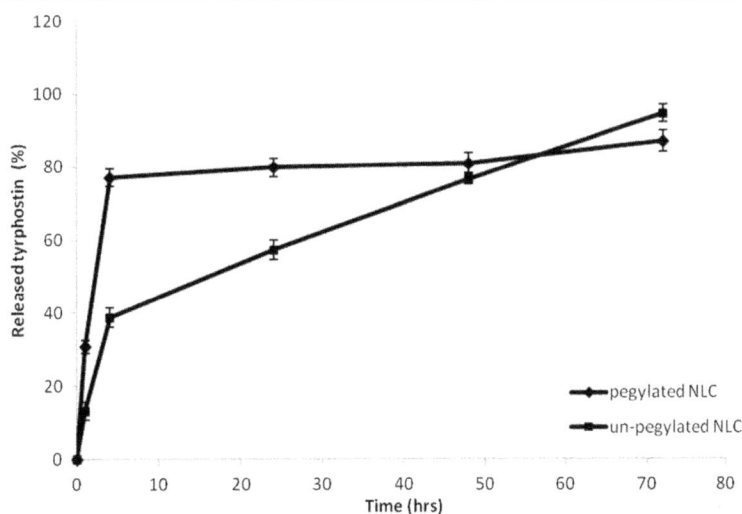

**Figure 1 Release profiles of tyrphostin AG-1478 from NLC-C and NLC-D samples in PBS pH 7.4/ethanol mixture (80:20 v/v) at 37 ± 0.1°C, expressed as percentage wt% of released drug as a function of incubation time.** Each value is the mean of three experiments.

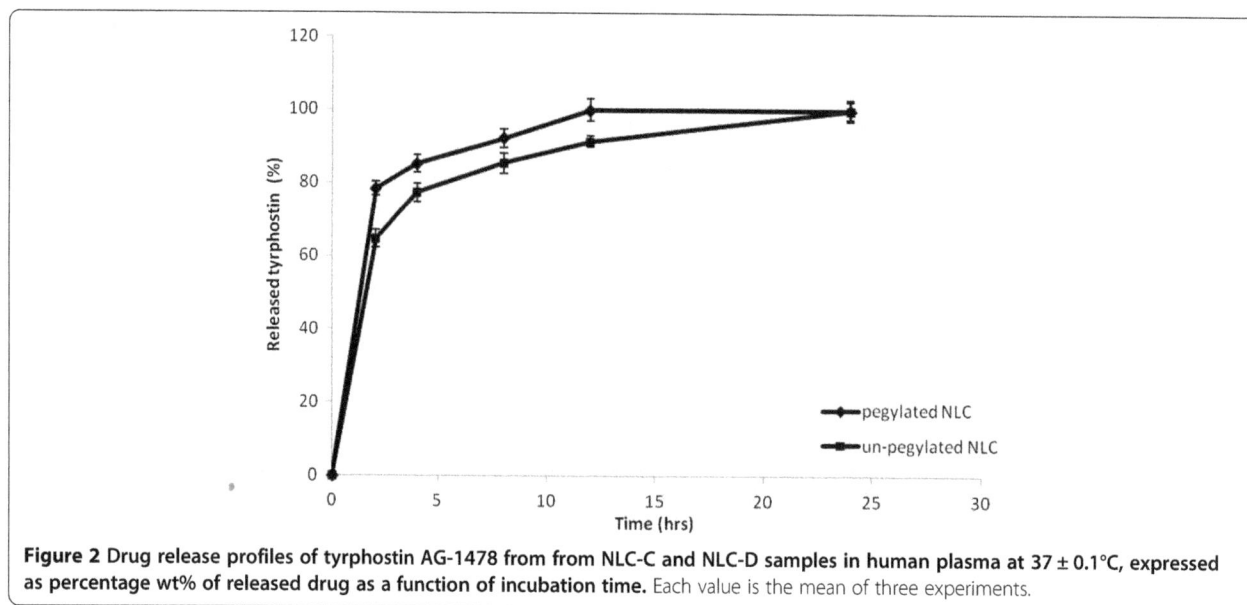

**Figure 2** Drug release profiles of tyrphostin AG-1478 from from NLC-C and NLC-D samples in human plasma at 37 ± 0.1°C, expressed as percentage wt% of released drug as a function of incubation time. Each value is the mean of three experiments.

the pegylated or the un-pegylated systems in human plasma, probably due to the different composition of the medium, such as the presence of proteins and enzymes in the medium. However, also in this case, the un-pegylated system released the drug slower than the pegylated one. This fact also in this case could be explained considering a higher affinity of the drug for the system obtained by using the un-pegylated liquid lipid mixed with tripalmitin (sample NLC-C).

Showing the NLC-C system the best surface charge and dimensional characteristics useful for parenteral administration and considering their capability to give a controlled release of tyrphostin AG-1478, a further *in vitro* biological characterization was carried out on this system.

In particular, the levels of EGFR protein expressed by the human hepatocellular carcinoma (HCC) cell line HA22T/VGH were evaluated by Western blot analysis. As shown in Figure 3A, the cell line intensely expressed the receptor.

Based on this result, HA22T/VGH cells were used for testing the inhibitory effects of tyrphostin AG-1478 free and loaded into the NLC on cell growth. In this regard, the clonogenic assay is currently considered the "gold standard" assay for the assessment of the ability of drugs in killing tumor cells *in vitro* experiments. In fact, this assay is a reliable method to measure the reproductive survival of tumor cells capable of clonal expansion.

In this regard, to evaluate the effect of tyrphostin AG-1478 free and loaded into NLC on the ability to form colonies, HA22T/VGH cells were subjected to clonogenic assay. As shown in Figure 3B, the ability of HA22T/VGH cells to form colonies was slightly inhibited after

treatment with free-tyrphostin AG-1478 up to a concentration of 25 µM, whereas, the delivery of tyrphostin AG-1478 from the NLC inhibited colonies formation to approximately 90% at 25 µM, therefore potentiating the activity of tyrphostin AG-1478 to inhibit HCC cell growth.

The results show that tyrphostin AG-1478 -loaded NLC maintain antitumor activity, demonstrating that the entrapment of tyrphostin AG-1478 into NLC does not cause an activity reduction of the drug, but even reduces cell colony survival much more than free drug.

Therefore, the results demonstrate an improved therapeutic efficacy of tyrphostin AG-1478 -loaded NLC compared to the free drug and suggest that lipid nanoparticles could have a great potential as tyrphostin AG-1478 targeted delivery systems.

Finally, considering that solid tumors present much more favorable conditions for preferential accumulation of colloidal sized drug delivery systems such as NLC, these systems can be useful for application in cancer therapy.

## Conclusion

In this paper, the realization of NLC with suitable characteristics for parenteral delivery of tyrphostin AG-1478 in the treatment of cancer was described. In particular, by using the precipitation technique, different lipid compositions were used to obtain the best NLC system in terms of drug loading, mean particle size, and zeta potential values. The amount of tyrphostin AG-1478 entrapped into NLC resulted to be higher into those systems obtained by using a mixture of solid and liquid lipids compared to those obtained by using only the solid lipid. Moreover, the un-pegylated nanoparticles

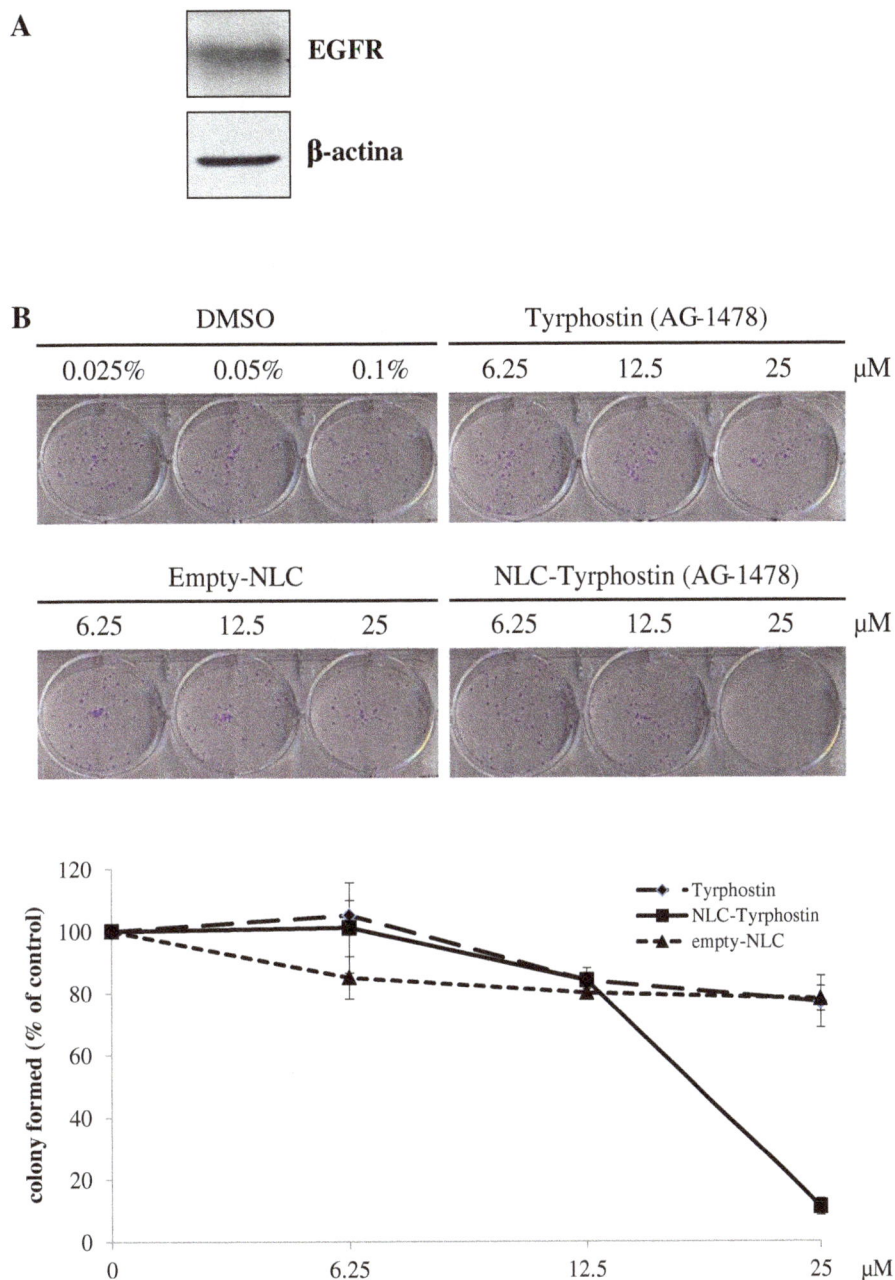

**Figure 3 A) Expression of EGFR in human hepatocellular carcinoma HA22T/VGH cells. B) Effects of free tyrphostin AG-1478, empty-NLC and tyrphostin AG-1478-loaded NLC on the ability of human hepatocellular carcinoma cell line HA22T/VGH to form colony.** Cells were plated overnight and exposed to the indicated concentration of solvent (DMSO), free tyrphostin, empty-NLC and tyrphostin-loaded NLC for 24 hours followed by growth in fresh culture media for 8 days, as described in Materials and Methods. Surviving colonies were stained (upper panel) and counted (lower panel). Data are expressed as a percentage of colony in untreated cells and are the mean ± SD of two determinations.

released the tyrphostin AG-1478 slower than the pegylated systems and the amount of unreleased drug was still inside of each nanoparticulate sample. This result supports the great potential of these nanostructures as drug delivery systems with a dispersing and protecting action on drugs, in aqueous media.

Finally, *in vitro* biological characterization was carried out and the HA22T/VGH cells were used for testing the inhibitory effects of tyrphostin AG-1478 free and loaded into the NLC on cell growth. The results show that after treatment with free-tyrphostin AG-1478 up to a concentration of 25 μM the ability of HA22T/VGH cells to form colonies was slightly inhibited, whereas, the delivery of tyrphostin AG-1478 from the NLC inhibited colonies formation to approximately 90% at 25 μM, therefore potentiating the activity of tyrphostin AG-1478 to inhibit HCC cell growth. In conclusion, tyrphostin AG-1478 - loaded NLC maintain antitumor activity, demonstrating that drug activity is not reduced in the presence of the nanoparticle carrier. Moreover, the results demonstrate an improved therapeutic efficacy of tyrphostin AG-1478 - loaded NLC compared to the free drug and suggest that solid lipid nanoparticles could have a great potential as tyrphostin AG-1478 targeted delivery systems for application in cancer therapy.

## Experimental
### Materials and methods
Tyrphostin AG-1478 was purchased from LC Laboratories (PKC Pharmaceuticals, Inc. USA). Tripalmitin (glyceryl tripalmitate) and acetonitrile for HPLC were purchased from Fluka (Milan, Italy). Compritol 888 ATO (mixture of approximately mono-, di- and tri-glycerides of behenic acid at 15, 35 and 50 wt%) and Compritol HD5 ATO (behenoyl polyoxyl-8 glycerides) were gift samples from Gattefossè (France). Captex 355 EP/NF (glyceryl tricaprylate/caprate medium chain triglycerides) and Acconon CC-6 (polyoxyethylene caprylic/capric glycerides) were gift samples from Abitec Corporation (Janesville, USA).

Epikuron 200 (soybean lecithin) was gift sample from Lucas Meyer Company (Germany). Sodium taurocholate was a gift from Prodotti Chimici e Alimentari S.P.A., Basaluzzo (Alessandria, Italy). Water of double distilled quality was obtained from MilliQ Plus systems (Millipore, Germany). The other chemicals, of analytical grade, were obtained from Sigma Aldrich (Milan, Italy).

HPLC (UFLC-Prominence system, Shimadzu Instrument, Kyoto, Japan) was equipped with two pumps LC-20 AD, an UV-visible detector SPD-20 AV, an autosample SIL-20A HT and a column Gemini® C18 Phenomenex (250 mm, 5 μm particle size, 110 Å pores size).

### Preparation of empty and drug-loaded nanostructured lipid carriers (NLC)
Un-pegylated and pegylated NLC, empty or drug-loaded, were prepared by the precipitation method, with appropriate modifications as described previously [9-11]. In particular, a solid lipid (Compritol 888 ATO, 230 mg) or a pegylated lipid (Compritol HD5 ATO, 230 mg) were used to obtain the lipid matrices, respectively named NLC-A or NLC-B; while a mixture between a solid lipid (Tripalmitin, 180 mg) with either un-pegylated (Captex 355EP/NF, 54 mg) or pegylated (Acconon CC-6, 54 mg) liquid lipid were used to obtain the lipid matrices,

respectively named NLC-C or NLC-D. As far as of drug-loaded samples preparation is concerned, tyrphostin AG-1478, under mechanical stirring, was added to the melted lipid phase. Preliminary studies were performed, in order to ensure the drug stability above the lipid melting point for a time period required to obtain the nanoparticles. No degradation process occurs on the drug at tested conditions (data not showed). After, an ethanolic solution of Epikuron 200 (48.4 mg/ml) was added and the organic outcome was dispersed into bidistilled water (100 ml) containing sodium taurocholate (177.4 mg) at 2-3°C and stirred by using an Ultraturrax T125 (IKA Labortechnik, Staufen, Germany) at 13,500 rpm for 10 minutes. Finally, the colloidal aqueous dispersion of NLC was purified by exhaustive dialysis in a dialysis tube with 12,000/14,000 Dalton cut-off (Spectra/Por®, California, USA), freeze-dried by a lyophilizer (FreeZone® Freeze Dry System, Labconco Corporation, Missouri, USA) and stored at 4 ± 1°C for successive characterization. Ethanol was completely removed from the aqueous dispersions during dialysis process.

### Particle size determination
The mean diameter and width of distribution (polydispersity index, PDI) of the obtained empty and drug-loaded nanoparticles in aqueous suspension, were determined by Photon Correlation Spectroscopy (PCS) using a Zetasizer Nano ZS (Malvern Instrument, Herrenberg, Germany), which utilizes Non-Invasive Back-Scattering (NIBS) technique. Each sample was appropriately diluted with filtered (0.2 μm) water, NaCl 0.9 wt% and PBS at pH 7.4, and the reading was carried out at 25° ± 1°C and at a 173° angle in respect to the incident beam. When the measurement was carried out in NaCl 0.9 wt%, the instrument setting conditions were: $\mu = 0.902$, RI =1.331; in PBS at pH 7.4, the setting conditions were: $\mu = 0.980$, RI =1.334. In all cases, the temperature of measurements was 25°C ± 1°C. Each suspension was kept in a cuvette and analyzed in triplicate. The deconvolution of the measured correlation curve to an intensity size distribution was accomplished by using a non negative least squares algorithm.

### Zeta potential measurements
The zeta potential values were measured by using principles of laser Doppler velocitometry and phase analysis light scattering (M3-PALS technique).

For this purpose, a Zetasizer Nano ZS Malvern Instrument equipped with a He-Ne laser at a power P = 4.0 mW and with $\lambda = 633$ nm was used. Each sample was dispersed in filtered (0.2 μm) bidistilled water, NaCl 0.9 wt% and in PBS at pH 7.4. Instrument setting conditions were equal to those described above for size measurements. Each sample was analyzed in triplicate.

Entrapment of an EGFR inhibitor into nanostructured lipid carriers (NLC) improves its antitumor activity...

155

## HPLC analysis and drug loading determination

An adequate HPLC method was developed to reveal tyrphostin AG-1478 and to study its stability in phosphate saline buffer (PBS) at pH 7.4, as well as Loading Capacity (LC%) and drug release profiles from drug-loaded systems. The HPLC analysis was performed at room temperature using the instrument described above. A $C_{18}$ column Gemini (Phenomenex, Hundsfield, UK) packed with 5 µm particles, with dimensions $250 \times 4.60$ mm i.d., was used for analysis. A mixture of acetonitrile and water (30:70 v/v) containing trifluoroacetic acid (0.1% v/v) with a flow rate of 0.1 ml/min was used as mobile phase.

The peak was measured at a wavelength of 254 nm and quantitatively determined by comparison with a standard curve obtained by using drug solutions in a mixture of acetonitrile:chloroform (1:1 v/v) at known concentrations ($t_r = 9.50$ min). The linearity of the method was studied in the range 5–20 µg/ml.

Loading capacity (LC%) was determined by solving each freeze dried NLC sample (5 mg) in 10 ml of an organic solution of acetonitrile:chloroform (1:1 v/v), filtered with 0.45 µm PTFE filters and analyzed by the HPLC method above described. The results are expressed as actual loading percent (LC%, mg of drug encapsulated per 100 mg of nanoparticles) and encapsulation efficiency (EE%, ratio of actual to theoretical loading). In order to ensure that the drug is not absorbed within the PTFE filters, several tyrphostin AG-1478 organic solutions at known concentrations were filtered and the concentrations values, before and after filtration, were evaluated by HPLC analysis. No significant differences in drug concentrations were evidenced.

## Storage stability

All lyophilised empty and tyrphostin AG-1478 -loaded NLC were stored at 0°C for 3 months in the dark. After this time, samples were dispersed in bidistilled water and characterized in terms of mean size, PDI and zeta potential. Moreover, chemical stability of tyrphostin AG-1478 loaded into the NLC was evaluated by HPLC analysis, as reported above.

## Drug release in PBS at pH 7.4/ethanol

Tyrphostin release was assayed on NLC samples at pre-fixed time intervals. For this purpose, dispersions of each batch containing 5 mg of each freeze-dried sample in a mixture of 9.6 ml of PBS 0.01 M at pH 7.4 and 2.4 ml of ethanol (80:20 v/v), were prepared and kept at $37 \pm 0.1$°C under mechanical stirring in a Benchtop 80°C incubator Orbital Shaker model 420 [16]. At scheduled time intervals, solution aliquots (1 ml) were taken out from the outside of the dialysis membrane and replaced with fresh PBS aqueous-ethanolic solution. Release profile was

determined by comparing the amount of released tyrphostin AG-1478 as a function of incubation time with the total amount of drug loaded into NLC. Data were corrected taking in account the dilution procedure. A control experiment to determine the release behavior of the free tyrphostin AG-1478 was also performed. A suspension of free tyrphostin AG-1478 in PBS aqueous-ethanolic solution at pH 7.4 was prepared at the same concentration of drug entrapped in the NLC, put into a dialysis tube (MWCO 5,000 Da) and immersed into the proper medium. The amount of tyrphostin AG-1478 was detected as reported above.

## Drug release in human plasma

Tyrphostin release was assayed on NLC samples at pre-fixed time intervals. For this purpose, dispersions of each batch containing 2.5 mg of each freeze-dried sample in 2 ml of human plasma were prepared and kept at $37 \pm 0.1$°C under mechanical stirring in a Benchtop 80°C incubator Orbital Shaker model 420. At suitable time intervals, samples were filtered through 0.45 µm nylon filters; then acetonitrile was added and the obtained blend was centrifuged at 4°C and 12,000 rpm for 15 min. Then the supernatant was filtered by 0.45 µm PTFE filters and analyzed by HPLC.

## Western blot analysis

For Western blot analysis whole cellular lysates were obtained using RIPA buffer (Cell Signaling Technologies Inc., Beverly, MA, USA). Protein concentrations of supernatants were determined with the Bio-Rad protein assay kit (Bio-Rad Laboratories SrL, Milan, Italy), and Western blotting were performed as previously described [17], with primary antibodies raised against β-actin (Sigma-Aldrich Srl, Milan, Italy) and EGFR (Cell Signaling Technologies Inc., Beverly, MA, USA).

## Cell culture and clonogenic assay

The human hepatocellular carcinoma HA22T/VGH cell line, a poorly differentiated human hepatocellular carcinoma cell line established from a surgical specimen of hepatocellular carcinoma obtained from a 56-year-old Chinese male was kindly provided by Professor Massimo Levrero (Laboratory of Gene Expression, Fondazione Andrea Cesalpino, University of Rome "La Sapienza", Rome, Italy) [18]. Cells were cultured in Roswell Park Memorial Institute (RPMI) medium (Sigma, Milan, Italy) supplemented with 10% heat-inactivated fetal calf serum (FCS) (Gibco, Milan, Italy), 2 mM L-glutamine, 1 mM sodium pyruvate, 100 units/ml penicillin and 100 µg/ml streptomycin (all reagents were from Sigma) in a humidified atmosphere at 37°C in 5% $CO_2$. Cells having a narrow range of passage number were used for all experiments.

The effect of different inhibitor concentrations on cell growth was assessed using a clonogenic assay. For this analysis, 200 cells were plated onto six-well plates in growth medium and after overnight attachment cells were exposed to various concentrations of solvent (DMSO), free tyrphostin AG-1478, empty NLC and NLC-loaded tyrphostin AG-1478 for 24 hrs. The cells were then washed with medium and allowed to grow for 8 days under inhibitor-free or nanoparticles-free conditions, after which the cell colonies were fixed with 70% ethanol at 4°C for 20 min and stained with crystal violet (0.1% in H$_2$O) for 5 min. The plates were rinsed with water, air-dried, photographed and evaluated for colony estimation. Colonies containing more than 50 cells were counted. Relative colony formation was determined by the ratio of the average number of colonies in cells treated with free-tyrphostin AG-1478, empty-NLC and NLC-loaded tyrphostin AG-1478 to the average number of colonies in cells treated with DMSO. All experiments were performed in duplicate and repeated twice.

### Abbreviations

NLC: Nanostructured lipid carriers; HCC: Hepatocellular carcinoma; EGFR: Epidermal growth factor receptor; MPS: Mononuclear phagocyte system; PDI: Polydispersity index; LC: Loading capacity; EPR: Enhanced permeability and retention; EE: Entrapment efficiency; DMSO: Dimethyl sulfoxide; PBS: Phosphate buffer solution.

### Competing interests

The authors declare that they have no competing interests.

### Authors' contributions

CB and EA are the PhD students who carried out the laboratory work. AA carried out the biological work in laboratory. MC was the supervisor of the biological study and helping to develop the study parameters and design. MLB was the principal, scientific supervisor of the study. She conceived the study, supervised the students in the laboratory, directed the analysis and wrote the manuscript. All authors read and approved the final draft of the manuscript. EFC and GG have revised the final version of manuscript.

### Acknowledgements

This work was supported by grants from the Italian "Ministero dell'Istruzione, dell'Università e della Ricerca (Ministry for Education, Universities and Research) – MIUR" FIRB-MERIT n. RBNE08YYBM to M.C. and M.L.B.

### Author details

[1]Istituto per lo Studio dei Materiali Nanostrutturati, U.O.S. Palermo, Consiglio Nazionale delle Ricerche, Via Ugo la Malfa 153, Palermo 90146, Italy. [2]Istituto di Biomedicina e Immunologia Molecolare "Alberto Monroy", Consiglio Nazionale delle Ricerche, Via Ugo la Malfa 153 Palermo 90146, Italy. [3]Lab. of Biocompatible Polymers, Dipartimento di Scienze e Tecnologie Biologiche Chimiche e Farmaceutiche (STEBICEF), via Archirafi 32, Palermo 90123, Italy.

### References

1. Cervello M, McCubrey JA, Cusimano A, Lampiasi N, Azzolina A, Montalto G: Targeted therapy for hepatocellular carcinoma: novel agents on the horizon. *Oncotarget* 2012, 3:236–260.
2. Ito Y, Takeda T, Sakon M, Tsujimoto M, Higashiyama S, Noda K, Miyoshi E, Monden M, Matsuura N: Expression and clinical significance of erb-B receptor family in hepatocellular carcinoma. *Br J Cancer* 2001, 84:1377–1383.
3. Kannangai R, Sahin F, Torbenson MS: EGFR is phosphorylated at Ty845 in hepatocellular carcinoma. *Mod Pathol* 2006, 19:1456–1461.
4. Kira S, Nakanishi T, Suemori S, Kitamoto M, Watanabe Y, Kajiyama G: Expression of transforming growth factor alpha and epidermal growth factor receptor in human hepatocellular carcinoma. *Liver* 1997, 17:177–182.
5. Foster J, Black J, LeVea C, Khoury T, Kuvshinoff B, Javle M, Gibbs JF: COX-2 expression in hepatocellular carcinoma is an initiation event; while EGF receptor expression with downstream pathway activation is a prognostic predictor of survival. *Ann Surg Oncol* 2007, 14:752–758.
6. Caja L, Sancho P, Bertran E, Ortiz C, Campbell JS, Fausto N, Fabregat I: The tyrphostin AG1478 inhibits proliferation and induces death of liver tumor cells through EGF receptor-dependent and independent mechanisms. *Biochem Pharmacol* 2011, 82:1583–1592.
7. Ellis AG, Doherty MM, Walker F, Weinstock J, Nerrie M, Vitali A, Murphy R, Johns TG, Scott AM, Levitzki A, McLachlan G, Webster LK, Burgess AW, Nice EC: Preclinical analysis of the analinoquinazoline AG1478, a specific small molecule inhibitor of EGF receptor tyrosine kinase. *Biochem Pharmacol* 2006, 71:1422–1434.
8. Bondì ML, Craparo EF, Picone P, Di Carlo M, Di Gesù R, Capuano G, Giammona G: Curcumin entrapped into lipid nanosystems inhibits neuroblastoma cancer cell growth and activate Hsp70 protein. *Curr Nanosci* 2010, 6:439–445.
9. Bondì ML, Azzolina A, Craparo EF, Capuano G, Lampiasi N, Giammona G, Cervello M: Solid lipid nanoparticles (SLNs) containing nimesulide: preparation, characterization and in cytotoxicity studies. *Curr Nanosci* 2009, 5(1):39–44.
10. Bondì ML, Craparo EF, Giammona G, Cervello M, Azzolina A, Diana P, Martorana A, Cirrincione G: Nanostructured lipid carriers-containing anticancer compounds: preparation, characterization, and cytotoxicity studies. *Drug Del* 2007, 14(2):61–67.
11. Bondì ML, Craparo EF, Picone P, Giammona G, Di Gesù R, Di Carlo M: Lipid nanocarriers containing esters prodrugs of Flurbiprofen. Preparation, physical-chemical characterization and biological studies. *J Biomed Nanotech* 2013, 9(2):238–246.
12. Levitzki A: Tyrosine kinases as targets for cancer therapy. *Eur J Cancer* 2002, 38(5):S11–S18.
13. Vonarbourg A, Passirani C, Saulnier P, Benoit JP: Parameters influencing the stealthiness of colloidal drug delivery systems. *Biogeosciences* 2006, 27:4356–4373.
14. Maeda H: The enhanced permeability and retention (EPR) effect in tumor vasculature: the key role of tumor-selective macromolecular drug targeting. *Adv Enzyme Regul* 2001, 41:189–207.
15. Singh R, Lillard JW: Nanoparticle-based targeted drug delivery. *Exp Mol Pathol* 2009, 86:215–223.
16. Craparo EF, Teresi G, Bondì ML, Licciardi M, Cavallaro G: Phospholipid-polyaspartamide micelles for pulmonary delivery of corticosteroids. *Int J Pharm* 2011, 406:135–144.
17. Cervello M, Giannitrapani L, La Rosa M, Notarbartolo M, Labbozzetta M, Poma P, Montalto G, D'Alessandro N: Induction of apoptosis by the proteasome inhibitor MG132 in human HCC cells: Possible correlation with specific caspase-dependent cleavage of beta-catenin and inhibition of beta-catenin-mediated transactivation. *Int J Mol Med* 2004, 13:741–748.
18. Chang C, Lin Y, O-Lee TW, Chou CK, Lee TS, Liu TJ, Peng FK, Chen TY, Hu CP: Induction of plasma protein secretion in a newly established human hepatoma cell line. *Mol Cell Biol* 1983, 3:1133–1137.

# 17

# The effects of multifunctional MiR-122-loaded graphene-gold composites on drug-resistant liver cancer

Yi Yuan[3†], Yaqin Zhang[4†], Bin Liu[5†], Heming Wu[3], Yanjun Kang[7], Ming Li[3], Xin Zeng[2,6*], Nongyue He[2*] and Gen Zhang[1,2*]

## Abstract

**Background:** Nano drugs have attracted increased attention due to their unique mode of action that offers tumor-inhibiting effects. Therefore, we have previously explored functionalized and drug-loaded graphene-gold nanocomposites that induced cancer cell apoptosis.

**Results:** In the present study, we developed a combination of monoclonal P-glycoprotein (P-gp) antibodies, folic acid (FA) and miR-122-loaded gold nanoparticles on graphene nanocomposites (GGMPN), which promoted drug-resistant HepG2 cell apoptosis with drug targeting and controlled release properties. We also investigated related apoptosis proteins and apoptosis signal pathways by GGMPN treatment in vitro and in vivo. Moreover, we further demonstrated the inhibition of tumor growth and the apoptosis-inducing effect by means of GGMPN with a semiconductor laser in a xenograft tumor model.

**Conclusion:** In conclusion, our results collectively suggested that GGMPN could serve as a novel therapeutic approach to control tumor cell apoptosis and growth.

**Keywords:** Graphene, Gold nanoparticles, Cell apoptosis, Control release, Target

## Background

Since its emergence, nanotechnology has been used in the medical field. Scientists foresee that nanotechnology has great potential in the research of cancer therapy development. Therefore, making excellent nano-material drugs with high drug loading, high targeting ability, controlled release capabilities, low toxicity, and tumor imaging functionality appears to be highly necessary [1,2].

One important component of miR-122-loaded gold nanoparticles on graphene nanocomposites (GGMPN) in this study was miRs, which were discovered in recent years as a class of 18–24 nucleotide non-coding small molecule RNA [3]. They are involved in life activities such as ontogeny regulation, cell proliferation, apoptosis and differentiation through complete or incomplete pairing of the 3′UTR, targeting gene mRNA degradation or inhibiting its translation. Various miRs related to the regulatory pathways of hepatoma cells are gradually being discovered. Many researchers have focused on differential miR expression in hepatoma cells. Expression of miR-122 is down-regulated in many hepatoma cells. As a tumor marker, miR-122 is involved in the regulation of the transfer of cancer cells in the liver and is significantly reduced or absent in liver intrahepatic metastasis. In the majority of liver cancer cells, miR-122 has low expression, and the expression level of miR-122 in the adjacent tissues is relatively high. There are differences between the expression of tumor cells and that of normal cells. The lower expression in high metastatic liver cancer cells in comparison with normal cells opens up the potential transport functionality for drug delivery [4-6].

Other important characteristics of GGMPN include the following: the gold nanoparticles can easily absorb

* Correspondence: august555482@hotmail.com; nyhe1958@163.com; zhanggen123@126.com
†Equal contributors
²The State Key Laboratory of Bioelectronics, Department of Biological Science and Medical Engineering, Southeast University, Nanjing 210096, China
¹Department of Cell Biology, Nanjing Medical University, Nanjing 210029, China
Full list of author information is available at the end of the article

small biological molecules and oligopeptides, lowering the chances of eliciting an immune response; the toxicity of nanomaterials is relatively low; they are not genotoxic because of their non-viral vectors; and specific molecules (such as the intracellular molecule GSH) can substitute for nucleic acid in certain concentrations [7]. The gold-gene nanoparticle vector is usually an amphiphilic substance (positive and negative electrical attraction) formed on the basis of a nano-polymer with the core-shell structure of RNA genetic drugs (miR-122). Folic acid (FA) receptor expression is highly overexpressed in cancers of epithelial origin [8]. The FA is loaded on the gold nanoparticles to provide a targeting function. The advantage of the gold gene vector is that with the effect of GSH, it can achieve controlled release of the nucleic acid, which is preferably more controllable than viral vectors and liposomes.

Graphene is characterized by its large specific surface area and can be fixed with a variety of substances, including antibody molecules, fluorescent molecules, and drugs (in this study, the P-gp antibody bound to graphene will play the role of targeting drug-resistant cancer cells) [9]. In addition, the size of graphene affects its role as a drug carrier and the effectiveness of the drug loaded on it. With regards to the selection aspect of the graphene, it should be in a range of more than 100 nm to ensure successful loading of the nano-drug onto it and to prevent it from being easily engulfed by phagocytic cells in the body. Nano-drugs can also make use of the enhanced permeability and retention (EPR) effect to locate tumor tissue [10-13].

As mentioned above, after the gold particles and miR-122 form a composite, the composite adheres onto the graphene that affects drug-resistant cancer cells (gold particles may be incorporated in the graphene). Chemotherapy is an important treatment method for liver cancer [14]. Most liver cancer patients often suffer from ineffective chemotherapy or from effective to gradually ineffective chemotherapy due to the multidrug resistance of cells [15]. Multidrug resistance occurs when tumor cells are exposed to certain anticancer drugs and evolve drug resistance; they have cross-resistance to other drugs with different structures and functions [16]. The mechanism of multidrug resistance formation is very complex, and the increased expression of the cell membrane P-gp and increased activity of GSH-transferase are two important factors [17]. The aim of this interdisciplinary study is to investigate how to use miR-122, the P-gp antibody and FA for cancer targeting, tumor imaging, and photo-thermal therapy. Size, surface charge, hydrophobicity and other surface properties will be used to enhance the killing of cancer cells by using GGMPN with a semiconductor laser. Furthermore, the toxicity profiles of the GGMPN on red blood cell (RBC) hemolysis

will be explored. Finally, the mechanisms of GGMPN-induced apoptosis and cytotoxicity were also investigated [18,19].

## Methods
### Cells, animals and chemicals
The animal studies were approved by the institutional animal care and committee of Nanjing Medical University. The female nude mice (6 weeks old) were purchased from the Animal Feeding Farm of the National Institute for the Control of Pharmaceutical and Biological Products (Beijing, China). All mice were housed in the animal facility, and the animal experiments were conducted following the guidelines of the Animal Research Ethics Board of Nanjing Medical University. The animals were kept in the facility with free access to food and water. The adriamycin-resistant HepG2 cell line was purchased from the Institute of Biochemistry and Cell Biology, Shanghai Institutes for Biological Sciences, Chinese Academy of Sciences (Shanghai, China) and was cultured in RPMI 1640 supplemented with 10% FBS (GIBCO) and penicillin (100 U/mL)/streptomycin (100 mg/mL) at 37°C in a 5% $CO_2$ and water-saturated atmosphere. MiR-122 was synthesized from GenePharma Biotechnology (Institute of Biochemistry and Cell Biology, Shanghai Institutes for Biological Sciences, Chinese Academy of Sciences).

### P-gp antibody-graphene oxide synthesis and characterization
Graphene oxide synthesis and collection: 1 g of graphene and 50 g of sodium chloride were milled together for 10 mins, and the polish was dissolved in water and filtered. The filtration residue was oxidized with 23 mL $H_2SO_4$ (98%) and stirred for 8 h. Then, 3 g of $KMnO_4$ was gradually added to the above mixture, and the reaction temperature was maintained at 20°C. After stirring the mixture at 38°C for 30 min and then stirring again for 45 min at 70°C, 46 mL of water was added to the above-mentioned mixture and was heated to 98°C for 30 min. Then, 140 mL of water and 10 mL of $H_2O_2$ (30%) was gradually added to the above mixture. After sufficient reaction product was recovered by filtration, the filtrate was dissolved in 10 mL HCl (5%). Gradient centrifugation was used on 1 mL of the above graphene (1.5 mg/mL) to separate it by size and type. The following centrifugation conditions were used, sequentially: 2 h, 10,000 rpm/min; 2 h, 20000 rpm/min; 2 h, 30,000 rpm/min; 2 h, 40,000 rpm/min; and 2 h, 50,000 rpm/min. After centrifugation, the sample was dried at room temperature, and a JEM-2100 transmission electron microscope (TEM) was used to observe the morphology of the sample. The hydroxyl group along the 500 nm side of the graphene oxide was replaced with a carboxylic acid. Then, 5 mL of

above-mentioned graphene oxide (2 mg/mL), 1.2 g NaOH (ultrasound 1 h) and 1.0 mL chloroacetic acid (Cl-CH$_2$-COOH) were added to the above solution and placed in ultrasound for 2 h. P-gp antibody (1 mg/mL) was added to the above-described oxidation graphene re-action system (v/v, 1:10) to react overnight. The product was dried under vacuum at room temperature, and protein electrophoresis analysis was performed. The antibody remaining in supernatant was checked using a Protein Assay kit (Thermo Scientific, USA). The same antibody without adsorption on GGMPN was used as the control.

### MiR-122-gold nanoparticles synthesis and control relase analysis

Briefly, 0.3 mL freshly prepared sodium borohydride (0.08%), 1 mL CTAB (2.15%) and 0.32 mL chloroauric acid (1%) were added dropwise to 30 mL of a FA (1 mg/mL) solution, which was stirred for 20 min at room temperature. Gold nanoparticles mixed with 0.5 mL miR-122 (0.001 mg/mL) were stirred for 0.5 h, and the gold nanoparticles were recovered by centrifugation. The OD value of the super-natant was used to quantify the amount of miR-122 loaded. The same amount of miR-122 of the gold nano-particles was loaded into the wells of an agarose gel to perform electrophoresis to detect GSH for miR-122 in the sustained-release experiment. For the well without GSH added, no nucleic acid showed bands. Similarly, we used miR-122 with added AO (acridine orange), which showed a fluorescence intensity change. After the disappear-ance of fluorescence, gold nanoparticles were added, and miR-122 was adsorbed onto the gold nanoparticles. Add-ing GSH (GSH replaced miR-122) enabled miR-122 to recombine with the AO. This experiment provided fur-ther evidence showing that GSH could control the release of miR-122.

Preparation and characterization of GGMPN compos-ites: 1 mL of P-g antibody-graphene oxide (1 mg/mL) was added to the chitosan solution (1% acetic acid, pH 5.0) and sonicated for 2 h. The final product was then mixed with 0.5 mL (0.001 mg/mL) of the miR-122-gold nanoparticles and stirred overnight. The reactant from vacuum drying was GGMPN, and a JEM-2100 trans-mission electron microscope was used for characterization of the GGMPN morphology.

### GGMPN biocompatibility assay

A SD rat (4 weeks, orbital vein blood) RBC hemolysis experiment was used to test the blood compatibility of GGMPN. Blood was collected in heparinized tubes and centrifuged for 10 min at 1,000 g using a cold centrifuge at 4°C. Samples were washed three times with PBS. The extent of hemolysis was determined under a microscope.

### HepG2 membrane permeability and intracellular miR-122 accumulation assay

The permeability of the adriamycin-resistant HepG2 (folate receptor FR(+)) cell membrane was measured by lactate dehydrogenase (LDH CytoTox 96 assay) treated with GGMPN. The intracellular fluorescence intensity of red fluorescence-labeled miR-122 of was used to detect and quantify the accumulation of miR-122 in cancer cells with confocal fluorescence microscopy.

### SEM analysis of morphological images of HepG2 cells

HepG2 cells were seeded on top of cover glass slips; GGMPN was then administered to these HepG2 cells. After 1 h of incubation, the cells were trypsinized and fixed using 2.5% glutaraldehyde overnight. The treated cells were washed with PBS for 5 min, after which they were washed again with 30%, 50%, 70%, 80%, 90%, 95% and 100% ethanol before being carefully dried for SEM experiments.

### TEM analysis of cellular distribution of gold nanoparticles

Drug resistant HepG2 cells were treated with GGMPN, washed with PBS, and then fixed in 2.5% glutaraldehyde. Ultrathin sections were cut and mounted on copper grids. These sections were viewed under a JEOL 1200-EX trans-mission electron microscope equipped with energy disper-sive X-ray spectroscopy (EDS). Gold nanoparticles were identified by EDS analysis, and their sub-cellular distri-bution was investigated from the transmission electron micrographs.

### MTT assay on cytotoxicity

Drug-resistant HepG2 cells were maintained in RPMI-1640 medium containing 10% FBS, 100 U/mL of penicil-lin, and 100 μg/mL of streptomycin at 37°C with 5% CO$_2$ before being plated in 96-well plates ($2 \times 10^3$ cells/well). After overnight incubation, various concentrations of GGMPN treatment were added into specified wells. After 36 h, a 20 μL MTT solution (5 mg/mL) aliquot was added to each well. After 4 h of incubation, the supernatant was removed, and 100 μL of DMSO was added to each well. The samples were then shaken for 15 min before the optical density (OD) was checked at a wavelength of 540 nm. All experiments were performed in triplicate. Relative inhibition of cell growth was calcu-lated as follows: Cell viability% = ([OD] test/[OD] con-trol) × 100%.

### *In vitro* GGMPN promote cancer cell apoptosis analysis

Staining detection of DNA fragments and flow cytome-try apoptosis rate determination was performed on the HepG2 cells treated with miR-122/Lipofectamine 2000 or GGMPN. Apoptotic DNA extraction of HepG2 cells was carried out by a Biovision apoptosis DNA ladder

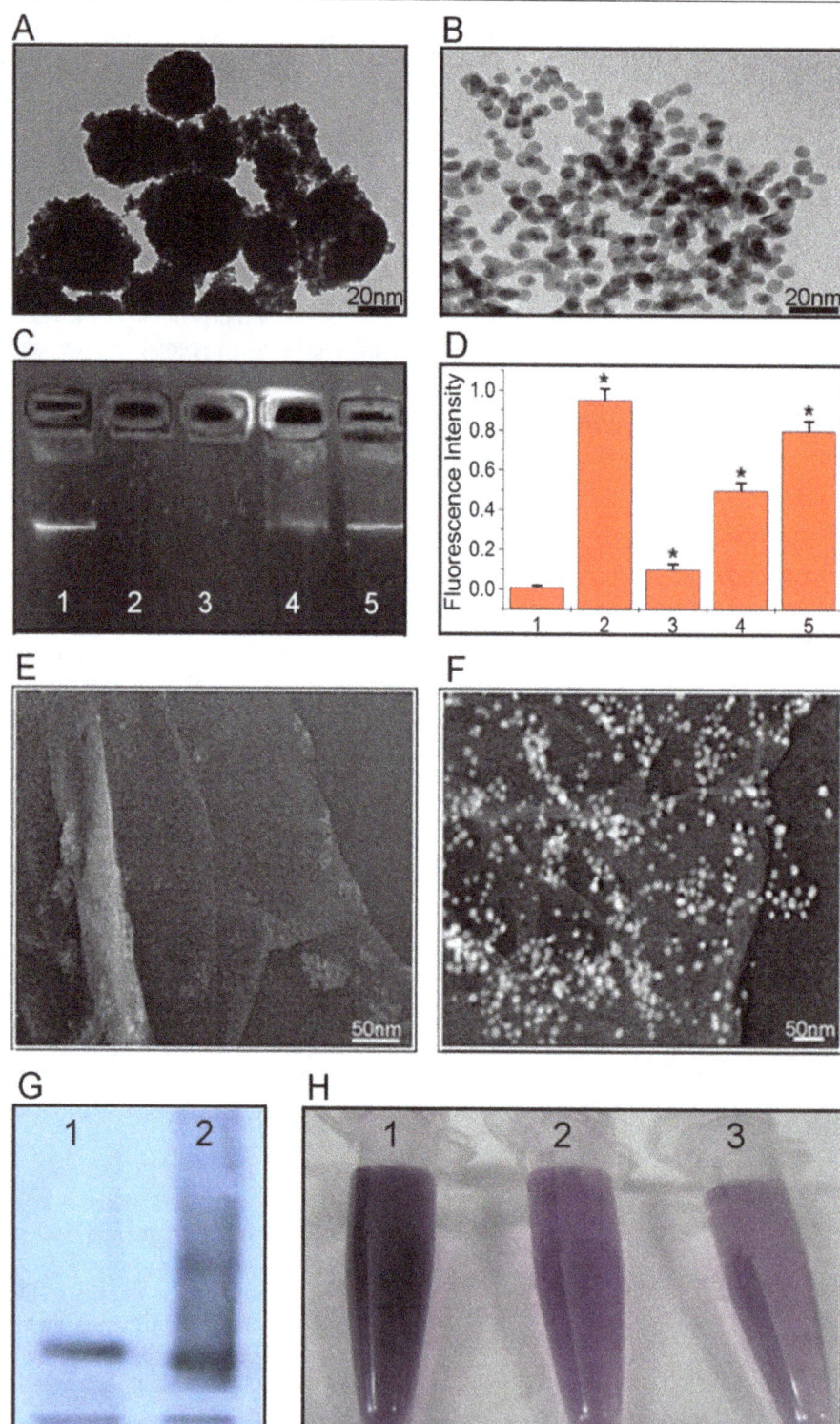

**Figure 1** (See legend on next page.)

**Figure 1 Synthesis and characterization of miR-122-loaded graphene-gold composites. A**: HRTEM image of miR-122-loaded graphene-gold composites (Scale bar =20 nm). **B**: Low magnification image of gold nanoparticles (Scale bar =20 nm). **C**: Confirmed function of miR-122 release by GSH through agarose gel electrophoresis assay; 1) 1 mg/L miR-122, 2) 10 mg/L GGMPN, 3) 10 mg/L GGMPN + 2 µM GSH, 4) 10 mg/L GGMPN + 2 mM GSH, 5) 10 mg/L GGMPN + 10 mM GSH. **D**: Verified function of miR-122 by GSH through AO fluorescence assay; 1) AO, 2) AO + miR-122, 3) AO + miR-122 + gold nanoparticles, 4) AO + miR-122 + 2 mM GSH, 5) AO + miR-122 + gold nanoparticle + 10 mM GSH. **E**: TEM image of graphene oxide (Scale bar =50 nm). **F**: TEM image of GGMPN nanocomplexes (Scale bar =50 nm). **G**: Protein electrophoresis analysis of P-gp antibody. P-gp antibody (lane 1), P-gp antibody-loaded GGMPN (lane 2). **H**: Quantification of P-gp antibody remaining in solution before (1) and after 1 h (2) or 24 h (3) exposure to graphene oxide.

reagent and then added into an agarose gel for electrophoresis analysis.

Western blot analysis: Antibodies against the following were used: Bcl-w, Caspase 9 (mitochondrial pathway), Caspase 3, PARP, p38, and JNK MAPK (involved in cell proliferation and differentiation). The proteins were detected by enhanced chemiluminescence.

## Photothermal therapy on HepG2 cells by GGMPN

GGMPN was used for HepG2 in vitro laser hyperthermia. The laser irradiation experiment involved choosing different wavelengths of semiconductor lasers. HepG2 cells were added to the GGMPN solution, exposed to a power density of 20 W/cm$^2$ of the semiconductor laser light source and irradiated for 1 min for trypan blue staining.

## GGMPN to target tumor cells image and promote apoptosis of HepG2 tumor in nude mice

HepG2 tumors in nude mice (*in vivo* model): HepG2 cells (10$^6$ cells in 200 µL DMEM culture) were injected in a logarithmic growth phase in nude mice and divided into 3 groups, each consisting of 5 nude mice: the first group was the saline control group, the second group was the 1 mg/kg miR-122/Lipofectamine 2000-treated group, and the third group was the 10 mg/kg GGMPN-treated group. One week after tumor cell inoculation, when the tumor had grown to approximately 50 mm$^3$ size, four groups of nude mice were injected in the tail vein with variety of drugs at 0, 2, 4, 6, 8, 10, 12, 14, 16, and 18 days. After the first 20 days, when the tumor was removed and fixed with formalin, the size of the tumor volume was calculated by the following formula: V = π/6 × [(A + B)/2]$^3$, where A was the maximum diameter of the tumor and B was the minimum diameter of the tumor.

Photothermal therapy experiments in vivo: nude mice were injected in the tail vein with GGMPN. The tumor was irradiated with the semiconductor laser light source 10 times for 10 min (every two days). Then, the tumor was removed, and its final volume was calculated.

For the tumor imaging study, biodistribution activities were induced to obtain enough activity to acquire the images. GGMPN was used for confocal microscopy 3D reconstruction imaging of HepG2 cells, and the detection of green, yellow, and red separately fluorescently labeled miR-122-GGMPN in HepG2 cells was carried out. The animals were anesthetized with pentobarbital sodium intraperitoneally and were placed on the table in a side position so that the detector was positioned on the tumor region of the animal. A small animal model *in vivo* imaging instrument (Carestream Multispectral) was used (Lumina XR).

Apoptosis was achieved by terminal deoxynucleotidyl transferase-mediated dUTP nick end labeling (TUNEL) detection of DNA fragments. When observed under a microscope, dark brown cell apoptosis was found in tumor cells, while blue cells were found in normal tumor cells. Three slices of each tumor were randomly selected, and 10 images of each slice were taken for statistical analysis. Apoptosis in vivo: pictures of nude mouse tumor tissue were taken, the tumor was lysed, and protein extracts were used for western blot analysis. The antibodies used included those against Bcl-w, Caspase 9 (mitochondrial pathway), and Caspase 3 to study the relationship of the signal transduction pathway and tumor proliferation.

## Detection of gold nanoparticles in nude mice' organs

Five mice from each group were sacrificed (carbon dioxide euthanasia) at 5 weeks to obtain organs (bone, skin, muscle, intestine, liver and tumor). The tissue was digested to measure Au levels. All of the organs were washed with distilled, deionized water and dried on paper towels. Samples were dried to constant weights at 105°C. The organs were then ground in an agate mortar and digested in aqua regia. After appropriate dilution with double-distilled H$_2$O, the metal concentrations of the samples were determined by atomic absorption spectrophotometry.

## Statistical analysis

Results were presented as Mean ± SD. A t-test was performed in each group for each time point. A value of P < 0.05 was considered statistically significant.

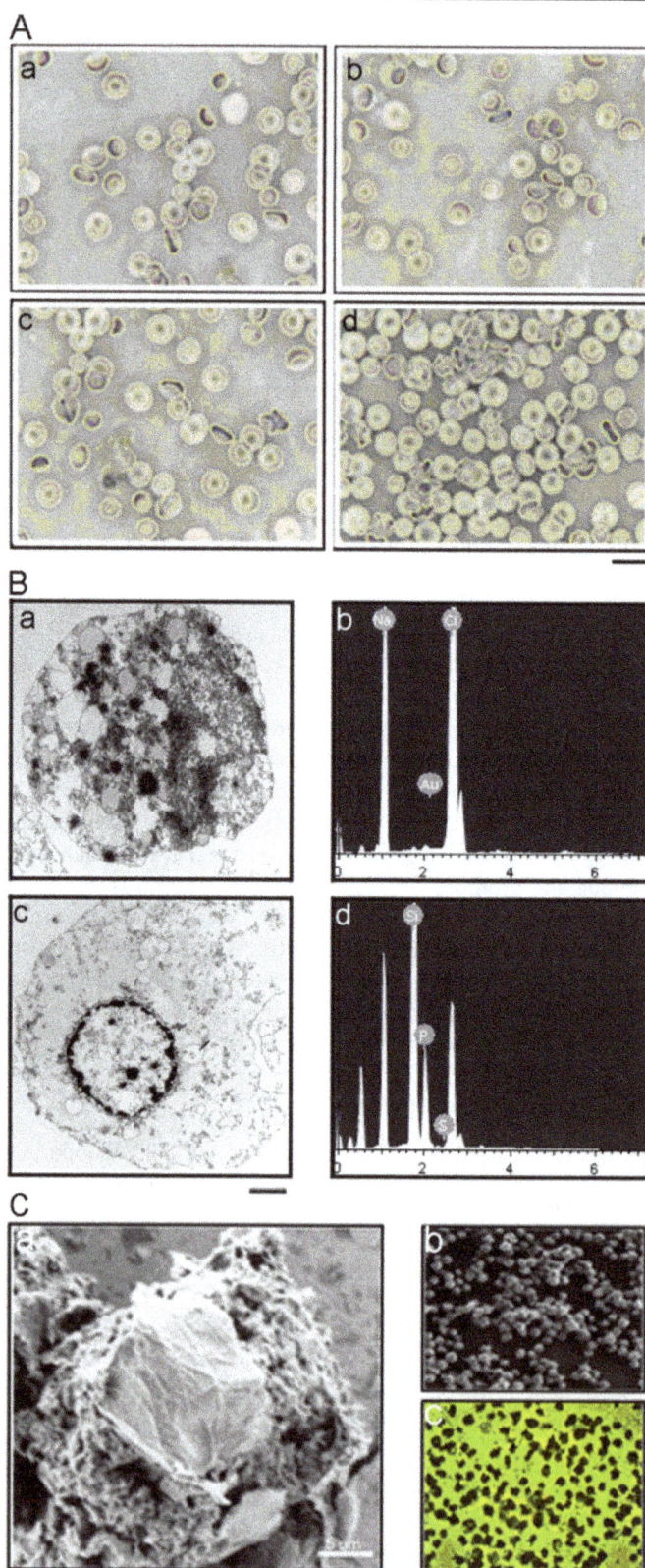

**Figure 2** (See legend on next page.)

(See figure on previous page.)

**Figure 2 Biocompatibility assay and TEM image of the cellular distribution of GGMPN. A:** Photographs of RBC suspensions in the presence of various reagents; **a)** 10 mg/L GGMPN for 1 h, **b)** 1 mg/L miR-122 (same concentration as loaded on GGMPN) was transfected with Lipofectamine 2000 for 1 h, **c)** untreated control, **d)** treated with 10 mg/L GGMPN for 5 h (Scale bar =20 µm). **B:** Characterization of sub-cellular distribution of gold nanoparticles by TEM and EDS; **a, c)** TEM image of gold nanoparticles in tumor cells treated with or without 10 mg/L GGMPN, **b, d)** EDS analysis of gold nanoparticles distributed in tumor cells treated with or without 10 mg/L GGMPN ( Scale bar =50 nm). **C: a)** SEM image of HepG2 cells after GGMPN treatment (during 1 h); **b)** SEM image of HepG2 cells transfected with miR-122 (1 mg/L, the same concentration as loaded on GGMNP) (during 1 h); **c)** Morphology of HepG2 cells after GGMPN treatments by microscope assays.

## Results

### Synthesis and identification of GGMPN

Gold nanoparticles loaded with miR-122, termed GGMPN, were synthesized and identified using TEM imaging. We found that the complex of gold nanoparticles and miR-122 was approximately 20 nm (Figure 1A). However, the average size of the gold nanoparticles was approximately 5 nm (Figure 1B). Thus, we speculated that an abundant amount of miR-122 could be combined with the gold nanoparticles. We already knew that some small molecules (e.g., RNA) could be flexibly released by GSH from the surface of the nanoparticles. We combined negatively charged miR-122 with positively charged gold nanoparticles. As shown in Figure 1, the release reactions between gold nanoparticles and miR-122 could be performed through electrophoresis assays (Figure 1C). We demonstrated that gold nanoparticles completely prevented miR-122 from moving to the positive electrode; thus, the gold nanoparticles/miR-122 remained in the sample well (Figure 1C, lane 2). It could be observed that the positively charged gold nanoparticles counteracted the negative charges of miR-122. As expected, a small amount of miR-122 was detected at the same site of pure miR-122 (Figure 1C, lane 1) when the concentration of GSH reached 2 mM (Figure 1C, lane 4). The mobility of miR-122 completely recovered when the final concentration of GSH reached 10 mM (Figure 1C, lane 5). Negatively charged GSH contained a thiol ligand, which had a stronger affinity to the gold nanoparticles. Herein, it was established that the addition of GSH might counteract the positive charge of gold nanoparticles to some extent by place exchange and resulted in the release of miR-122 from the gold nanoparticles (Figure 1D).

As shown in Figure 1E and F, graphene oxide and GGMPN nanocomposites (500 nm) were synthesized and characterized. The TEM image demonstrated a homogeneous distribution of gold nanoparticles on the P-gp antibody-graphene oxide surface with chitosan functionality. Moreover, we also illustrated that the P-gp antibody could be effectively absorbed by graphene oxide (Figure 1H) and separated from GGMPN (Figure 1G). The results suggested that P-gp antibody-graphene oxide and GSH might play a critical role in combining miR-122 with GGMPN to enhance the targeting of miR-122 to

cancer cells. The relevant miR-122 loading efficiency was further determined by OD analysis, which indicated that the miR-122 loading onto GGMPN was approximately 10%.

### Biocompatibility and cellular distribution analysis of GGMPN

We next assessed the hemolytic effect of GGMPN in cells subjected to various treatments. For RBCs (red blood cells) treated with 10 mg/L GGMPN for 5 h (Figure 2A, d), there was no hemolysis of RBCs co-cultured with 10 mg/L GGMPN for 1 h (Figure 2A, a), of those transfected with miR-122 (Figure 2A, b), or of the untreated control (Figure 2A, b). Furthermore, it was expected that slight hemolysis would occur when RBCs were treated with GGMPN for 5 h (Figure 2A, d). The results showed that GGMPN had a low hemolytic effect when treated with cells for 5 h.

We next observed the morphological changes on sub-HepG2 cells after treatment with or without GGMPN. TEM characterization showed the typical distribution of gold nanoparticles in HepG2 cells treated with GGMPN (Figure 2B, a) compared with the untreated control (Figure 2B, c). Meanwhile, both dispersive nanoparticles and clusters of gold nanoparticles were observed in tumor cells (Figure 2B, a). Additionally, the results (Figure 2B, b) of EDS analysis remarkably demonstrated gold content in the cells, which was consistent with the above TEM study (Figure 2B, a), suggesting that gold nanoparticles could be readily internalized by cells for drug delivery. In contrast, the images (Figure 2B, d) from EDS analysis showed no gold content in HepG2 cells (not treated with GGMPN). These results suggested that GGMPN was biologically safe and could deliver miR-122 into targeted cancer cells.

Based on the above study, bio-imaging of GGMPN or miR-122 alone in HepG2 cell lines was performed with a scanning electron microscope (SEM). As shown in Figure 2C, a, the morphology of HepG2 cells was changed when treated with GGMPN. The treatment also caused stronger adsorption of GGMPN on the cell membrane compared with miR-122 transfected with Lipofectamine 2000 (Figure 2C, b). GGMPN induced the morphological changes in HepG2 cells (Figure 2C, c).

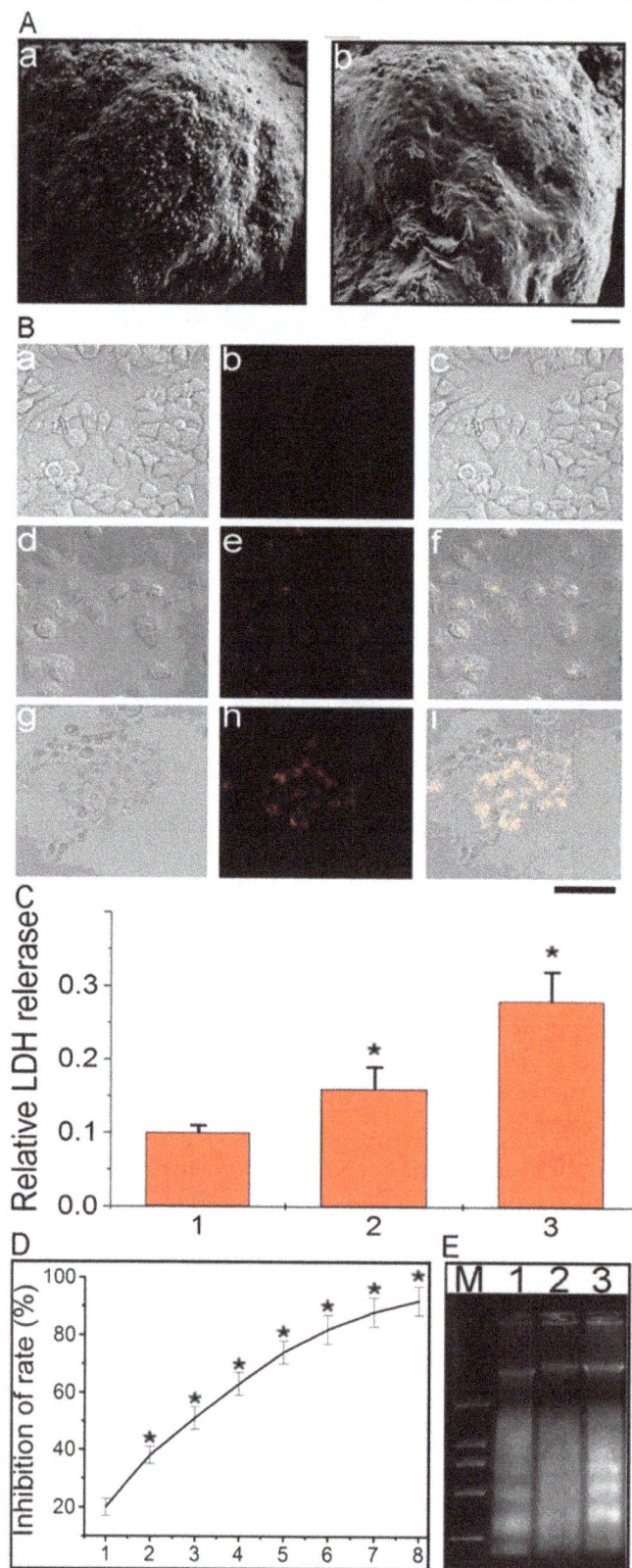

**Figure 3** (See legend on next page.)

(See figure on previous page.)
**Figure 3 Morphological and intracellular miR-122 accumulation assay. A**: SEM image of HepG2 cells incubated with 10 mg/L GGMPN **(a)**, or without treatment **(b)** for 1 h (Scale bar =3 μm). **B**: GGMPN delivered miR-122 into resistant HepG2 cells as imaged through laser confocal fluorescence microscopy; **a-c)** untreated cells, **d-f)** cells transfected with red fluorescent-modified miR-122 (1 mg/L, same concentration as loaded on GGMPN), **g-i)** cells combined with 10 mg/L GGMPN-loading red fluorescent-modified miR-122 (Scale bar = 50 μm). **C**: Quantitative assay of GGMPN on cell membrane permeability based on the CytoTox 96 assays; 1) untreated control, 2) resistant HepG2 cells transfected with miR-122 (1 mg/L, same concentration as loaded on GGMPN), 3) resistant HepG2 cells incubated with 10 m/L GGMPN. **D**: MTT assay for evaluation of the growth of cells treated with GGMPN. HepG2 cells were treated with 0.001, 0.01, 0.1, 1, 10, 100, 1000, or 10000 mg/L of GGMPN. *P < 0.05 indicates a significant difference in comparison to untreated control. E: DNA fragmentation of HepG2 cells after different treatments. Genomic DNA was isolated from HepG2 cells, which were treated as follows: 5 mg/L GGMPN (lane 1), 2 mg/L GGMPN (lane 2), or 10 mg/L GGMPN (lane 3); DNA marker (M).

## SEM image and intracellular miR-122 accumulation assay

FA on miR-122 of gold nanoparticles caused more miR-122 adherence with the gold nanoparticles on the surface of the cell membranes (Figure 3A, a) compared with cancer cells (unloaded FA on gold nanoparticles) (Figure 3A, b). We demonstrated that the miR-122 on the gold nanoparticles could precisely target the cancer cells with the FA functionality.

Next, we further determined the location of GGMPN in HepG2 cells with laser confocal fluorescence microscopy. For the control cells without treatment, we observed almost no intracellular fluorescence in the HepG2 cells (Figure 3B, a,b,c). However, the intracellular fluorescence in HepG2 cells increased dramatically upon treatment with GGMPN containing the red fluorescent-modified miR-122 (Figure 3B, g,h,i) compared with miR-122-transfected cells (Figure 3B, d,e,f). The results indicate that the intracellular content of miR-122 increased after treatment with GGMPN. These results demonstrated that GGMPN carrying miR-122 could be effectively taken in by drug-resistant HepG2 cells. They also showed that GGMPN had an impact on cell permeability compared with cells transfected with miR-122 (Figure 3C). Moreover, when increasing the concentration of GGMPN, we also demonstrated that the growth of HepG2 cells was strongly suppressed (Figure 3D), and the intensity of fragmented chromosomal DNA bands of treated HepG2 cells became much stronger (Figure 3E).

## Analysis of apoptosis in GGMPN treated cells

In order to further determine the apoptotic effect of GGMPN in HepG2 cells, the AO/EB staining assay was used. Apoptotic nuclei were identified by their characteristic features such as chromosomal condensation, with distinct margination and fragmentation under fluorescence microscopy. In the present study, we also found that the apoptotic nuclei of HepG2 cells (Figure 4A (d,h,l), later apoptosis nuclei) treated with GGMPN for 48 h could be clearly identified by their distinctively marginated and fragmented appearance compared with early stage of apoptosis in cells treated

for 24 h (Figure 4A (b,f,j), early apoptosis nuclei) and normal dead cells (Figure 4A (c,g,k)). For the control cells without treatment, cell nuclei were normal, as shown in Figure 4A (a,e,i).

It was shown using Annexin-V-FITC apoptosis detection that GGMPN induced a much higher apoptosis rate in resistant HepG2 cells (Figure 4B, c) than that of cells transfected with miR-122 (Figure 4B, b) or the untreated control (Figure 4B, a). Meanwhile, we also found that the percentage of apoptotic cells was 60.1%, 47.8%, and 5% for those treated with GGMPN, miR-122 and no treatment, respectively (Figure 4B, d). Furthermore, we further confirmed the apoptosis of cells induced by GGMPN treatment using a DNA fragmentation assay. When HepG2 cells were treated with GGMPN, the intensity of fragmented chromosomal DNA bands (Figure 4C, lane 3) was much higher than that observed from cells treated with miR-122 (Figure 4C, lane 2) or the untreated control (Figure 4C, lane 1).

In order to explore the molecular mechanisms underlying the GGMPN-induced DNA fragmentation, we examined the expression of apoptosis-related proteins in the cells. As shown in Figure 4D, we found that the protein level of Bcl-w, which was a target gene of miR-122, was reduced in HepG2 cells after treatment with GGMPN. Moreover, the cleaved Caspase 9 signals were much stronger in cells treated with miR-122 (Figure 4D, lane 2) than in the untreated control cells (Figure 4D, lane 1). The strongest activation of Caspase 9 occurred after GGMPN treatment (Figure 4D, lane 3). Similar results were obtained for cleaved Caspase 3 and cleaved PARP because they are the downstream elements of the Caspase 9 pathway. The MAPK signal was weaker after GGMPN treatment than after miR-122 treatment as a result of the drug-resistant nature of the cells (Figure 4D, lanes 3 and 2, respectively). The same trend of protein expression was not obtained for P38 and JNK. These data suggested that GGMPN treatment involved the inhibition of activation of anti-apoptosis proteins and caused apoptosis by activation of the Caspase-9, Caspase-3 and MAPK pathways in resistant HepG2 cells.

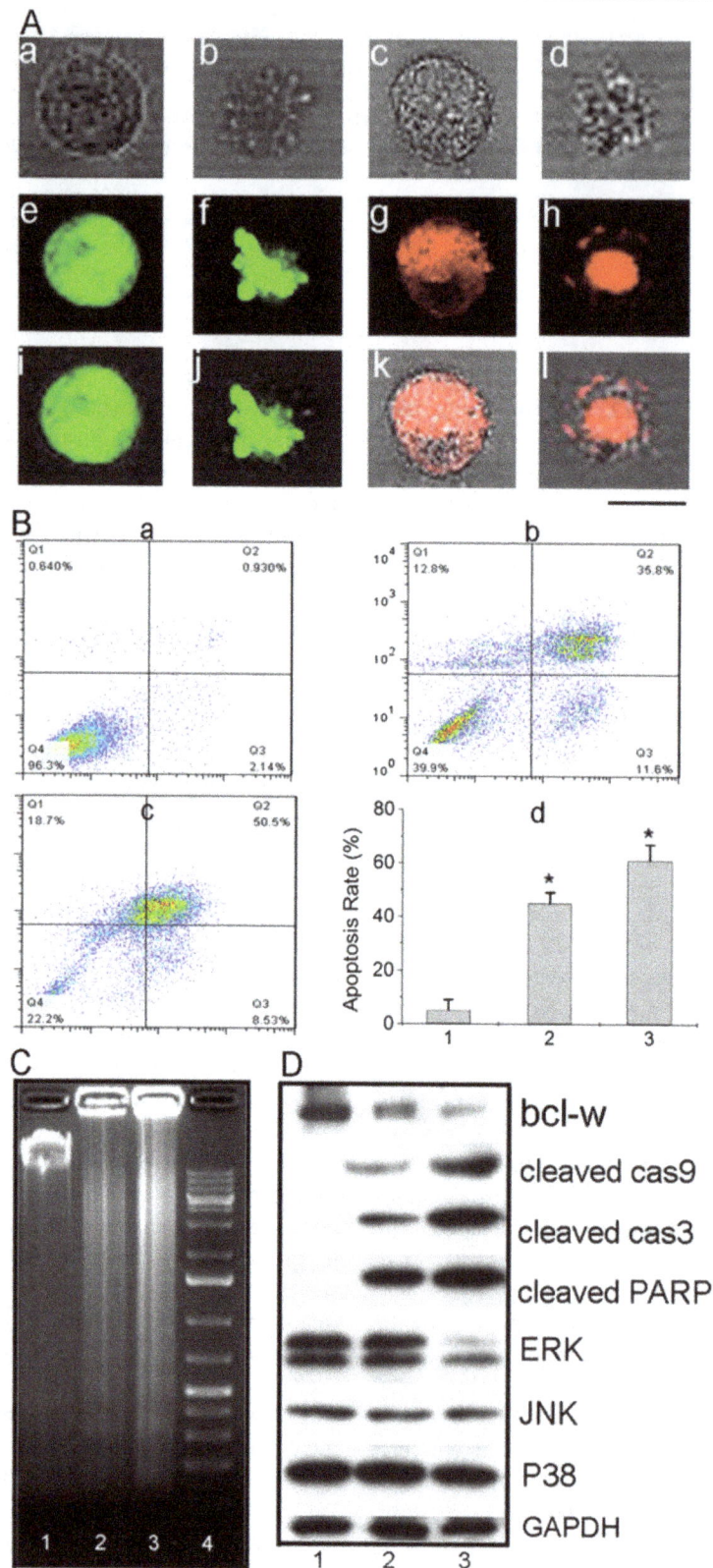

**Figure 4** (See legend on next page.)

**Figure 4 Apoptotic assay of HepG2 cells induced by GGMPN. A**: HepG2 cells were treated with 10 mg/L GGMPN, and their apoptotic level was detected by AO/EB staining; **(a, e, i)** image of normal cells, **(b, f, j)** image of early apoptotic cells, **(c, g, k)** normal dead cells, **(d, h, l)** image of late apoptotic cells (Scale bar =10 μm). **B**: Flow cytometric measurement of cellular apoptosis of resistant HepG2 cells treated with various reagents; **a)** untreated control, **b)** transfected cells with miR-122 (1 mg/L, same concentration as loaded on GGMPN), **c)** treatment of cells with 10 mg/L GGMPN for 36 h, **d)** quantitative analysis of apoptotic cells after various treatments shown in a), b) and c), *P < 0.05, compared with the control treatment. **C**: DNA fragmentation in resistant HepG2 cells after different treatments; 1) untreated cells, 2) transfected cells with miR-122 (1 mg/L, same concentration as loaded on GGMPN), 3) treatment of cells with 10 mg/L GGMPN, 4) DNA marker. **D**: Western blot analysis of activated Caspase levels after various treatments; 1) without treatment cells, 2) cells transfected with miR-122, 3) cells treated with GGMPN.

## Photothermal therapy on HepG2 cells treated with GGMPN

To further explore the multifunctional anti-cancer effect of HepG2 cells treated with GGMPN, we probed the GGMPN with a semiconductor laser to perform a hyperthermia experiment. As shown in Figure 5, we found that HepG2 cells treated with GGMPN were severely damaged at a laser power threshold of 20 W/cm² for 10 min (Figure 5A, d) compared with other treatments (Figure 5A, a,b,c). However, no photo-thermal destruction was observed for HepG2 cells treated with miR-122 (Figure 5A, b). Quantitative analysis also showed that the percentages of dyed cells (blue cells) were 2% (control), 3.1% (miR-122 treated), 77.4% (10 mg/L GGMPN at a laser power threshold of 20 W/cm² for 1 min), and 95.8% (for 10 min) (Figure 5C).

To further identify the function of GGMPN in vivo, we established a method to estimate the effect of GGMPN in tumor tissue (Figure 5D-G). In this experiment, 6-week-old mice were subcutaneously implanted with 10⁶ HepG2 tumor cells. After 10 days post-implantation, the mice were divided to 3 groups with 5 mice in each group (Figure 5D). The mice were intravenously injected with various reagents every other day. Combined GGMPN with a 2 W/cm² power semiconductor laser for 10 min every two days (Figure 5E, c) effectively reduced the size and volume (Figure 5D, c) (Figure 5F, 3) of the implanted tumors compared with the untreated group (Figure 5D, a) (Figure 5F, 1) or the miR-122 treatment group (Figure 5D, b) (Figure 5F, 2).

We then further examined the effects of treatment with GGMPN on apoptotic signals. In this experiment, we examined the expression of apoptosis-related proteins in mouse-implanted tumors. As shown in Figure 5G, we found that the protein level of Bcl-w was reduced in mice tumors after treatment with GGMPN (lane 3) compared with miR-122 (lane 2) or the untreated group (lane 1). Moreover, the cleaved Caspase 9 and 3 signals were much stronger in tumors treated with GGMPN with photothermal therapy (lane 3) than with miR-122 (lane 2) or the untreated group (lane 1). These results further provided evidence that GGMPN with photothermal therapy could reduce the apoptosis and inhibit the growth of tumor *in vivo*.

## Analysis of target tumor cell image *in vivo*

Finally, we detected the fluorescent effect of GGMPN labeled by different fluorescent dyes in vitro and in vivo. As shown in Figure 6, 3D reconstruction of HepG2 cells with GGMPN treatment demonstrated a higher intracellular distribution and target function of miR-122 (Figure 6A). Six-week-old nude mice were subcutaneously implanted with 10⁶ HepG2 tumor cells that were treated with labeled GGMPN. We found that the tumors of mice treated with labeled GGMPN could produce fluorescence spontaneously (Figure 6B, b and c). We also found that the percentage of apoptotic cells was 75.9%, 39.7% and 9.1% for treatment with 10 mg/kg GGMPN, miR-122 (transfected cells with miR-122) and the untreated control, respectively (Figure 6C). These results further indicated that GGMPN was good carrier to effectively deliver miR-122 into cancer cells. Moreover, Au concentration in nude mice injected with GGMPN was significantly higher in tumor tissues than in the other groups, as shown in Figure 6D.

## Discussion

As a novel delivery tool, gold nanoparticles (positively charged) could easily absorb small biological molecules (FA) and non-coding RNAs (miR-122). The rationale was that gold nanoparticles, FA and miR-122 were amphiphilic substances (both positive and negative electrical attraction) formed on the core-shell structure of the FA and miR-122 genetic drugs (Figure 1). Gold nanoparticles-miR-122 were formed in nanocomposites, which were further adhered onto graphene. P-gp antibody combined with graphene (Figure 1G,H) performed the targeting of drug-resistant HepG2 cells (Figure 2C). In reality, the size of the graphene is a factor that affects its functioning as a drug carrier. If the size of graphene is too large, it will affect the drug transport in the blood stream. If it is too small, it will affect the drug loading and be easily phagocytosed. Thus, we concluded that the size of graphene should be in the range of approximately 500 nm (through gradient centrifugation) to ensure the graphene drug loading and to avoid phagocytosis by phagocytic cells in vivo. As mentioned above, the nano-drug size range could use

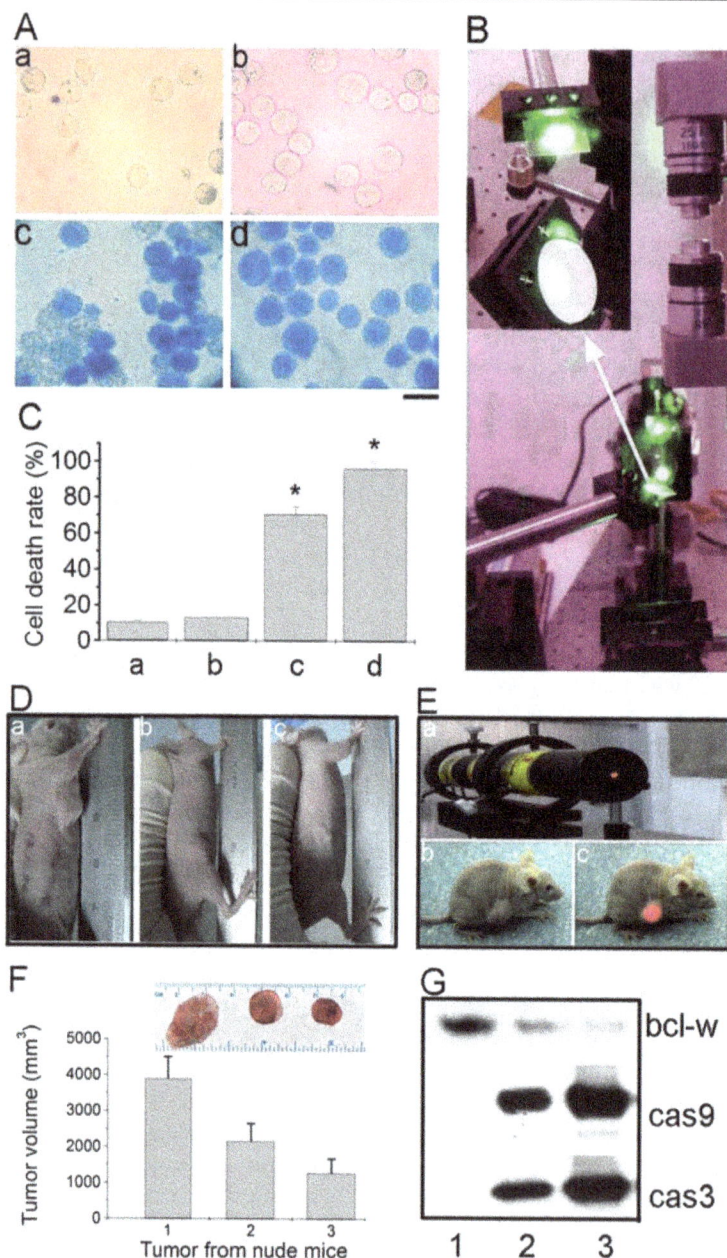

**Figure 5 Photothermal therapy assay of HepG2 cells treated with GGMPN. A**: Images of photothermal therapy of cells with various treatments; **a)** control experiment, **b)** transfected with miR-122, **c)** treated 10 mg/L GGMPN with laser power threshold of 20 W/cm$^2$ for 1 min, **d)** or 10 min. (Scale bar = 20 μm). **B**: Photo of photothermal therapy with semiconductor laser light. **C**: Quantitative analysis of apoptotic cells after various treatments as shown in **A**, * P < 0.05, compared to the control treatment. **D**: Laser hyperthermia with laser irradiation light for inhibition of tumor growth in HepG2 nude mice with different treatments, **a)** untreated used as control, **b)** transfected with miR-122 (1 mg/kg, same concentration as loaded on GGMPN), **c)** treated 10 mg/L GGMPN with laser power threshold of 2 W/cm$^2$. **E**: Photo of tumor irradiated for by laser hyperthermia; **a)** photo of laser hyperthermia, **b)** untreated control, **c)** tumor irradiated by laser hyperthermia. **F**: Quantitative analysis of tumor volume after various treatments as in **(D)**. **G**: Western blot analysis of apoptosis-related protein in tumors of mice treated as in **(D)**.

the enhanced permeability and retention (EPR) effect to target the tumor.

GSH could control the miR-122 release from the gold nanoparticles by replacing the function, which allowed the realization of sustained, controlled release of miR-122 in cancer cells. As a result of our study, the concentration of GSH in erythrocytes was 2 mM, while it was 10 mM in the resistant HepG2 cells (Figure 1C). FR was highly over-expressed in the HepG2 cell line that we selected. Due to the P-gp antibody and FA, the GGMPN could target the

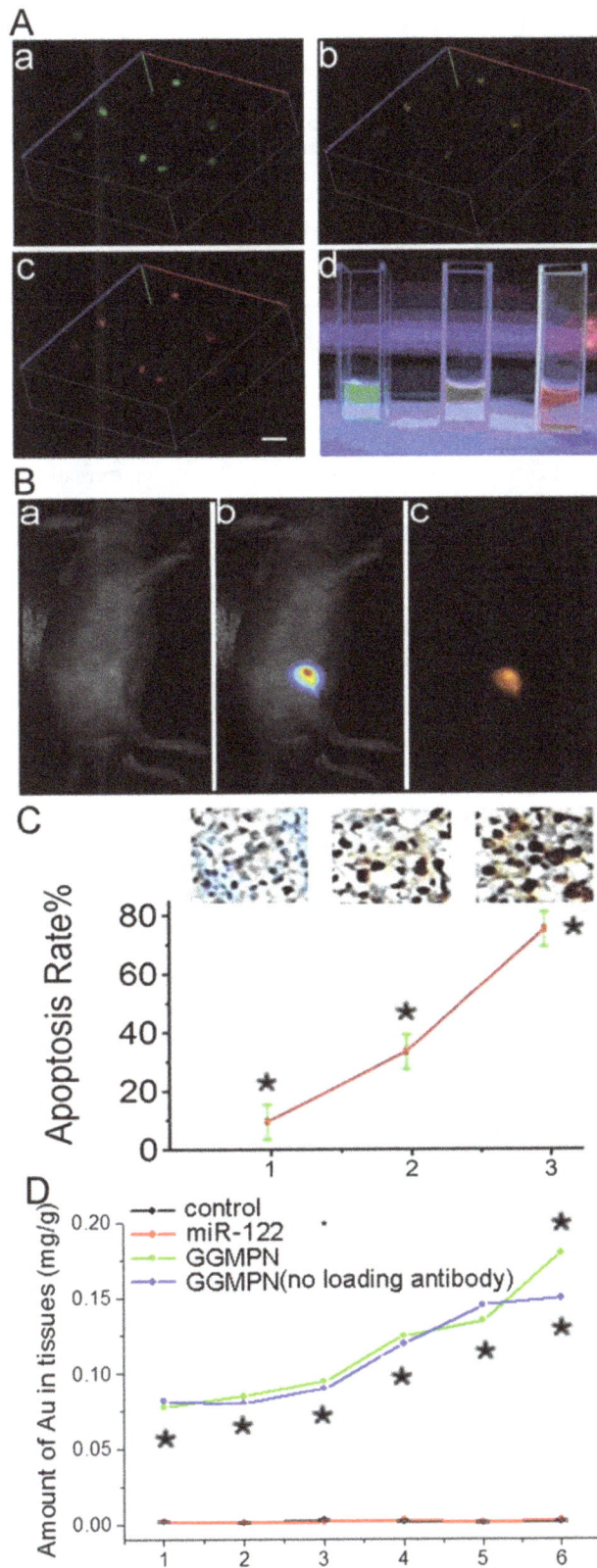

**Figure 6** (See legend on next page.)

(See figure on previous page.)
**Figure 6 Images of tumor cells in vitro and *in vivo*. A**: 3D reconstruction of HepG2 cells treated with 10 mg/L GGMPN with green **(a)**, yellow **(b)**, and red **(c)** fluorescence separately to analyze intracellular distribution (Scale bar = 100 μm), image of HepG2 cells treated with GGMPN labeled with green, yellow and red fluorescence **(d)**. **B**: Fluorescence image of tumor after intravenous injection of 10 mg/L GGMPN (miR-122 with red fluorescent) solution for 2 h; **a)** bright mouse image, **b)** fluorescence intensity scan of xenograft tumor, **c)** red fluorescence near the tumor. **C**: TUNEL staining of HepG2 xenograft tumors after various treatments; 1) untreated control, 2) transfected cells with miR-122, 3) treatment cells with GGMPN, quantitative analysis of apoptotic rate after various treatments **(C)**. **D**: Distribution of Au levels in the liver, the brain, the bone, the muscle, the intestines, and the tumor, respectively. The group numbers for the mouse organs are as follows: (1) bone, (2) skin, (3) muscle, (4) intestine, (5) liver and (6) tumor.

HepG2 cell membrane. Cellular uptake of FA is mediated by both the membrane FR and the reduced folate carrier [20,21]. In this study, we targeted cancer cells via two pathways. As mentioned above, gold nanoparticles loaded with miR-122 were formed as nanocomposites, and the nanocomposite was adhered onto graphene to induce the apoptosis of drug-resistant cancer cells (gold nanoparticles incorporated in the graphene with chitosan activity). Therefore, the nanoparticles could enter the cell by absorbing and puncturing the cancer cell membrane when miR-122-loaded gold nanoparticles were absorbed by HepG2 cells (Figure 3A). The GSH effect provided a potential environment for miR-122 entry into HepG2 cells. In fact, we selected miR-122 instead of chemical drugs for two reasons: to avoid the high toxicity of chemical drugs and to attempt to avoid the multi-drug resistance mechanism of hepatocellular carcinoma in chemotherapy.

HepG2 membrane permeability and intracellular miR-122 accumulation assays were performed. After GGMPN treatment, an increase in the intracellular intensity of the amount of miR-122 was observed in the HepG2 cells. The results demonstrated that cell membrane permeability was significantly increased by GGMPN that then induced the intake of miR-122 in HepG2 cells (Figure 3B). Consistent with this result, gold nanoparticles were also found in the HepG2 cells by TEM characterization and EDS analysis (Figure 2B). These results suggested that gold nanoparticles could be readily internalized by cells for drug delivery.

Next, we further investigated the apoptotic effect of GGMPN on cancer cells by the use of an MTT assay, nuclei staining, and a DNA fragment assay. The results demonstrated that GGMPN elicited an anti-proliferative effect in a dose-dependent manner in HepG2 cells. The apparent IC50 value for GGMPN was estimated as 10 mg/L for HepG2 cells (Figure 3D). Using AO/EB staining for apoptotic cells, apoptotic nuclei were identified by their distinctively marginated and fragmented appearance. The apoptotic nuclei of HepG2 cells (Figure 4A) at 48 h could be identified by their distinctively marginated and fragmented appearance. For the control cells without treatment, cell nuclei were normal. In effect, this was the reason why DNA extracting methods were used to produce apoptosis DNA ladders. Next, it was determined whether cell growth inhibition was caused by the apoptotic response, and the results in Figure 4B show that relevant GGMPN induced a much higher cell apoptosis rate than the untreated control using the Annexin-V-FITC, PI apoptosis detection method. The apoptosis DNA ladders were examined by agarose gel electrophoresis. HepG2 cells were treated with GGMPN, and the intensity of the apoptosis DNA ladders were much higher than that observed from untreated cells or those treated with miR-122. Our observations supported the hypothesis that the remarkable enhancement of apoptosis was induced by the synergistic effect of GGMPN. We carried out anti-cancer research on the GGMPN apoptosis signaling pathway. According to previous studies, miR-122 could induce apoptosis through the Bcl-w pathway. However, the underlying molecular mechanisms of graphene-gold materials and miR-122-induced cancer cell apoptosis were still not very clear. This study highlighted the mechanism of apoptosis in drug-resistant HepG2 cells by GGMPN treatment. We found that GGMPN treatment activates Bcl-w and Caspase 9 pathways to induce apoptosis in HepG2 cells. Cleaved Caspase-9 activated Caspase-3, which correlated with the increased cleaved PARP expression after GGMPN treatments (Figure 4D). Apoptosis DNA ladders were induced during the cell apoptosis by cleaved PARP expression.

Analysis of fluorescent bio-images of the tumors indicated that GGMPN enhanced the treated group, and the image showed features of HepG2 tumors in vivo (Figure 6B). This was expected to improve target volume consistency for treatment. The image results also indicated evidence of photothermal activity. Photothermal activity could deposit a sufficient amount of energy into the tissue under appropriate conditions to raise the temperature above a certain threshold so that cellular cancer destruction could occur. The GGMPN-enhanced photothermal killing of tumor cells by laser had been proven to be effective both in vitro and in vivo. As shown in Figure 5, cancer cells treated with GGMPN were destroyed with the laser, and the growth of the tumor was suppressed. This result was indeed consistent with the earlier observations regarding laser treatment for photothermal therapy in vitro. Meanwhile, the possibility of a tumor inhibition effect on cellular metabolism that increased the apoptosis of tumor cells was analyzed in vivo. The anticancer effect of GGMPN was then evaluated by investigating the extent of apoptosis induction by TUNEL staining in vivo (Figure 6C). In agreement with in vitro signal expression results, HepG2 tumors considerably induced apoptosis protein expression in mice treated with GGMPN. We also found that the Au concentration in the nude mice injected with GGMPN was significantly higher in tumor tissues than in the other groups (Figure 6D). In summary, these results demonstrated that the delivery of miR-122 by the multifunctional effect of GGMPN provided a novel and effective strategy to induce apoptosis and inhibit the growth of tumor cells.

## Conclusions

Taken together, GGMPN has the following advantages: (1) due to the high proportion of specific surface area of graphene, the drug loading capacity of the nanocomposite is greatly improved; (2) the properties of graphene and gold nanoparticles result in low toxicity; (3) bound P-gp antibody and FA has preferred targeting ability; (4) the nano-composite can increase the permeability of a drug-resistant cancer cell membrane, promote the gold particle uptake by the cancer cells and enhance intracellular drug accumulation; (5) the nano-composites have good properties to promote drug-resistant cancer cell apoptosis; (6) the nano-composites attach to tumor cells, resulting in efficient photothermal therapy for killing cancer cells; and (7) the nano-composites allow specific fluorescent bio-marking of the tumors.

### Abbreviations
GGMPN: Monoclonal P-glycoprotein (P-gp) antibodies, folic acid (FA) and miR-122 loaded gold nanoparticles on graphene nanocomposites; MTT: 3-(4,5-dimethylthiazol-2-yl)-2,5-diphenyl tetrazolium bromide; PARP: Proteolytic cleavage of poly-(ADP-ribose) polymerase; TUNEL: Terminal deoxynucleotidyl transferase-mediated dUTP nick end-labeling.

### Competing interests
The authors declare that they have no competing interests.

### Authors' contributions
YY, YQZ, BL, HMW synthesized GGMPN; YJK, YY, ML performed the cell and the animal studies; GZ, XZ, NYH wrote the manuscript. All authors read and approved the final manuscript.

### Acknowledgements
This research was financially supported by NSFC 31201003, 81301305, 61401217, 863 project of China (2012AA022703), funding from the state key laboratory of bioelectronics of southeast university (2012F12, 2012F13, 2014HX12), and science and technology innovation supporting fund (JX10131801149, JX10131801147, JX10131801154), Natural Science Foundation of Jiangsu Province (BK20130892, BK20140900, 13KJB320013, SBK201342972, 13KJB310008).

### Author details
[1]Department of Cell Biology, Nanjing Medical University, Nanjing 210029, China. [2]The State Key Laboratory of Bioelectronics, Department of Biological Science and Medical Engineering, Southeast University, Nanjing 210096, China. [3]Institute of Stomatology, Nanjing Medical University, Nanjing 210029, China. [4]Department of Biochemistry and Molecular Biology, Nanjing Medical University, Nanjing 210029, China. [5]Department of Biomedical Engineering, Nanjing Medical University, Nanjing 210029, China. [6]Maternal and Child Health Institute, Nanjing Maternity and Child Health Care Hospital, Nanjing 210029, China. [7]Jiangnan University Medical School, Wuxi, Jiangsu 214122, China.

### References
1. Pathak A, Vyas SP, Gupta KC. Nano-vectors for efficient liver specific gene transfer. Int J Nanomedicine. 2008;3:31–49.
2. Ruan J, Song H, Li C, Bao C, Fu H, Wang K, et al. DiR-labeled Embryonic Stem Cells for Targeted Imaging of in vivo Gastric Cancer Cells. Theranostics. 2012;2:618–28.
3. Basu S, Bhattacharyya SN. Insulin-like growth factor-1 prevents miR-122 production in neighbouring cells to curtail its intercellular transfer to ensure proliferation of human hepatoma cells. Nucleic Acids Res. 2014;42(11):7170–85.
4. Filipowicz W, Grosshans H. The liver-specific microRNA miR-122: biology and therapeutic potential. Prog Drug Res. 2011;67:221–38.
5. Hou W, Bukong TN, Kodys K, Szabo G. Alcohol facilitates HCV RNA replication via up-regulation of miR-122 expression and inhibition of cyclin G1 in human hepatoma cells. Alcohol Clin Exp Res. 2013;37:599–608.
6. Li W, Abu Samra D, Merzaban J, Khashab NM. P-glycoprotein targeted nanoscale drug carriers. J Nanosci Nanotechnol. 2013;13:1399–402.
7. van Vlerken LE, Amiji MM. Multi-functional polymeric nanoparticles for tumour-targeted drug delivery. Expert Opin Drug Deliv. 2006;3:205–16.
8. Chiappetta DA, Sosnik A. Poly(ethylene oxide)-poly(propylene oxide) block copolymer micelles as drug delivery agents: improved hydrosolubility, stability and bioavailability of drugs. Eur J Pharm Biopharm. 2007;66:303–17.
9. Hayama A, Yamamoto T, Yokoyama M, Kawano K, Hattori Y, Maitani Y. Polymeric micelles modified by folate-PEG-lipid for targeted drug delivery to cancer cells in vitro. J Nanosci Nanotechnol. 2008;8:3085–90.
10. Sahu A, Choi WI, Lee JH, Tae G. Graphene oxide mediated delivery of methylene blue for combined photodynamic and photothermal therapy. Biomaterials. 2013;34:6239–48.
11. Yoshida GJ, Fuchimoto Y, Osumi T, Shimada H, Hosaka S, Morioka H, et al. Li-Fraumeni syndrome with simultaneous osteosarcoma and liver cancer: increased expression of a CD44 variant isoform after chemotherapy. BMC Cancer. 2012;12:444.
12. Stark GR. Cancer chemotherapy. Progress in understanding multidrug resistance. Nature. 1986;324:407–8.
13. Solarska K, Gajewska A, Bartosz G, Mitura K. Induction of apoptosis in human endothelial cells by nanodiamond particles. J Nanosci Nanotechnol. 2012;12:5117–21.
14. Long Q, Xiel Y, Huang Y, Wu Q, Zhang H, Xiong S, et al. Induction of apoptosis and inhibition of angiogenesis by PEGylated liposomal quercetin in both cisplatin-sensitive and cisplatin-resistant ovarian cancers. J Biomed Nanotechnol. 2013;9:965–75.
15. Gui C, Cui DX. Functionalized gold nanorods for tumor imaging and targeted therapy. Cancer Biol Med. 2012;9:221–33.
16. Khlebtsov N, Bogatyrev V, Dykman L, Khlebtsov B, Staroverov S, Shirokov A, et al. Analytical and theranostic applications of gold nanoparticles and multifunctional nanocomposites. Theranostics. 2013;3:167–80.
17. Bellamy WT. P-glycoproteins and multidrug resistance. Annu Rev Pharmacol Toxicol. 1996;36:161–83.
18. Hou Z, Zhan C, Jiang Q, Hu Q, Li L, Chang D, et al. Both FA- and mPEG-conjugated chitosan nanoparticles for targeted cellular uptake and enhanced tumor tissue distribution. Nanoscale Res Lett. 2011;6:563.
19. Zhao R, Hanscom M, Chattopadhyay S, Goldman ID. Selective preservation of pemetrexed pharmacological activity in HeLa cells lacking the reduced folate carrier: association with the presence of a secondary transport pathway. Cancer Res. 2004;64:3313–9.
20. McGuire JJ, Haile WH, Yeh CC. 5-amino-4-imidazolecarboxamide riboside potentiates both transport of reduced folates and antifolates by the human reduced folate carrier and their subsequent metabolism. Cancer Res. 2006;66:3836–44.
21. Lin CJ, Gong HY, Tseng HC, Wang WL, Wu JL. miR-122 targets an anti-apoptotic gene, Bcl-w, in human hepatocellular carcinoma cell lines. Biochem Biophys Res Commun. 2008;375:315–20.

# 18

# Mutation of arginine residues to avoid non-specific cellular uptakes for hepatitis B virus core particles

Izzat Fahimuddin Bin Mohamed Suffian[1,3], Yuya Nishimura[2], Kenta Morita[1], Sachiko Nakamura-Tsuruta[1], Khuloud T Al-Jamal[3], Jun Ishii[2], Chiaki Ogino[1] and Akihiko Kondo[1*]

## Abstract

**Background:** The hepatitis B virus core (HBc) particle is known as a promising new carrier for the delivery of drugs and nucleic acids. However, since the arginine-rich domain that is located in the C-terminal region of the HBc monomer binds to the heparan sulphate proteoglycan on the cell surface due to its positive charge, HBc particles are introduced non-specifically into a wide range of cells. To avoid non-specific cellular uptake with the intent to control the ability of cell targeting, we individually replaced the respective arginine (R) residues of the arginine-rich domain located in amino acid positions 150–159 in glycine (G) residues.

**Results:** The mutated HBc particles in which R154 was replaced with glycine (G) residue (R154G) showed a drastic decrease in the ability to bind to the heparan sulphate proteoglycan and to avoid non-specific cellular uptake by several types of cancer cells.

**Conclusions:** Because this mutant particle retains most of its C-terminal arginine-rich residues, it would be useful in the targeting of specificity-altered HBc particles in the delivery of nucleic acids.

## Background

Hepatitis B virus core (HBc) particles have been studied as promising virus-like particles (VLPs) to serve as carriers in drug delivery systems (DDSs) [1,2]. HBc particles consist of 180 (T = 3) or 240 (T = 4) units of HBc monomers that have the ability to form an icosahedral capsid [3,4]. Coordinating salt and urea concentrations enable control of the phases between assembly and disassembly of the HBc capsid [5]. HBc monomers are composed of two distinct domains: i) an assembly domain (amino acid residues (aa) 1–149) that drives particle formation, and ii) an arginine-rich domain (aa 150–183) that recognizes the cell surface heparan sulphate proteoglycan with an electrostatic interaction [6]. The heparan sulphate proteoglycan is known as a major physiological ligand for many heparin-binding proteins [7]. Additionally, the arginine-rich domain behaves as a binding site for nucleic acids, because of its positively charged residues [8,9].

It has been demonstrated that the engineered HBc monomer deleting the entire arginine-rich domain (aa 150–183) could associate and form a particle structure but it could not bind the cells [10,11]. In particular, the aa 150–162 of HBc is necessary, whereas the aa 163–183 is dispensable for heparan sulphate proteoglycan-mediated cell attachment, even though the aa 160–183 is useful as the binding site to nucleic acid medicine [12]. Thus, there is no doubt that the arginine residues in aa 150–159 serve the cell binding and the uptake. However, the question remains as to which of the aa 150–159 in the arginine-rich domain will bind to the heparan sulphate proteoglycan. To employ HBc particles for the targeted cell-specific delivery of nucleic acids, it is important to understand the arginine residues involved in the non-specific cellular uptake of HBc particles.

In this research, we performed site-directed mutagenesis for the HBc monomer to identify the amino acid residues concerned in the binding to the heparan sulphate proteoglycan. Each arginine (R) residue among aa 150–159 of the arginine-rich domain in the HBc monomer was individually replaced with a glycine (G) residue, and the cellular uptakes of the mutated HBc particles were evaluated. The HBc particle introducing the R154G mutation showed a drastic decrease in all capacities of cellular uptake for HeLa, NuE and A431

* Correspondence: akondo@kobe-u.ac.jp
[1]Department of Chemical Science and Engineering, Graduate School of Engineering, Kobe University, Kobe, Japan
Full list of author information is available at the end of the article

cells. Our results would be useful in the engineering of HBc particles to serve as carriers with cell-specific targeting for nucleic acid delivery.

## Results and discussion

Wild-type and singly mutated (respectively replacing R with G among aa 150–159 in the arginine-rich domain) HBc monomers (Additional file 1) were expressed in *E. coli*, and the proteins were extracted with lysis buffer as well as with dissociation buffer. HBc dimers were then purified by affinity chromatography. It has been proved that the C-terminal histidine-tag on HBc monomer had no significant adverse effect on the particle formation and the cell binding [11]. The expression of each HBc monomer (21 kDa) was confirmed by western blot analysis using anti-His6 antibody (data not shown). The particle formation was confirmed by atomic force microscopy (AFM), scanning electron microscope (SEM) and dynamic light scattering (DLS) (Figure 1). These results indicated that point-mutations replacing R with G in the arginine-rich domain (150–159 aa) did not affect the self-assembly capacity of the HBc dimers.

To evaluate the cell-binding capability of singly mutated HBc particles, each HBc particle was labelled with Alexa Fluor 488. HeLa, A431 and NuE cells were then treated with the labelled HBc particles. After washing the cells to remove the non-bound HBc, the green fluorescence of the cells was analyzed using a flow cytometer. The fluorescence intensity of the cells treated with wild-type HBc particles was measured in relative fluorescence units (RFUs) (Figure 2). Although the relative ability of all singly mutated HBc particles to bind with NuE cells was lower than the ability to bind to HeLa and A431 cells, the relative binding of wild-type HBc and the mutants was consistent among different cell types. The replacement of the R residues at aa 157, 158 and 159

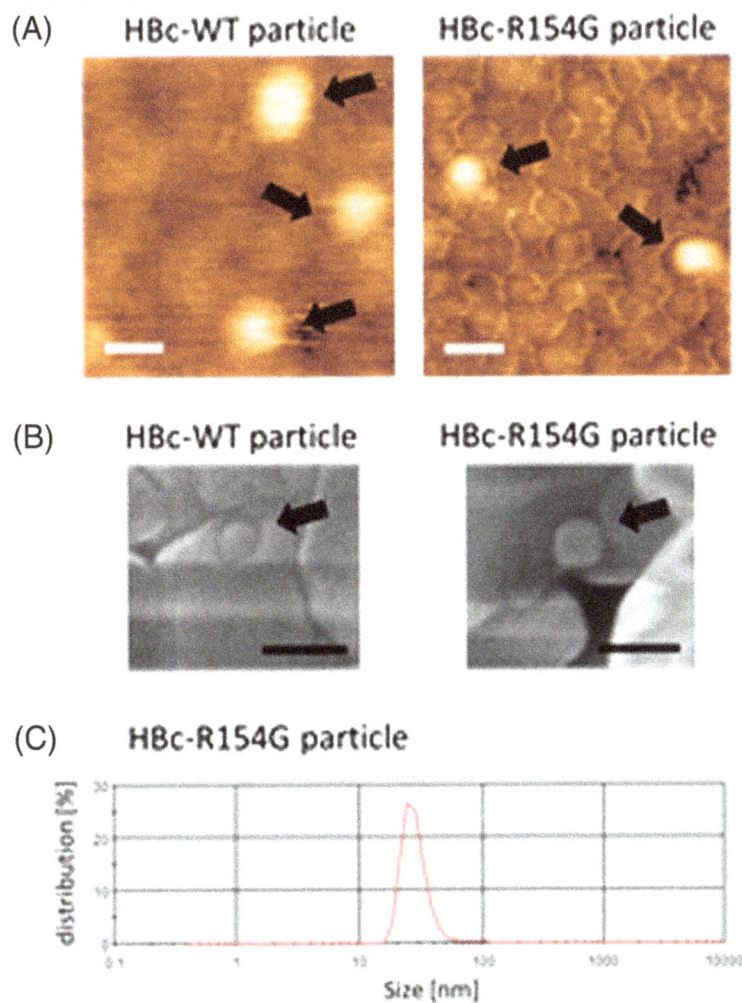

**Figure 1 Analyses of purified HBc particles. (A)** Atomic force microscope images of HBc-WT particle (left) and HBc-R154G particle (right). Scale bar: 50 nm. **(B)** Scanning electron microscope images of HBc-WT particle (left) and HBc-R154G particle (right). Scale bar: 100 nm. **(C)** Size distribution using DLS analysis. The average size of the HBc-R154G particle was 28.7 nm.

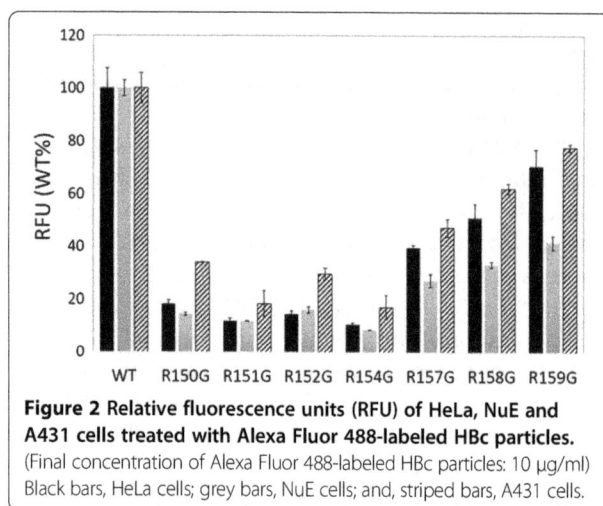

**Figure 2 Relative fluorescence units (RFU) of HeLa, NuE and A431 cells treated with Alexa Fluor 488-labeled HBc particles.**
(Final concentration of Alexa Fluor 488-labeled HBc particles: 10 μg/ml)
Black bars, HeLa cells; grey bars, NuE cells; and, striped bars, A431 cells.

(R157G, R158G and R159G) showed a comparatively higher cell binding ability compared with other HBc mutants. The mutations of R residues at aa 150, 151, 152 and 154 (R150G, R151G, R152G and R154G) in HBc considerably decreased the cell binding ability. Among them, the R154G mutation of HBc was the most effective in decreasing the cell binding ability to all three cell types, while its potency was fairly close to those of R150G, R151G and R152G. Thus, the R154 residue and its peripheral R residues (aa 150–152) in the arginine-rich domain are critical to the cell binding ability of HBc particles, and the HBc-R154G particles would be useful in the development of an engineered HBc particles for the targeted cell-specific delivery of nucleic acids.

Proteins possessing either an arginine-rich domain or a protein transduction domain (PTD) will bind to the heparan sulfate proteoglycan on a cell surface [13,14]. To examine the binding affinity of mutated HBc particles with a heparan sulfate proteoglycan, we performed surface plasmon resonance (SPR) analysis (Figure 3). The binding curve of the HBc-R154G particle was lower than that of wild-type HBc particles, which agreed with the results found using a flow cytometer. The value of $k_a$ showed a 1.5-fold difference between WT-HBc ($1.45 \times 10^7$) and HBc-R154G ($9.44 \times 10^6$) particles. These results indicated that the arginine residue at aa 154 is surely involved in binding to the cell surface of a heparan sulfate proteoglycan.

To evaluate the effect of R154G mutation on cellular uptake, HeLa, NuE and A431 cells were treated with HBc-WT and HBc-R154G particles labelled with Alexa Fluor 488. After incubation for 3 h, the cells were observed by confocal laser-scanning microscope (CLSM) (Figure 4). Green fluorescent signals of HBc-WT particles were observed clearly in all three cell types. In contrast, the green fluorescence of HBc-R154G particles was little observed in any three cell types. This result indicated that the HBc-

R154G particles showed the decrease of the non-specific cellular uptake ability for three different cell types.

## Conclusions

Wild-type HBc particles have the ability to bind to a wide range of cells due to the C-terminal arginine-rich domain that interacts with the cell surface of a heparan sulfate proteoglycan. Arginine residues located within aa 150–159 among the arginine-rich domain were thought to be related to the interaction [12]. Therefore, singly mutated HBc particles in which each arginine residue (aa 150–159) was replaced with glycine residues were prepared. As a result, the cell-binding abilities of most of the mutated HBc particles were decreased compared with wild-type HBc particles. In particular, the HBc-R154G particles displayed the lowest degree of cell binding ability. The HBc-R154G particles showed a clear decrease in the binding ability to a heparan sulfate proteoglycan, as well as a decrease in the cellular uptake capacity. Therefore, the replacement of an arginine residue at the aa 154 position was critical to avoid non-specific cellular binding and uptake. Thus, the R154-mutated HBc particles would be useful in the development of specificity-altered HBc for targeted nucleic acid delivery.

## Methods

### Plasmid construction of wild-type and singly mutated HBc

The plasmid pET-22b-HBc [15] was used to prepare a wild-type HBc particle containing a histidine-tag (His6) at the C-terminus (HBc-WT-His6). To prepare HBc particles with a single mutation (HBc-R15XG-His6, X = 0, 1, 2, 4, 7, 8, 9), each arginine residue was replaced with glycine residue in plasmids expressing singly mutated HBc monomers that were constructed as follows. DNA fragments encoding HBc-R15XG-His6 (X = 0, 1, 2, 4, 7, 8, 9) were amplified by polymerase chain reaction (PCR) from pET-22b-HBc with the the following primers: (5′- TAA TCT CGA GTC TAG AGA ATT AGT AGT CAG CTA TGT -3′ and 5′- CCC CCG CGG CGA GGG AGT TCT TCT TCT AGG GGA CCT GCC TCG TCG TCT AAC AAC AGT AGT TTC -3′ replacing each R with G) based on Additional file 1. The amplified fragments and pET-22b-HBc were digested with XbaI/SacII, and were ligated at the same sites. The resultant plasmids were designated as pET-22b-HBc-R15XG-His6 (X = 0, 1, 2, 4, 7, 8, 9).

### Expression of HBc monomers in Escherichia coli

Each plasmid expressing wild-type and singly mutated HBc monomers was introduced into Escherichia coli BL21 (DE3). The cultures of the transformants (4 ml) were inoculated into 1 L of fresh LB-media (1% tryptone, 0.5% yeast extract, 0.5% NaCl) containing 100 μg/ml ampicillin and grown at 37°C with shaking at 150 rpm until the $OD_{600}$ reached 0.7 ~ 0.8. Then, protein production was

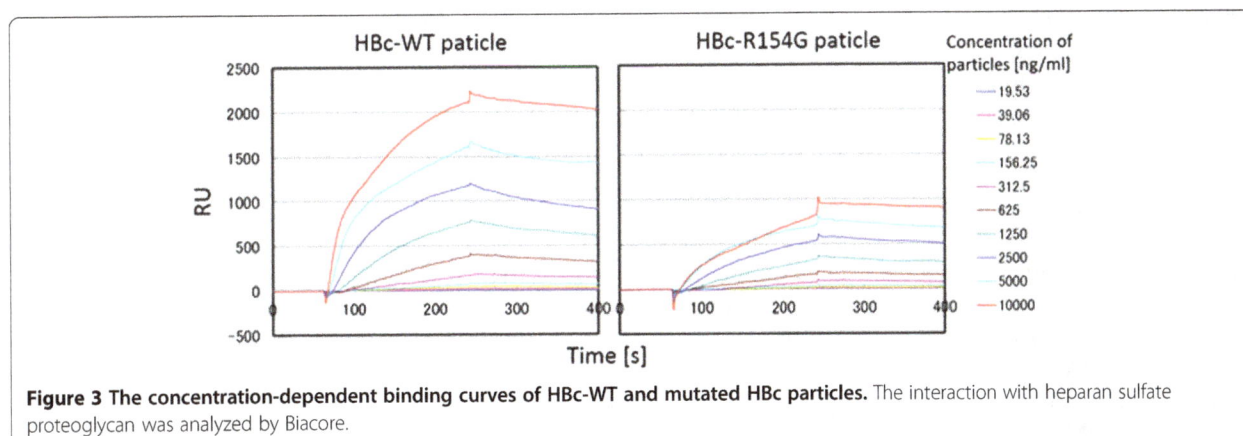

**Figure 3 The concentration-dependent binding curves of HBc-WT and mutated HBc particles.** The interaction with heparan sulfate proteoglycan was analyzed by Biacore.

induced by adding isopropyl-β-thiogalactopyranoside (IPTG) with a final concentration of 100 μM at 25°C overnight. Cells were collected at 3,000 rpm for 15 min, and the sediment was used for purification.

### Purification of HBc particles

Each HBc particle was purified as reported previously [16]. Briefly, a cell pellet was suspended in 30 ml of lysis buffer (pH 8.0) (50 mM Tris–HCl, 100 mM NaCl, 5 mM EDTA, 0.2% Triton X-100, 10 mM β-mercaptoethanol, 10 mg/ml DNAse I, 10 mg/ml RNAse A) with a vortex. The cells were lysed on ice by 3 cycles of sonication for 1 min each at 1 min intervals to avoid heating of the material. The supernatant was removed by centrifugation at 15,000 rpm and 4°C for 30 min. The HBc particles in the pellet were twice washed in 50 ml of lysis buffer and each time collected by centrifugation at 12,000 rpm and 4°C for 15 min. The HBc particles and contaminating *E. coli* proteins were dissolved in 25 ml of dissociation buffer (pH 9.5) (4 M urea, 200 mM NaCl, 50 mM sodium carbonate, 10 mM β-mercaptoethanol) by overnight incubation in a refrigerator at 4°C. After the addition of 10 ml of dissociation buffer, the preparation was incubated for an additional 2 h on ice.

Contaminating proteins were separated from HBc proteins using denaturing affinity chromatography. A column with 10 ml of Ni-agarose (COSMOGEL His-Accept; Nacalai Tesque, Kyoto, Japan) was equilibrated with 5 ml of dissociation buffer in 3 cycles. The preparation was loaded onto the equilibrated column and washed with 5 ml of dissociation buffer in 3 cycles. Bound proteins were eluted with 10 ml of elution buffer (pH 9.5) (dissociation buffer containing 1 M imidazole), and the elution was collected into 1 ml fractions. Each fraction was separated by 15% sodium dodecyl sulphate-polyacrylamide gel electrophoresis (SDS-PAGE), and stained with Coomassie brilliant blue (CBB) to analyse its purity. Fractions containing the pure proteins were polymerized to HBc particles by removal of the urea in the dialysis buffer (pH 7.0) (500 mM NaCl, 50 mM Tris–HCl, 0.5 mM EDTA) overnight. Dialysed HBc particles were obtained through a 0.22 μm filter in 3 cycles. The concentration was measured using a Protein Assay Bicinchoninate Kit (BCA Protein Assay) (Nacalai Tesque).

### Western blotting

The expression of each HBc particle was determined by western blot analysis using a polyvinilidene fluoride (PVDF) membrane. Rabbit anti-6-His antibody (Bethyl Laboratories, Montgomery, TX, USA) was used for the immunoblotting,

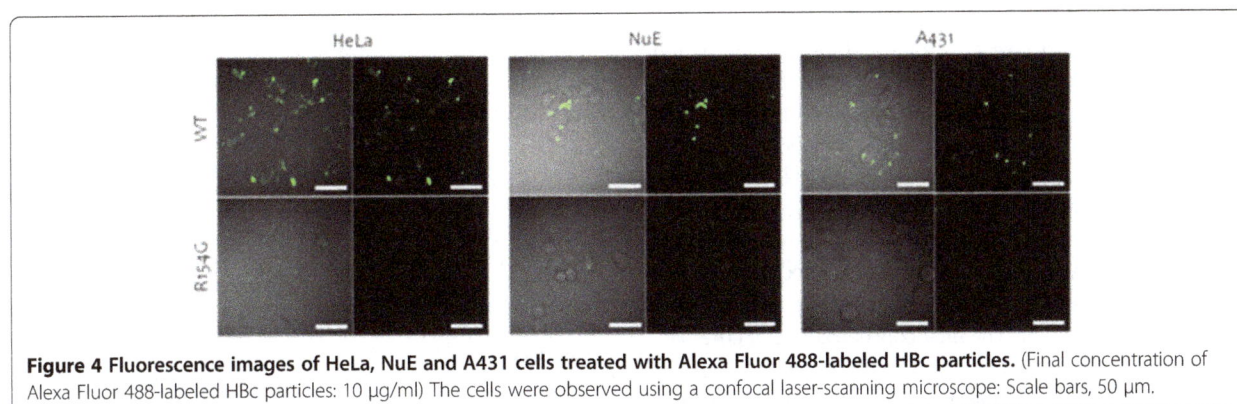

**Figure 4 Fluorescence images of HeLa, NuE and A431 cells treated with Alexa Fluor 488-labeled HBc particles.** (Final concentration of Alexa Fluor 488-labeled HBc particles: 10 μg/ml) The cells were observed using a confocal laser-scanning microscope: Scale bars, 50 μm.

followed by alkaline phosphatase (AP) conjugated anti-rabbit IgG antibody (Promega, Madison, WI, USA). The membrane was stained with 5-bromo-4chloro-3-indolyl phosphate (BCIP) and nitro blue tetrazolium (NBT) (Promega).

### Atomic force microscope (AFM)

One hundred microliter solution containing HBc particles was deposited on mica surfaces (11 mm × 11 mm × 0.15 mm) at room temperature for 5 minutes, and then flushed with air. Tapping mode AFM analysis (TM-AFM) was carried out in air at 25°C using a Bruker Dimension ICON with ScanAsyst® (Bruker UK Ltd, Coventry, United Kingdom). The surface was imaged with a tapping tip mode by MikroMasch in Estonia (NSC15/no Al, tip radius < 10 nm; tip height = 20–25 µm; cone angle < 40°, cantilever thickness = 3.5-14.5 µm; cantilever width = 28–32 µm; cantilever length = 120–130 µm; frequency $f_0$ = 265–400 kHz; force constant k = 20–75 N m$^{-1}$, VEECO, USA). The statistical analysis of the AFM images was carried out using WSxM v5.0 Developed 6.2 software (Nanotec Electronica S.L., Madrid, Spain).

### Scanning electron microscope (SEM)

The freeze-dried HBc particles were analyzed using a JSM-7500 F (JEOL, Munchen, Germany), following the manufacturer's procedure.

### Dynamic light scattering (DLS)

The diameter of HBc particles was measured using a Zetasizer Nano ZS (Malvern Instruments, Worcestershire, UK), following the manufacturer's procedure.

### Cell culture

HeLa and A431 cells were cultured in Dulbecco's modified Eagle's medium (DMEM) (Nacalai Tesque) containing 10% fetal bovine serum (FBS) (Nacalai Tesque), 5% penicillin and streptomycin in the presence of 5% of $CO_2$ at 37°C. NuE cells were cultured in RPMI1640 medium (Nacalai Tesque) containing 10% fetal bovine serum (FBS), 5% penicillin and streptomycin in the presence of 5% of $CO_2$ at 37°C.

### Evaluating the cell binding ability of HBc particles

Purified HBc particles were reacted with Alexa Fluor 488 succinimidyl esters (Molecular Probes/Life Technologies, Carlsbad, CA) for 1 h at room temperature under shading. The mixture then was dialyzed with dialysis buffer overnight to remove the free Alexa Fluor 488 [17]. Approximately $1 \times 10^5$ units of HeLa, A431 and NuE cells were seeded per well into 12-well plates and cultured overnight. The cells were washed with phosphate-buffered saline (PBS) (Nacalai Tesque) and treated with each particle in serum-free medium at 37°C for 1 h. The final concentrations of core particles were 10 µg/ml for each cell. The cells were then washed twice with serum-free medium and treated with fresh-serum

medium at 37°C for 2 h. After washing with PBS, the green-fluorescence was analyzed using a BD FACSCanto II flow cytometer (BD Biosciences, San Jose, CA, USA).

### Surface Plasmon resonance (SPR) analysis

The interaction between HBc particles and heparan sulfate proteoglycan was measured using a Biacore 3000 (GE Healthcare, Piscataway, NJ, USA) [13]. A sensor chip SA (GE Healthcare) immobilizing heparin sodium salt from porcine intestinal mucosa (Sigma-Aldrich, St. Louis, MO, USA) was prepared using an amine coupling method, according to the manufacturer's procedure. Each HBc particle was dissolved in running buffer (HBS-EP buffer: 0.01 M HEPES, 0.15 M NaCl, 3 mM EDTA, 0.005% Surfactant P20, pH 7.4) (GE Healthcare) and loaded onto the sensor chip. The chip was regenerated in 1 M NaCl buffer. As the experimental curve-fitting methodology, a 1:1 Langmuir binding model was used. Each HBc particle was dissolved in running buffer and loaded onto the sensor chip. The signal data were collected using Biacore 3000 Control Software.

### Evaluating the cellular uptake of HBc particles

Approximately $2 \times 10^4$ units of HeLa, A431 and NuE cells were seeded in 35 mm glass-based dishes (Iwaki/AGC Techno Glass, Tokyo, Japan). After incubation for 24 h, the cells were washed with PBS and treated either with HBc-WT or HBc-R154G in serum-free medium at 37°C for 1 h. The final concentration of the particles was 10 µg/ml. The cells were then washed twice with serum-free medium and treated with fresh-serum medium at 37°C for 2 h. The cells were observed using a CLSM 5 PASCAL (Carl Zeiss, Oberkochen, Germany) confocal laser-scanning microscope.

## Additional file

Additional file 1: Base and amino acid sequences of HBc particles.

### Competing interests

The authors declare that they have no competing interests.

### Authors' contributions

Conceived and designed the experiments: IFMS, YN, JI and CO. Performed the experiments: IFMS, YN, KM, SNT and KTAJ. Analyzed the data: IFMS and YN. Wrote the paper: IFMS, YN and JI. Supervised the whole work: AK. All authors have read and approved the final manuscript.

### Acknowledgements

This work was supported in part by a Special Coordination Fund for Promoting Science and Technology, Creation of Innovative Centers for Advanced Interdisciplinary Research Areas (Innovative Bioproduction Kobe) from the Ministry of Education, Culture, Sports and Technology (MEXT), and by Science Research Grants from the Ministry of Health, Labor and Welfare, Japan.

### Author details

[1]Department of Chemical Science and Engineering, Graduate School of Engineering, Kobe University, Kobe, Japan. [2]Organization of Advanced

Science and Technology, Kobe University, Kobe, Japan. [3]Institute of
Pharmaceutical Science, Faculty of Life Sciences and Medicine, King's College
London, London, UK.

### References

1. Garcea RL, Gissmann L. Virus-like particles as vaccines and vessels for the delivery of small molecules. Curr Opin Biotechnol. 2004;15:513–7.
2. Sominskaya I, Skrastina D, Dislers A, Vasiljev D, Mihailova M, Ose V. Construction and Immunological Evaluation of Multivalent Hepatitis B Virus (HBV) Core Virus-Like Particles Carrying HBV and HCV Epitopes. Clin Vaccine Immunol. 2010;17:1027–33.
3. Machida A, Ohnuma H, Tsuda F, Yoshikawa A, Hoshi Y, Tanaka T, et al. Phosphorylation in the carboxyl-terminal domain of the capsid protein of hepatitis B virus: evaluation with a monoclonal antibody. J Virol. 1991;65:6024–30.
4. Lewellyn EB, Loeb DD. The arginine clusters of the carboxy-terminal domain of the core protein of hepatitis B virus make pleiotropic contributions to genome replication. J Virol. 2011;85:1298–309.
5. Beterams G, Bottcher B, Nassal M. Packaging of up to 240 subunits of a 17 kDa nuclease into the interior of recombinant hepatitis B virus capsids. FEBS Lett. 2000;481:169–76.
6. Crowther RA, Kiselev NA, Bottcher B, Berriman JA, Borisova GP, Ose V, et al. Three-dimensional structure of hepatitis B virus core particles determined by electron cryomicroscopy. Cell. 1994;77:943–50.
7. Osmond RI, Kett WC, Skett SE, Coombe DR. Protein-heparin interactions measured by BIAcore 2000 are affected by the method of heparin immobilization. Anal Biochem. 2002;310:199–207.
8. Weigand K, Knaust A, Schaller H. Assembly and export determine the intracellular distribution of hepatitis B virus core protein subunits. J Gen Virol. 2010;91:59–67.
9. Cooper A, Shaul Y. Recombinant viral capsids as an efficient vehicle of oligonucleotide delivery into cells. Biochem Biophys Res Commun. 2005;327:1094–9.
10. Nassal M. The arginine-rich domain of the hepatitis B virus core protein is required for pregenome encapsidation and productive viral positive-strand DNA synthesis but not for virus assembly. J Virol. 1992;66:4107–16.
11. Nishimura Y, Mimura W, Mohamed Suffian IF, Amino T, Ishii J, Ogino C, et al. Granting specificity for breast cancer cells using a hepatitis B core particle with a HER2-targeted affibody molecule. J Biochem. 2013;153:251–6.
12. Cooper A, Shaul Y. Clathrin-mediated endocytosis and lysosomal cleavage of hepatitis B virus capsid-like core particles. J Biol Chem. 2006;281:16563–9.
13. Rusnati M, Tulipano G, Urbinati C, Tanghetti E, Giuliani R, Giacca M, et al. The Basic Domain in HIV-1 Tat Protein as a Target for Polysulfonated Heparin-mimicking Extracellular Tat Antagonists. J Biol Chem. 1998;273:16027–37.
14. Console S, Marty C, García-Echeverría C, Schwendener R, Ballmer-Hofer K. Antennapedia and HIV Transactivator of Transcription (TAT) "Protein Transduction Domains" Promote Endocytosis of High Molecular Weight Cargo upon Binding to Cell Surface Glycosaminoglycans. J Biol Chem. 2003;278:35109–14.
15. Nishimura Y, Shishido T, Ishii J, Tanaka T, Ogino C, Kondo A. Protein-encapsulated bio-nanocapsules production with ER membrane localization sequences. J Biotechnol. 2012;157:124–9.
16. Wizemann H, von Brunn A. Purification of E. coli-expressed HIS-tagged hepatitis B core antigen by Ni2+ –chelate affinity chromatography. J Virol Methods. 1999;77(2):189–97.
17. Green I, Christison R, Voyce CJ, Bundell KR, Lindsay MA. Protein transduction domains: are they delivering? Trends Pharmacol Sci. 2003;24:213–5.

# 19

# Microfluidic biosensor for β-Hydroxybutyrate (βHBA) determination of subclinical ketosis diagnosis

Xuan Weng[1], Wenting Zhao[2], Suresh Neethirajan[1*] and Todd Duffield[3]

## Abstract

**Background:** Determination of β-hydroxybutyrate (βHBA) is a gold standard for diagnosis of Subclinical Ketosis (SCK), a common disease in dairy cows that causes significant economic loss. Early detection of SCK can help reduce the risk of the disease progressing into clinical stage, thus minimizing economic losses on dairy cattle. Conventional laboratory methods are time consuming and labor-intensive, requiring expensive and bulky equipment. Development of portable and robust devices for rapid on-site SCK diagnosis is an effective way to prevent and control ketosis and can significantly aid in the management of dairy animal health. Microfluidic technology provides a rapid, cost-effective way to develop handheld devices for on-farm detection of sub-clinical ketosis. In this study, a highly sensitive microfluidics-based biosensor for on-site SCK diagnosis has been developed.

**Results:** A rapid, low-cost microfluidic biosensor with high sensitivity and specificity was developed for SCK diagnosis. Determination of βHBA was employed as the indicator in the diagnosis of SCK. On-chip detection using miniaturized and cost-effective optical sensor can be finished in 1 minute with a detection limit of 0.05 mM concentration. Developed microfluidic biosensor was successfully tested with the serum samples from dairy cows affected by SCK. The results of the developed biosensor agreed well with two other laboratory methods. The biosensor was characterized by high sensitivity and specificity towards βHBA with a detection limit of 0.05 mM.

**Conclusions:** The developed microfluidic biosensor provides a promising prototype for a cost-effective handheld meter for on-site SCK diagnosis. By using microfluidic method, the detection time is significantly decreased compared to other laboratory methods. Here, we demonstrate a field-deployable device to precisely identify and measure subclinical ketosis by specific labeling and quantification of β-hydroxybutyate in cow blood samples. A real-time on-site detection system will maximize convenience for the farmers.

**Keywords:** β-hydroxybutyrate (βHBA), Microfluidic biosensor, On-site diagnostics, Subclinical ketosis

## Background

Subclinical ketosis (SCK) is characterized by the increase in the concentration of circulating ketone bodies without the presence of clinical signs of ketosis [1]. SCK is a common disease in high-producing dairy cows and typically occurs in early lactation [2]. It is reported that the incidence of SCK may be as high as 40 ~ 60% herds, which is much higher than the 2 ~ 15% incidence of clinical ketosis [2,3]. SCK has been found to be associated with decreased milk production, impaired reproductive performance, displaced abomasum and higher risk of clinical ketosis, thus causing huge economic losses [4,5]. To prevent SCK from becoming a clinical disease and to minimize economic losses, it must be identified at an early stage for cows so that effective treatment can begin. However, it is difficult to identify SCK due to the lack of clinical signs and it may be undetected by regular clinical ketosis tests.

β-hydroxybutyrate (βHBA) is considered a gold standard for diagnosing of SCK due to its stability in blood. A cut-off value of 1.2 to 1.4 mM of βHBA in blood samples is used to distinguish between cows with and without SCK [6-8]. Conventional quantitative determination for βHBA is conducted in a laboratory by using special equipment

* Correspondence: sneethir@uoguelph.ca
[1]BioNano Laboratory, School of Engineering, University of Guelph, Guelph, ON N1G 2W1, Canada
Full list of author information is available at the end of the article

and requires time-consuming, labor-intensive procedures and skilled personnel [9,10]. Current available commercially kits for βHBA determination (Cayman Chemical® β-Hydroxybutyrate (Ketone Body) Colorimetric Assay Kit; Abcam's beta Hydroxybutyrate (beta HB) Assay; BHBA ELISA Kit from antibodies-online Cow (Bovine); typically based upon an enzymatic catalysis followed by fluorescence, absorbance or electrochemical detection which still involve complex procedures and depend on special and expensive optical instrument for signal detection. Usually, a relatively high sample volume and reagent amount is used, resulting in a lengthy assay time. Although the methods achieve high sensitivity and specificity, all of the aforementioned limitations prevent field deployable and on-site applications.

Recently, numerous "cowside" tests for diagnosis of ketosis based on βHBA determination have been developed. Although some of the cowside diagnostic tests have been commercially available for ketosis by detecting βHBA (e.g., Ketolac, Biolab, München, Germany), they can only provide semi-quantitative results [11,12]. More recently, human ketosis detector has been used as cowside ketosis test [7,13-18]. Evaluation of human ketosis handheld devices in the determination of βHBA in cow's blood samples provided moderate to excellent levels of agreement with the laboratory tests. However, the results of the evaluation of Optimum Xceed human ketosis hand-held meter by Voyvoda and Erdogan [12] showed that the sensitivity for βHBA detection in comparison with laboratory test was less than 85%. Furthermore, since these tests are designed specifically for use on humans, veterinary application may not be supported and the use of these tests could be lost if the manufacturer decides the human market does not support sales. Hence, it is clear that the human ketosis detector may not be applicable for consistently accurate and reliable measurement of βHBA in cow's blood and animal samples. The study by Mahrt et al. [18] states that the Novavet biosensor provided only 82% specificity in βHBA in comparison to the lab tests, with significant false-positive results indicating that this biosensor may not be suitable for on-farm detection of sub-clinical ketosis.

Therefore, motivated by the limitations of current devices for cowside SCK diagnosis, we have developed a high performance microfluidic biosensor to meet the market needs. The uniqueness of the presented biosensor is that it is based on a microfluidic system with superior specificity and sensitivity along with the higher accuracy for determination of βHBA in serum samples of cows. Microfluidics and lab-on-a-chip technology have been widely used in biosensor applications, enhancing analytical performance by miniaturization. Microfluidic biosensors present distinctive advantages such as significantly increasing sensitivity with reduced

assay time and reduced sample and reagent consumption [19]. In order to make a cost-effective biosensor, expensive, bulky and complex optical instruments such as FTIR, (NMR) spectroscopy spectrometry and gas chromatography-mass spectrometry (GC-MS) have to be avoided. The objective of this study was to develop a low-cost, highly sensitive and miniaturized microfluidic biosensor as a handheld device capable of rapid, accurate detection of βHBA for SCK diagnosis in dairy cows.

## Materials and methods
### Reagents and materials
The reagents and materials were obtained as a commercial kit (Cayman Chemical® β-Hydroxybutyrate (ketone Body) Colorimetric Assay kit, Cedarlane labs, Burlington, ON, Canada) which consisted of βHBA assay buffer, reconstitute βHBA standard, βHBA enzyme solution and βHBA colorimetric detector. The βHBA standard solution ranging from 0.05 mM to 1.0 mM was made by diluting the reconstituted βHBA Standard with βHBA assay buffer to prepare the βHBA standard curve. The βHBA enzyme solution and colorimetric detector were mixed to make the detector mixture buffer at a ratio of 24:1 before each test.

### Preparation of serum sample
Blood samples collected from periparturient Holstein dairy cows from 4 dairy farms in South West Ontario were utilized for analysis. The detailed sample preparation procedure can be found elsewhere [20]. Briefly, cow's blood was first collected from the coccygeal blood vessels in a vacuum tube without anticoagulant and stored in a cool place. Collected blood sample was centrifuged at 4°C within 6 h after collection at $2990 \times g$ to harvest serum and stored at -20°C for further use. Before assaying, the serum sample was thawed at room temperature and diluted 1:6 with the βHBA assay buffer.

### Principle of the colorimetric assay
The method for βHBA determination in this study is based upon the enzymatic conversion of βHBA to acetoacetate (AcAc) by βHBA dehydrogenase, and concomitantly the cofactor nicotineamide adenine dinucleotide ($NAD^+$) is converted to its reduced form β-nicotinamide adenine dinucleotide (NADH). In the presence of diaphorase, NADH reacts with the colorimetric detector WST-1 to produce a formazan dye with a maximum absorbance at 445 nm to 455 nm, proportional to the βHBA concentration. Figure 1 shows the principle of βHBA determination based upon the enzymatic reaction.

### Design and fabrication of microfluidic PDMS chip
The microfluidic chip design was created using AutoCAD software and made by following the standard soft lithography protocol as detailed by Biddiss et al. [21]. The layout

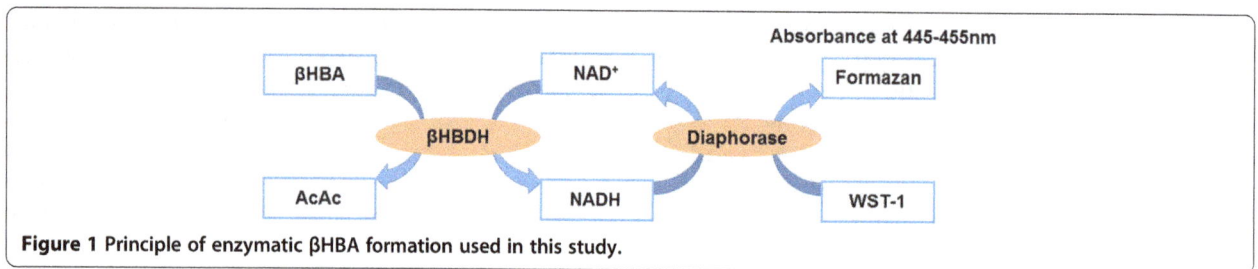

**Figure 1** Principle of enzymatic βHBA formation used in this study.

of the microfluidic chip is shown in Figure 2a. The microfluidic chip consists of the mixing channel housing hundreds of posts, incubation channel, sensing well, two inlets and one outlet. A silicon wafer master mold was fabricated by first spin-coating a thin layer of SU-8 2025 negative photoresist (MicroCHEM, US) on the surface of the wafer. After the prebaking, a photomask with the designed microchannel geometry was placed onto the coated silicon wafer and exposed to UV using a UV exposure system (UV-KUB, Kloé, France). After the post-baking and developing, it was used as a mold for creating the PDMS chip. A 10:1 (w/w) mixture of PDMS prepolymer and the curing agent (Sylgard, Dow Corning, Burlington, ON, Canada) was stirred thoroughly and degassed under vacuum. Then the mixture was poured onto the master mold and cured at 75°C for 4 h. After curing, the PDMS replica was peeled off from the master, punched with holes to provide inlets and outlet and bonded onto a glass slide ($25 \times 75 \times 1$ mm, VWR International, Suwanee, GA, USA) after oxygen plasma treatment for 40 s. A position marker was used to facilitate the alignment between the sensing well and the sensing window of the photodiode mounted in a custom design box when conducting the bonding. A picture of microfluidic chip is shown in Figure 2b.

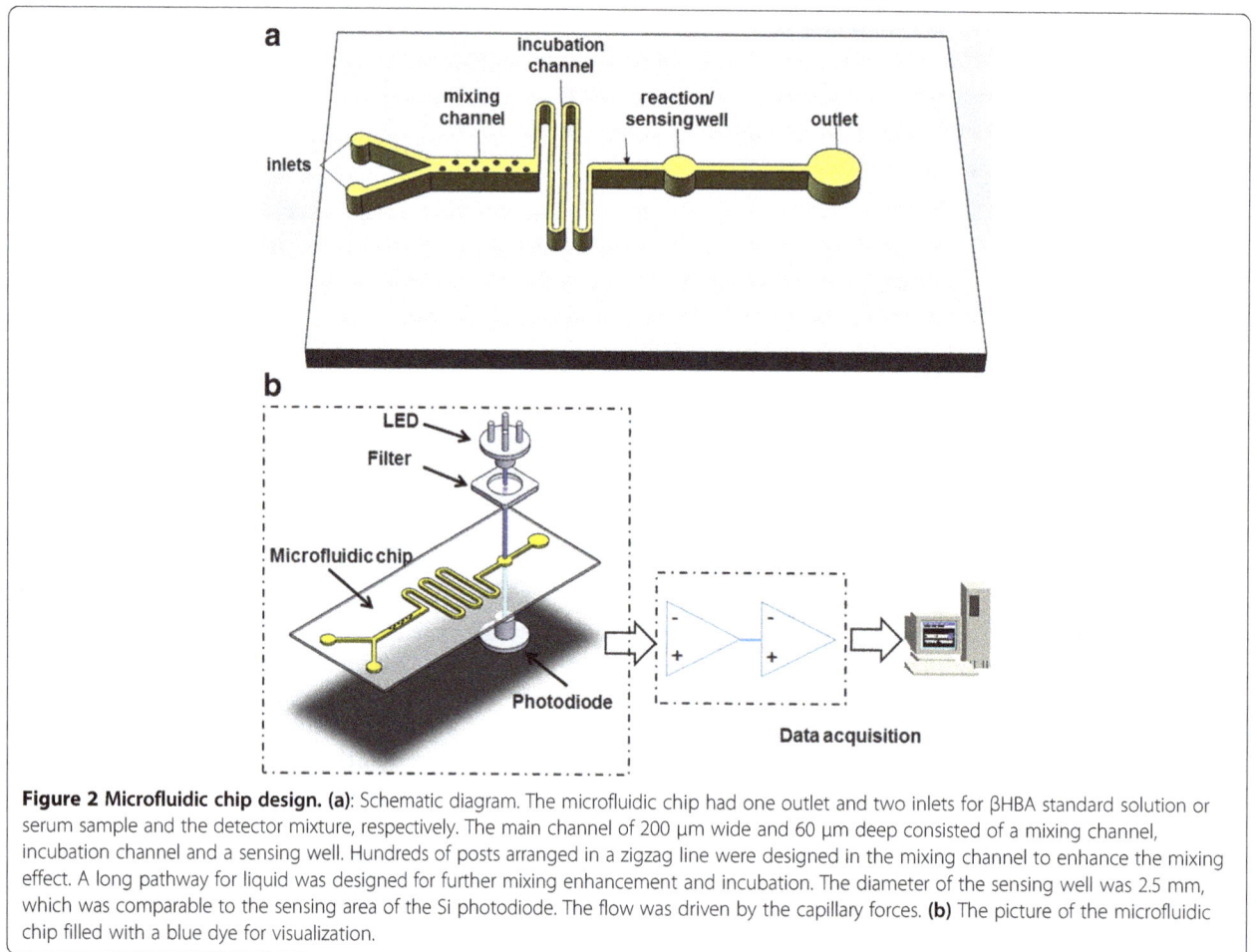

**Figure 2 Microfluidic chip design. (a)**: Schematic diagram. The microfluidic chip had one outlet and two inlets for βHBA standard solution or serum sample and the detector mixture, respectively. The main channel of 200 µm wide and 60 µm deep consisted of a mixing channel, incubation channel and a sensing well. Hundreds of posts arranged in a zigzag line were designed in the mixing channel to enhance the mixing effect. A long pathway for liquid was designed for further mixing enhancement and incubation. The diameter of the sensing well was 2.5 mm, which was comparable to the sensing area of the Si photodiode. The flow was driven by the capillary forces. **(b)** The picture of the microfluidic chip filled with a blue dye for visualization.

## Miniaturized, low-cost optical biosensor

The principle of the biosensor is based upon the property of the resulting complex to absorb UV in the 445 to 455 nm range. The transmitted light intensity signal acquired by the Si photodiode is dependent on the βHBA concentration in the samples.

The light absorption analysis was performed by a custom-built miniaturized and low-cost optical biosensor. The schematic diagram of the optical sensor is shown in Figure 3a. The biosensor used a LED (447.5 nm, Luxeon Rebel, Luxeon Star LEDs, Brantford, ON, Canada) with a single-band bandpass filter (435 nm, semrock, Rochester, NY, USA) as the illumination light source and a low-noise, high-sensitivity Si photodiode (Hamamatsu, Bridgewater, NJ, USA) with preamp as the detector for light absorption analysis. The collected light intensity signal by the Si photodiode was then digitized and transferred to a PC for storage by a programmable microcontroller (Arduino Uno, SparkFun Electronics, Niwot, CO, USA) through an interface circuit. Optical and electrical components were assembled in a sensor packaging assembly to block ambient light, as shown in Figure 3b. The LED and filter were mounted in the lid and on the top of the microfluidic chip platform to illuminate the sensing micro-well. The Si photodiode was placed at the bottom of the platform aligned to the sensing well.

## Detection procedure

As mentioned previously, βHBA determination was based upon an enzymatic reaction. First, a 1:1 ratio volume of βHBA standard solution or diluted serum sample and the detector mixture containing βHBA enzyme solution and βHBA colorimetric detector were loaded into the respective inlets of the microfluidic chip placed on the chip platform. The two solutions underwent full mixing in the mixing channel and then passed through the incubation channel and the sensing well to the outlet. After the incubation time of 1 min, the power supply and the Arduino microcontroller were activated for signal recording. All experiments were conducted at room temperature.

The light signal was recorded for 5 s. For each experiment, the standard deviation (SD) for signals from 3 duplicate tests was calculated, and is indicated by the error bars (Figures 4, 5, and 6). The detection limit, sensitivity and specificity of the biosensor were evaluated based on the experiments.

The βHBA concentration of the serum sample was detected by three different approaches to evaluate the performance of the presented biosensor. Same samples of serum were analyzed using a Roche Cobas 6000 c501 automated chemistry analyzer (Roche Canada, Laval, QC, Canada), a Synergy H4 Hybrid Multi-Mode Microplate Reader (Biotek, Winooski, VT, USA) and the developed microfluidic Lab-on-a-Chip biosensor, respectively. The values of βHBA in a sample were calculated using the linear regression equations of their own standard curves obtained by each approach.

## Determination of the operating parameters

The principle of the biosensor is based upon light absorption analysis. The LED served as the illumination light source to the biosensor. The transmitted light intensity signal is dependent on the βHBA concentration, was captured by a Si photodiode. It was found that the parameters of applied LED intensity, the volume of the resultant complex and the incubation time were interconnected, and optimization of these parameters was performed in order to obtain a stable, effective and reliable outcome with high sensitivity. A series of experiments using standard βHBA solution ranging from 0 ~ 1.0 mM were performed to study and optimize the operating parameters. A different light intensity from LED was obtained by adjusting the voltage applied on LED. A series of

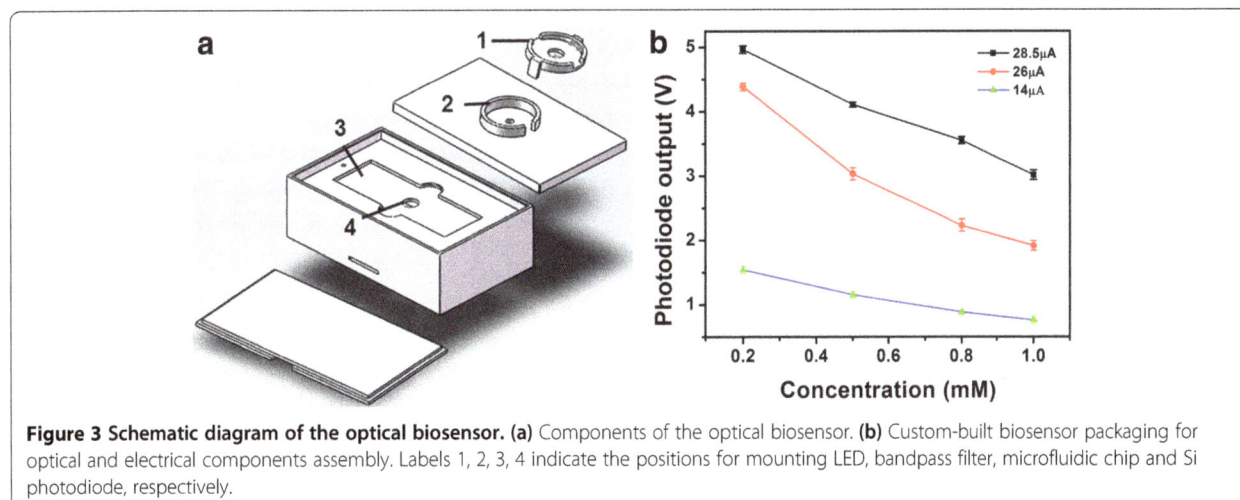

**Figure 3 Schematic diagram of the optical biosensor. (a)** Components of the optical biosensor. **(b)** Custom-built biosensor packaging for optical and electrical components assembly. Labels 1, 2, 3, 4 indicate the positions for mounting LED, bandpass filter, microfluidic chip and Si photodiode, respectively.

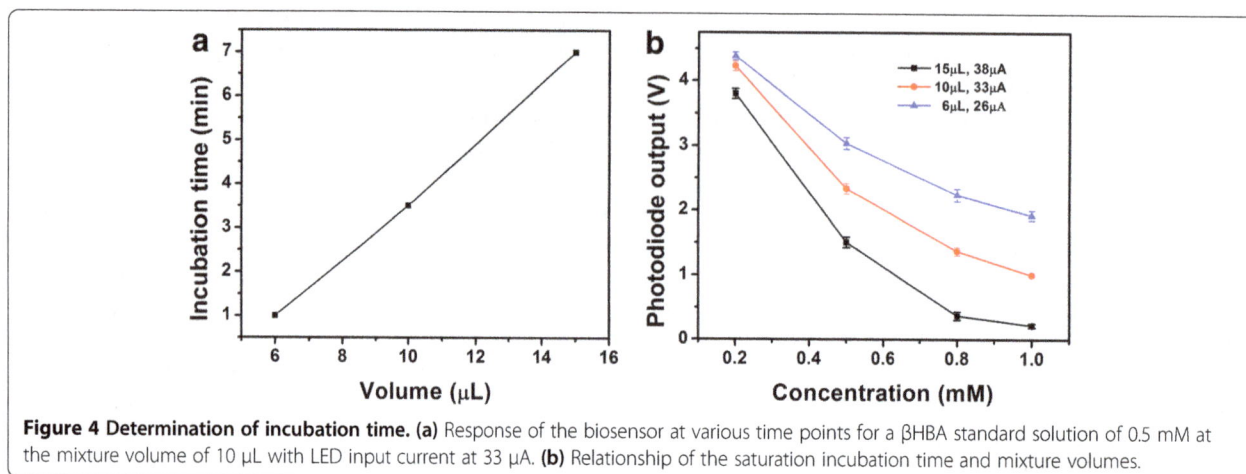

**Figure 4 Determination of incubation time. (a)** Response of the biosensor at various time points for a βHBA standard solution of 0.5 mM at the mixture volume of 10 μL with LED input current at 33 μA. **(b)** Relationship of the saturation incubation time and mixture volumes.

volumes of resultant complex associated with the optimized incubation time for each one were studied. Well-based tests with relatively big volumes (15 μL, 10 μL and 6 μL) of reaction mixture were first evaluated to investigate the feasibility and performance of the biosensor. Based on the initial optimization experiments, on-chip tests using the microfluidic chip were then conducted.

## Results and discussion
### Optimization of operating parameters based on well-based tests

Three operating parameters: illumination light intensity, sample/reagent volume and incubation time were optimized. Figure 7 shows the determination of illumination light intensity generated by LED. The volume of reaction mixture with a series of sample concentrations was fixed and illumination light intensity was varied to investigate the response of Si photodiode. The illumination light

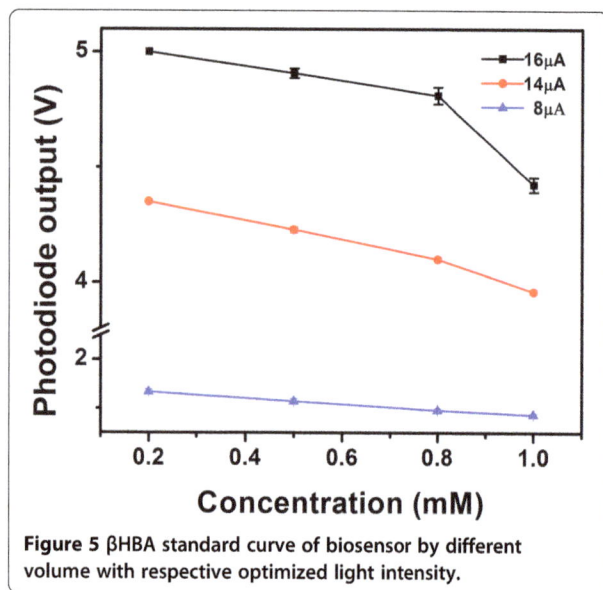

**Figure 5 βHBA standard curve of biosensor by different volume with respective optimized light intensity.**

intensity was adjusted by regulating the current applied to the LED. The magnitude of the current was directly proportional to the light intensity of the LED. For a mixture solution volume of 6 μL, 3 light intensities were applied; the output of the photodiode is shown in Figure 7a. It was found that the signal of Si photodiode was proportional to the input light intensity and a wide linear range was obtained when the applied current was 14 μA. Too low and too high light intensity produced poor resolution. Therefore, it was determined that for a mixture volume of 6 μL, the LED intensity under 14 μA was appropriate. Similarly, a relationship of the mixture volume and the individually optimized LED intensities were investigated which is shown in Figure 7b.

Once the LED light intensity was determined, incubation time was studied. Since the sample and reagent volume were reduced significantly compared to the 100 μL applied by the associated commercial kit, the time could be reduced accordingly. An example is given in Figure 4a, a reaction mixture volume of 10 μL with the βHBA concentration at 0.5 mM was tested. A current of 33 μA was applied to the LED for determining the optimized light intensity for the working reagent volume (Figure 7b). The output of Si photodiode was recorded every minute to investigate the reaction rate of the enzyme reaction. The readout of the photodiode was monitored until no further variation with time was noted. The time point at that moment was then considered as the saturation time based on the enzyme kinetics for the enzyme reaction under the associated volume. Seven minutes, three minutes and one minute time points were investigated as the saturation time for the volume of 15 μL, 10 μL and 6 μL, respectively, as shown in Figure 4b.

After determination of the optimized illumination light intensity and the incubation time, standard curves for three representative volumes, 15 μL, 10 μL and 6 μL, were built (Figure 5). A series of βHBA standard solutions with the concentration ranging from 0.2 mM to

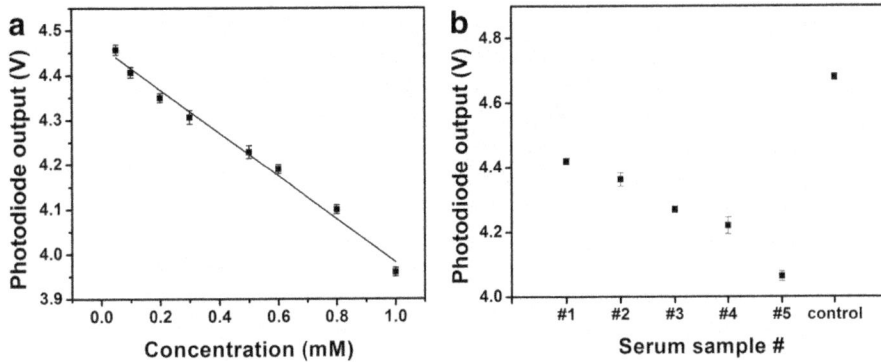

**Figure 6 Response of biosensor for the on-chip test at a volume of 0.2 μL. (a)** Determination of LED light intensity by detecting different concentration of βHBA standard solution. **(b)** βHBA standard curve of the microfluidic biosensor.

1.0 mM were measured by the presented biosensor. An overall lower photodiode signal was investigated with the change in the volume of the reagent mixture. For example, at the concentration of 0.5 mM, the outputs of the photodiode were 1.5 V, 2.3 V and 3.0 V for the volume of 15 μL, 10 μL and 6 μL, respectively. This result can be explained due to the linear relationship between the light absorption and the amount of absorbing substance.

## Optimization of operating parameters based on chip-based tests

The feasibility and detection performance of the microfluidic biosensor has been proved based on the results obtained by the well-based tests. One microliter of βHBA standard solution and detector mixture was loaded into the inlets on the microfluidic chip, simultaneously. The actual detected volume of mixture sample solution in the sensing well was 0.2 μL. Similarly, the appropriate LED intensity was determined for this 0.2 μL volume. As shown in Figure 6a, a relative higher or lower light intensity would result in a poor resolution and lead to decrease in

the sensing range of samples. A current of 14 μA was determined as the appropriate LED intensity for the on-chip tests. After 1 min incubation time, the βHBA standard solution with a series of concentrations ranging from 0.05 mM to 1.0 mM was tested on chip to create the calibration curve for the microfluidic biosensor. The standard curve (Figure 6b) of the output of the microfluidic biosensor had good linearity with the βHBA at concentrations of 0.05 mM to 1.0 mM. The regression model was determined to be $y = -0.4858x + 4.467$ with $R^2 = 0.991$. The detection limit of the microfluidic biosensor was 0.05 mM. The detection limit and the upper range tested are more than sufficient to distinguish healthy from SCK cows, particularly with sample dilution.

## βHBA determination in serum sample

The detection performance of the microfluidic biosensor was compared to the other two laboratory methods, namely a chemistry analyzer and microplate reader. A series of serum samples and a control were assayed by the three methods on the same day. The serum samples were diluted to 1:6 ratio before conducting the assay

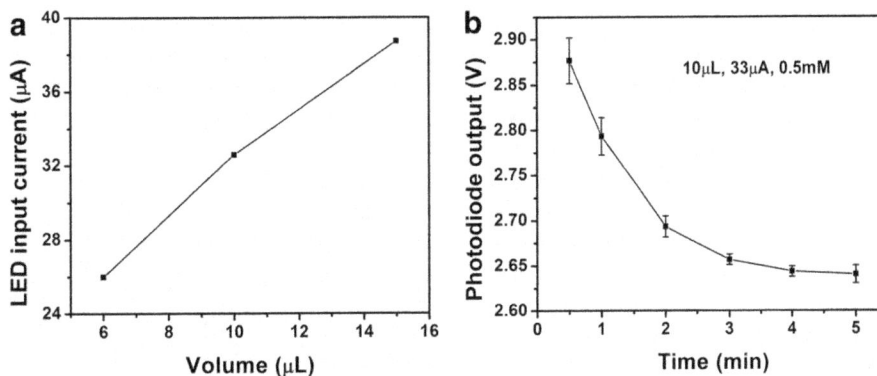

**Figure 7 Determination of optimized LED light intensity. (a)** Response of biosensor with different LED light intensity for different concentration of βHBA standard solution at a volume of 6 μL. **(b)** Optimized LED light intensity for different volumes.

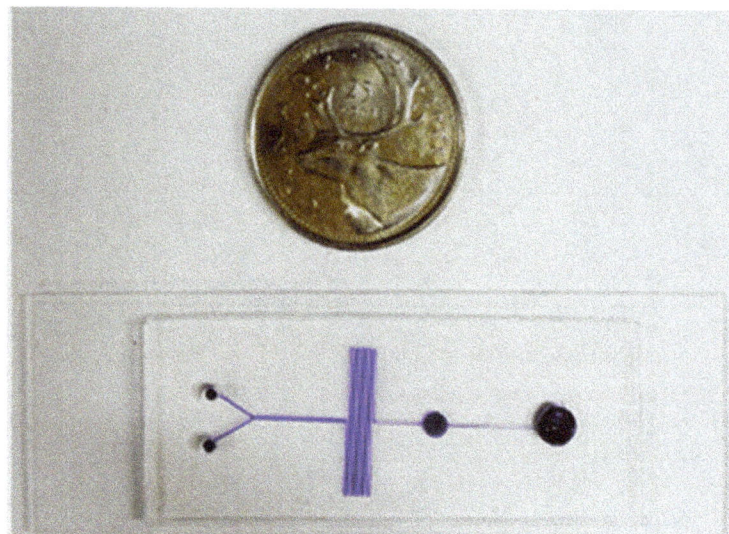

**Figure 8** Response of biosensor in determination of the βHBA concentration in serum samples.

experiments. The results of light signal captured by Si photodiode are shown in Figure 8. The values of the βHBA concentration in serum samples were then calculated using the obtained standard curve as shown in Figure 6b. The results of the detection of BHBA in blood samples using our developed microfluidic biosensor are in agreement with the microplate reader assay and the chemistry analyzer tests (Table 1). In addition, the microfluidic biosensor showed a good performance in assaying samples with βHBA concentration varying over a wide range, 0 mM to 5 mM, (Figure 6b) as the photodiode was able to sense higher concentration (>1.0 mM) with effective outputs (0 V to 3.9 V).

Evaluation of human medicine hand-held devices [7,13,16] in the determination of βHBA in cow's blood samples provided acceptable level of agreement with the laboratory tests but with significant false positive tests. Cows and humans are both mammals with considerable differences in their physiology. Cows have 11 major blood group systems (A, B, C, F, J, L, M, R, S, T

and Z) unlike 4 groups in human system owing to different antigen expressions, which makes it complex and inaccurate to determine βHBA in cows using human medicine ketosis detector. Hence, human ketosis detector cannot be efficiently deployed for accurate and reliable measurement of βHBA in cow's blood and animal samples.

Since the diagnosis and the determination of βHBA are dependent on a variety of body fluids, the hand-held commercially available human ketosis detectors are limited in its function. The uniqueness of the developed lab on a chip system is that the sensor has been built based on microfluidic systems with higher specificity and sensitivity along with higher accuracy for measurement in blood samples of cows. Unlike the human ketosis detection system, the developed microfluidic optical biosensing system is specific for determining βHBA in cow blood samples. The cross-reactivity detection between the target antigen and the analogues for other species is considered low due to the specificity and the sensitivity 0.95 nmol/mL sensitivity. The reagents and solutions used for the sensing event can be stored over 2 months upon refrigeration @ -80°C to avoid the loss of bioactivity and contamination.

## Conclusions

Conventional laboratory methods for βHBA determination are time-consuming, labour-intensive and requiring high sample/reagent consumption. Owing to the differences in the blood types and the antigen expression differences between the humans and cows, the commercially available human ketosis detection system cannot be efficiently employed for veterinary applications. A clear need exists in the miniaturization and simplification of the

**Table 1 Comparison of βHBA determination in serum sample by three approaches**

| Serum sample # | Method | | |
| --- | --- | --- | --- |
| | Chemistry analyzer [μM] | Microplate reader [μM] | Microfluidic biosensor [μM] |
| 1 | 627 | 530 | 580 |
| 2 | 1224 | 1277 | 1280 |
| 3 | 2399 | 2784 | 2433 |
| 4 | 3005 | 3093 | 3051 |
| 5 | 5152 | 4541 | 4985 |
| Control | 0 | 0.03 | <0 |

detection devices for βHBA. The developed microfluidic biosensor prototype overcomes the above limitations. Sample/ reagent consumption and incubation time were significantly reduced to 1 min and 0.2 μL respectively through microfluidic method. A miniaturized, low-cost optical sensor has been developed for the photometric detection and incorporated in the biosensor with 0.05 mM LOD. The presented microfluidic biosensor prototype in this study have its distinct advantages such as low cost, lower sample consumption and lower detection limit, which serves as an alternative for the development of rapid, accurate, highly sensitive and specific portable devices for on-farm and cowside diagnosis of SCK.

## Competing interests
The authors declare that they have no competing interests.

## Authors' contributions
SN conceptualized the idea for this study. SN and XW designed the project. XW and WZ built-up the instrumentation system and performed the experiments. XW wrote the manuscript with SN. TD prepared the serum samples and detected the sample by chemical analyzer. All authors read and approved the manuscript.

## Acknowledgements
The authors sincerely thank the Natural Sciences and Engineering Research Council of Canada, Canada Foundation for Innovation and the Dairy Farmers of Ontario for funding this study.

## Author details
[1]BioNano Laboratory, School of Engineering, University of Guelph, Guelph, ON N1G 2W1, Canada. [2]Department of Industrial Engineering, South China University of Technology, Guangzhou, Guangdong 510640, China. [3]Department of Population Medicine, Ontario Veterinary College, University of Guelph, Guelph, ON N1G 2W1, Canada.

## References
1. Andersson L. Subclinical ketosis in dairy cows. Vet Clin North Am Food Anim Pract. 1988;4:233–51.
2. Gordon JL, LeBlanc SJ, Duffield TF. Ketosis treatment in lactating dairy cattle. Vet Clin North Am Food Anim Pract. 2013;29:433–45.
3. McArt JA, Nydam DV, Oetzel GR. Epidemiology of subclinical ketosis in early lactation dairy cattle. J Dairy Sci. 2012;95:5056–66.
4. Ospina PA, Nydam DV, Stokol T, Overton TR. Associations of elevated nonesterified fatty acids and β-hydroxybutyrate concentrations with early lactation reproductive performance and milk production in transition dairy cattle in the northeastern United States. J Dairy Sci. 2010;93:1596–603.
5. Seifi HA, LeBlanc SJ, Leslie KE, Duffield TF. Metabolic predictors of post-partum disease and culling risk in dairy cattle. Vet J. 2011;188:216–20.
6. Duffield TF. Subclinical ketosis in lactating dairy cattle: metabolic disorders of ruminants. Vet Clin North Am Food Anim Pract. 2000;16:231–53.
7. Iwersen M, Falkenberg U, Voigtsberger R, Forderung D, Heuwieser W. Evaluation of an electronic cowside test to detect subclinical ketosis in dairy cows. J Dairy Sci. 2009;92:2618–24.
8. Ospina PA, Nydam DV, Stokol T, Overto TR. Evaluation of nonesterified fatty acids and β-hydroxybutyrate in transition dairy cattle in the northeastern United States: critical thresholds for prediction of clinical diseases. J Dairy Sci. 2010;93:546–54.
9. Townsend J. Cowside tests for monitoring metabolic disease. 2011. http://tristatedairy.osu.edu/Proceedings%202011/Townsend%20paper.pdf. Accessed 10 Jan 2015.
10. Larsen T, Nielsen NI. Fluorometric determination of β-Hydroxybutyrate in milk and blood plasma. J Dairy Sci. 2005;88:2004–9.
11. Samiei A, Liang JB, Ghorbani GR, Hirooka H, Yaakub H, Tabatabaei M. An evaluation of beta-hydroxybutyrate in milk and blood for prediction of subclinical ketosis in dairy cows. Pol J Vet Sci. 2010;13:349–56.
12. Larsen M, Kristensen NB. Effect of a lucerne feeding strategy in the first week postpartum on feed intake and ketone body profiles in blood plasma, urine, and milk in Holstein cows. Acta Agr Scand Sect A -Anim SC. 2010;60:239–49.
13. Voyvoda H, Erdogan H. Use of a hand-held meter for detecting subclinical ketosis in dairy cows. Res Vet Sci. 2010;89:344–51.
14. Panousis N, Kritsepi-Konstantinou M, Karagiannis I, Kalaitzakis E, Lafi S, Brozos C. Evaluation of Precision Xceed® for on-site monitoring of blood β-hydroxybutyric acid and glucose in dairy cows. J Hell Vet Med Soc. 2011;62:109–17.
15. Mahrt A, Burfeind O, Heuwieser W. Effects of time and sampling location on concentrations of β-hydroxybutyric acid in dairy cows. J Dairy Sci. 2014;97:291–8.
16. Iwersen M, Klein-Jöbstl D, Pichler M, Roland L, Fidlschuster B, Schwendenwein I, et al. Comparison of 2 electronic cowside tests to detect subclinical ketosis in dairy cows and the influence of the temperature and type of blood sample on the test results. J Dairy Sci. 2013;96:7719–30.
17. Zhang Z, Liu G, Wang H, Li X, Wang Z. Detection of subclinical ketosis in dairy cows. Pak Vet J. 2012;32:156–60.
18. Mahrt A, Burfeind O, Voigtsberger R, Müller A, Heuwieser W. Evaluation of a new electronic handheld meter for measurement of β-hydroxybutyric acid in dairy cows. Tierarztl Prax Ausg G Grosstiere Nutztiere. 2014;42:5–10.
19. Mairhofer J, Roppert K, Ertl P. Microfluidic systems for pathogen sensing: a review. Sensors. 2009;9:4804–23.
20. Gohary K, LeBlanc SJ, Lissemore KD, Overton MW, Von Massow M, Duffield TF. Effect of prepartum administration of recombinant bovine somatotropin on health and performance of lactating dairy cows. J Dairy Sci. 2014;97:6231–41.
21. Biddiss E, Erickson D, Li D. Heterogeneous surface charge enhanced micromixing for electrokinetic flows. Anal Chem. 2004;76:3208–13.

# 20

# Characterization of interaction of magnetic nanoparticles with breast cancer cells

Macarena Calero[1,5†], Michele Chiappi[2†], Ana Lazaro-Carrillo[1,5], María José Rodríguez[2], Francisco Javier Chichón[2], Kieran Crosbie-Staunton[3], Adriele Prina-Mello[3,4], Yuri Volkov[3,4], Angeles Villanueva[1,5*] and José L Carrascosa[2,5*]

## Abstract

**Background:** Different superparamagnetic iron oxide nanoparticles have been tested for their potential use in cancer treatment, as they enter into cells with high effectiveness, do not induce cytotoxicity, and are retained for relatively long periods of time inside the cells. We have analyzed the interaction, internalization and biocompatibility of dimercaptosuccinic acid-coated superparamagnetic iron oxide nanoparticles with an average diameter of 15 nm and negative surface charge in MCF-7 breast cancer cells.

**Results:** Cells were incubated with dimercaptosuccinic acid-coated superparamagnetic iron oxide nanoparticles for different time intervals, ranging from 0.5 to 72 h. These nanoparticles showed efficient internalization and relatively slow clearance. Time-dependent uptake studies demonstrated the maximum accumulation of dimercaptosuccinic acid-coated superparamagnetic iron oxide nanoparticles after 24 h of incubation, and afterwards they were slowly removed from cells. Superparamagnetic iron oxide nanoparticles were internalized by energy dependent endocytosis and localized in endosomes. Transmission electron microscopy studies showed macropinocytosis uptake and clathrin-mediated internalization depending on the nanoparticles aggregate size. MCF-7 cells accumulated these nanoparticles without any significant effect on cell morphology, cytoskeleton organization, cell cycle distribution, reactive oxygen species generation and cell viability, showing a similar behavior to untreated control cells.

**Conclusions:** All these findings indicate that dimercaptosuccinic acid-coated superparamagnetic iron oxide nanoparticles have excellent properties in terms of efficiency and biocompatibility for application to target breast cancer cells.

**Keywords:** MCF-7 cells, Superparamagnetic iron oxide nanoparticles, Intracellular trafficking, Transmission electron microscopy, Cellular uptake, Endocytosis, Cytotoxicity

## Background

Although huge efforts have led to worldwide advances in cancer treatment, this multifactorial and heterogeneous disease is still one of the major causes of death in developed countries [1,2]. In the recent years, several reports have focused on the potential use of superparamagnetic iron oxide nanoparticles (SPION) in cancer research. These reports have raised great expectations because SPION are a promising tool for biomedical applications, including diagnosis by magnetic resonance imaging (MRI) and targeted therapy of cancer by hyperthermia and/or releasing anti-cancer molecules, which can be combined in theranostic approaches [3-5].

Factors such as size, shape and surface charge of nanoparticles (NPs) can determine their cellular internalization and distribution and, thus, their effective performance [6,7]. Furthermore, colloidal stability can be achieved, which is essential to ensure reproducibility, as well as to influence the amount of cellular loading and toxicity. The possibility to modify the surface of these particles with biologically active compounds enables transport of therapeutic agents into specific target cells, increasing specificity and avoiding the access of cytotoxic agents to non-target tissues during the delivery process [8]. Different SPION have been tested for potential use in cancer treatment by hyperthermia, as they enter into cells with high effectiveness and without any cytotoxicity,

---

* Correspondence: angeles.villanueva@uam.es; jlcarras@cnb.csic.es
†Equal contributors
[1]Departamento de Biología, Universidad Autónoma de Madrid, Cantoblanco, 28049 Madrid, Spain
[2]Department of Macromolecular Structure, Centro Nacional de Biotecnología, Consejo Superior de Investigaciones Científicas, 28049 Madrid, Spain
Full list of author information is available at the end of the article

and they are retained for relatively long periods of time inside the cells [3]. The evaluation of the potential use of these nanoparticles requires a precise knowledge of surface modified SPION internalization mechanisms at the ultrastructural level and resulting intracellular pathways, as well as on the fate of SPION inside the cells. Factors such as uptake rate and internalization dynamics are the key to understand how an insufficient cellular accumulation of nanoparticles can lead to usage limitations, for example as imaging probes [9].

In the past few years, there has been a great interest in applying nanotechnology for biomedical studies, in particular for diagnostic and therapeutic purposes. However, the possible toxicity of nanoparticles to humans and environment has become a question of absolute priority in Nanomedicine [4-6,10].

In this regard, cell cultures are important first line tools to screen therapeutic efficiency and safety of drugs (nanoparticles included) and provide essential information to understanding cell-nanoparticle interactions, before moving to *in vivo* analysis [11]. Hence, any new magnetic nanoparticle formulation with potential biomedical applications should be accompanied by a detailed study that ensures both its effectiveness and safety. In this sense, several specific parameters and experimental protocols for assessing nanomaterial toxicity have been developed [10].

We have studied the interaction of dimercaptosuccinic acid-coated superparamagnetic iron oxide nanoparticles (DMSA-SPION) with breast cancer cells (MCF-7) in culture. Monodisperse nanoparticles (around 15 nm in diameter) with a high saturation magnetization value, were surface modified by *meso*-2,3-dimercaptosuccinic acid (DMSA) to ensure their dispersion and stability in aqueous buffers and media [12]. Interaction, uptake of the particles ($0.05-0.4$ mg ml$^{-1}$), as well as their accumulation and persistence inside cells after prolonged incubation (up to 72 h), were assessed by combining optical light and electron microscopy methods. This approach allowed us to correlate the overall cell visualization with the precise localization of SPION inside the cell, their relationship to cell organelles and the analysis of particle shapes and sizes. Furthermore, several cytotoxicity assays, including cell morphology, analysis of cytoskeleton and adhesion proteins, cell cycle distribution, measurement of intracellular reactive oxygen species (ROS) levels and two viability tests, have been carried out to evaluate biocompatibility of these nanoparticles.

## Results and discussion
### DMSA-SPION uptake and internalization in cultured cells
Size, shape and charge of iron oxide nanoparticles, as well as cell type, are important parameters which affect effective internalization of nanoparticles into cells in culture [13-16]. It has been well documented that positively charged magnetic nanoparticles (MNP) showed a higher degree of internalization than neutral and negatively charged MNP due to their effective attachment to negatively charged cell-membrane surface [3,14,16]. Although there are somewhat contradictory findings about cytotoxicity levels between positively or negatively charged nanoparticles [3,17-19], the latter ones are favored due to their overall lower toxicity levels.

Incorporation of DMSA-SPION into MCF-7 cells can be followed by bright field microscopy after 24 h incubation (Figure 1A), where SPION are observed inside living cells, distributed as brown cytoplasmic spots of different sizes, always outside of the nucleus. Similar results have been previously described for iron oxide nanoparticles with different coatings and different sizes in HeLa (human cervical adenocarcinoma) cell line [3,17].

In depth qualitative and quantitative studies on the internalization of DMSA-SPION in MCF-7 cancer cells were performed by both Prussian blue staining and ferrozine-based assay. Figure 1B shows cells incubated with DMSA-SPION for different times ($0.5-72$ h) by Prussian blue staining. An increase of intracellular DMSA-SPION accumulation was visualized as blue cytoplasmic granular stain within cells directly correlating with incubation times. However, the uptake of nanoparticles seems to reach a saturation point at 24 h. It is important to note that 100% cell labeling efficiency (Prussian blue positive staining) was achieved after 12 h nanoparticles incubation.

These results were confirmed by colorimetric ferrozine-based assay, a widely recognized test to quantify iron in cultured cells [20]. Figure 1C shows intracellular iron concentrations after 24 and 48 h incubation at 0.4 mg ml$^{-1}$ DMSA-SPION (20.67 pg cell$^{-1}$ and 28 pg cell$^{-1}$, respectively). There is abundant literature with regard to SPION-labeling efficiency, although results are difficult to compare because the experimental protocols are different (size and surface coating of the SPION, incubation time, concentration, cell line type, etc.). Generally, prolonged incubation times, as well as elevated iron doses enable to reach higher intracellular loading of SPION and increase labeling efficiency [21,22]. However, overexposure to high concentrations of SPION for extended times may cause cytotoxicity [23]. Therefore, sufficient intracellular uptake of nanoparticles for efficient diagnosis and/or treatment must be balanced with their biocompatibility [17]. In this sense, our results with ferrozine assay indicate that DMSA-SPION accumulate effectively (20.67 pg cell$^{-1}$) within MCF-7 cells. Previously, we had detected 37.1 pg cell$^{-1}$ (into HeLa cells), after 24 h of incubation at 0.5 mg ml$^{-1}$ DMSA magnetic nanoparticles with lower core diameter (9 nm). The small difference in the amount of accumulated iron could be either due to different of SPION diameters (15 *vs* 9 nm) or to the type of cell line (HeLa *vs* MCF-7) [17]. Much lower amounts

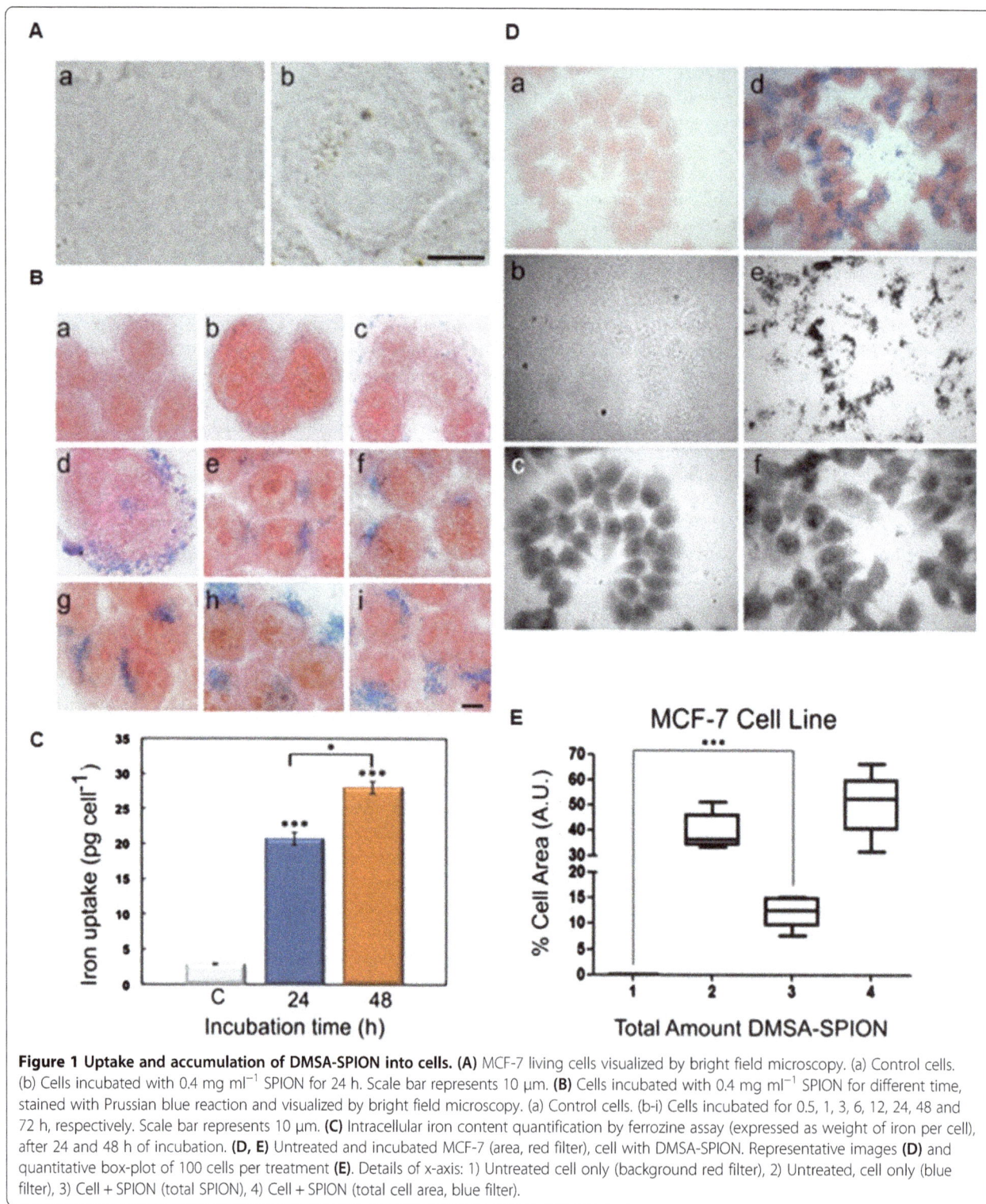

**Figure 1 Uptake and accumulation of DMSA-SPION into cells. (A)** MCF-7 living cells visualized by bright field microscopy. (a) Control cells. (b) Cells incubated with 0.4 mg ml$^{-1}$ SPION for 24 h. Scale bar represents 10 μm. **(B)** Cells incubated with 0.4 mg ml$^{-1}$ SPION for different time, stained with Prussian blue reaction and visualized by bright field microscopy. (a) Control cells. (b-i) Cells incubated for 0.5, 1, 3, 6, 12, 24, 48 and 72 h, respectively. Scale bar represents 10 μm. **(C)** Intracellular iron content quantification by ferrozine assay (expressed as weight of iron per cell), after 24 and 48 h of incubation. **(D, E)** Untreated and incubated MCF-7 (area, red filter), cell with DMSA-SPION. Representative images **(D)** and quantitative box-plot of 100 cells per treatment **(E)**. Details of x-axis: 1) Untreated cell only (background red filter), 2) Untreated, cell only (blue filter), 3) Cell + SPION (total SPION), 4) Cell + SPION (total cell area, blue filter).

$(5.3 \pm 1.1 \text{ pg cell}^{-1})$ have been detected over 48 h of incubation with SPION (Feridex®) at 0.075 mg ml$^{-1}$ in labeled NPC (neural progenitor cells) [24].

Quantitative and statistical population analysis of total iron oxide area per total cell area of 100 MCF-7 cells

was carried out by automated epifluorescence imaging with multichannel acquisitions (bright field, blue and red channels). From the overlapping and thresholding against the iron content it was possible to identify and quantify the ratio of inorganic iron content versus the total cell area. Figure 1D shows representative microscopy images of untreated and exposed MCF-7 cells to 0.4 mg ml$^{-1}$.

Samples from the same experiments were processed for observation by electron transmission microscopy (Figure 2). Even after very short incubation times (0.5 h), it was possible to detect SPION clusters within cell cytoplasm (Figure 2a). DMSA-SPION were found surrounded by a membrane and no free cytoplasmatic nanoparticles were detected. Incubations of 1 and 3 h revealed a small increment in the presence of vesicles containing DMSA-SPION (Figure 2b, c). During longer incubation times (6, 12 and 24 h), the number of vesicles with larger DMSA-SPION aggregates increased and they were accumulated close to the nuclei (Figure 2d-f and inset in f). Together with an increment in the number of vesicles, prolonged incubation time also resulted in important morphological changes of DMSA-SPION containing vesicles. While analysis of sectioned cells revealed a small increment in their size, the most important change however was related to their morphology, where a clear evolution from translucent vesicles with nanoparticles towards a much denser and multivesicular aspect has been detected (Figure 2 a-f).

As MCF-7 cells are derived from a human breast adenocarcinoma, we decided to study also DMSA-SPION uptake and accumulation in a non-malignant breast cell line MCF-10A. Cells were incubated with DMSA-SPION under the same conditions as MCF-7 cells. Analysis by bright field microscopy showed that uptake and accumulation of nanoparticles in MCF-10A cells was equivalent to MCF-7 cancer cells (see Additional file 1). This was confirmed by Prussian blue staining. Analysis by electron microscopy clearly revealed that aggregates of particles were accumulated inside MCF-10A cells near nucleus with similar kinetics to that found in carcinoma cells (Additional file 1). The overall response of these non-cancerous cells was similar to carcinoma cells (see Additional file 1).

Results obtained for nanoparticles internalization in malignant (MCF-7) and non-malignant (MCF-10A) cell lines are not entirely surprising. It is important to recall that all established cell lines, including non-malignant cells, have alterations in their genome, which make them different from healthy cells of an organism. Therefore, MCF-10A cannot be considered as a fully "normal" human cell line [25,26]. In this sense, quantum dot (QD) nanoparticles with different surface coatings can be internalized within human mammary non-tumorigenic epithelial cell line MCF-10A as well as in human mammary adenocarcinoma epithelial cell line MCF-7 [27]. Zhang *et al.* [28] have described that both (MCF-7 and MCF-10A) cells can internalize iron oxide nanoparticles by vesicular transport after incubation for different times (30 min, 4 and 24 h). This research was carried out using commercial iron oxide nanoparticles (maghemite $\gamma$-Fe$_2$O$_3$ with diameter around 30 nm) from Alfa Aesar® (Karlsruhe, Germany) without any coating.

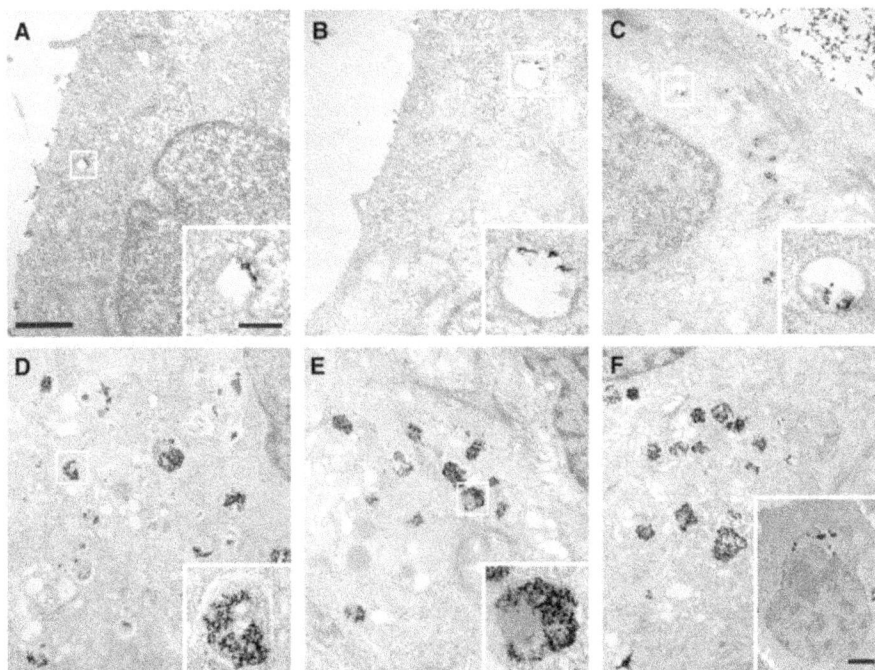

**Figure 2 Electron microscopy analysis of uptake kinetics.** Images from thin sections of MCF7 cells incubated with DMSA-SPION. **(a)** Cells incubated for 0.5 h, **(b)** 1 h, **(c)** 3 h, **(d)** 6 h, **(e)** 12 h and **(f)** 24 h. The inset in **(f)** shows the overall cell shape and morphology. Scale bars represent 1 μm for each image, 200 nm for insets in a to e, and 2 μm for the inset in f, respectively.

In summary, it is rather difficult to compare our results with those reported in the literature previously, because nanoparticles used in other studies have very different characteristics. It is well known that parameters such as nanoparticle size and particle surface coating are crucial on nanoparticle-cell interactions [3,8,17,29].

### Internalization mechanism and accumulation of DMSA-SPION inside cells

To analyze internalization mechanism, cells were incubated with particles at different temperatures. At 4°C, internalization of DMSA-SPION was inhibited and nanoparticles were attached at the cell surface, while uptake was developed successfully after 3 h at 37°C (Figure 3A). This result indicated that an active energy-dependent transport was implicated in the SPION internalization process [13,14,17,21].

To get insight into these nanoparticles subcellular localization, MCF-7 cells were incubated with DMSA-SPION for 24 h and then incubated with LysoTracker Red to stain the lysosomal compartment and finally visualized by bright field and fluorescence microscopy. Figure 3B show SPION into MCF-7 living cells using fluorescence microscopy. As can be seen in the same figure lysosomes were labeled with LysoTracker Red. Merged images displayed a substantial fraction of red fluorescence from LysoTracker which colocalizes with internalized nanoparticles, strongly suggesting that DMSA-SPION were accumulated in endosome/lysosome fraction.

To identify the precise mechanism of endocytosis (phagocytosis, pinocytosis, macropinocytosis, clathrin-mediated endocytosis, or caveolae-mediated endocytosis), we performed transmission electron microscopy (TEM) studies. The high contrast of the magnetic particles allowed for their clear identification (Figure 4). Small groups of particles were seen near cell membranes. Actually, SPION incubated in culture media present a relatively wide size distribution (ranging between 50 to more than 400 nm, see Additional file 2). Although we did not make an attempt to sort the SPION by size, we found significant differences in the way the SPION were incorporated in the cells according to the aggregate size. Smaller aggregates were seen adjacent to distinct clathrin-coated patches (Figure 4A). Closed clathrin vesicles containing small DMSA-SPION aggregates (smaller than 200 nm) were seen in the cytoplasm, near membrane. Larger DMSA-SPION aggregates were seen near cell periphery, in most cases engulfed by cell membrane extensions, indicating the existence of a macropinocytic DMSA-SPION uptake process (Figure 4B a, b). Other studies have also proposed a macropinocytic process for cationic iron oxide nanoparticles internalization [30], as well as for other nanoparticles [31].

Following short incubation times, particles were found near the cell membrane, showing SPION-containing vesicles closely resembling early endosomes (Figure 4C a). At later incubation stages, there were denser SPION-containing vesicles resembling multi-vesicular bodies containing intraluminal vesicles (Figure 4C b). Subsequently, the vesicles adopted a multi-lamellar lysosome aspect containing large numbers of DMSA-SPION clusters (Figure 4C c,d).

The same type of analysis has been carried out with the non-malignant MCF10-A cells. The results clearly

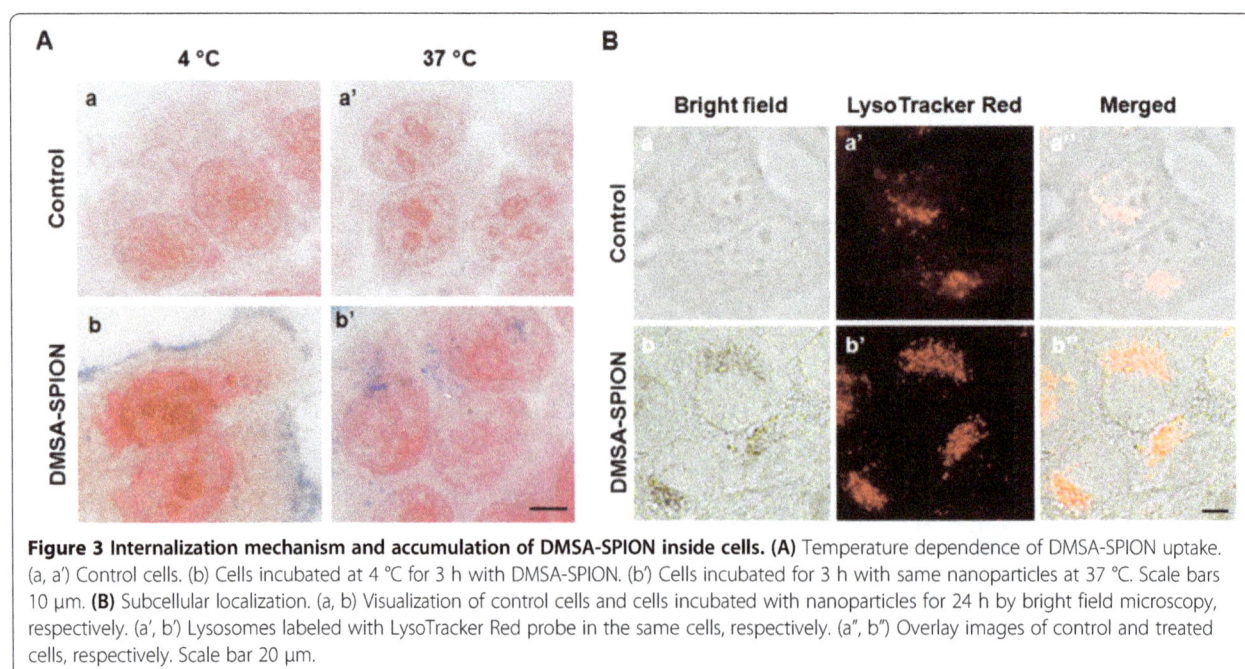

**Figure 3 Internalization mechanism and accumulation of DMSA-SPION inside cells. (A)** Temperature dependence of DMSA-SPION uptake. (a, a') Control cells. (b) Cells incubated at 4 °C for 3 h with DMSA-SPION. (b') Cells incubated for 3 h with same nanoparticles at 37 °C. Scale bars 10 μm. **(B)** Subcellular localization. (a, b) Visualization of control cells and cells incubated with nanoparticles for 24 h by bright field microscopy, respectively. (a', b') Lysosomes labeled with LysoTracker Red probe in the same cells, respectively. (a", b") Overlay images of control and treated cells, respectively. Scale bar 20 μm.

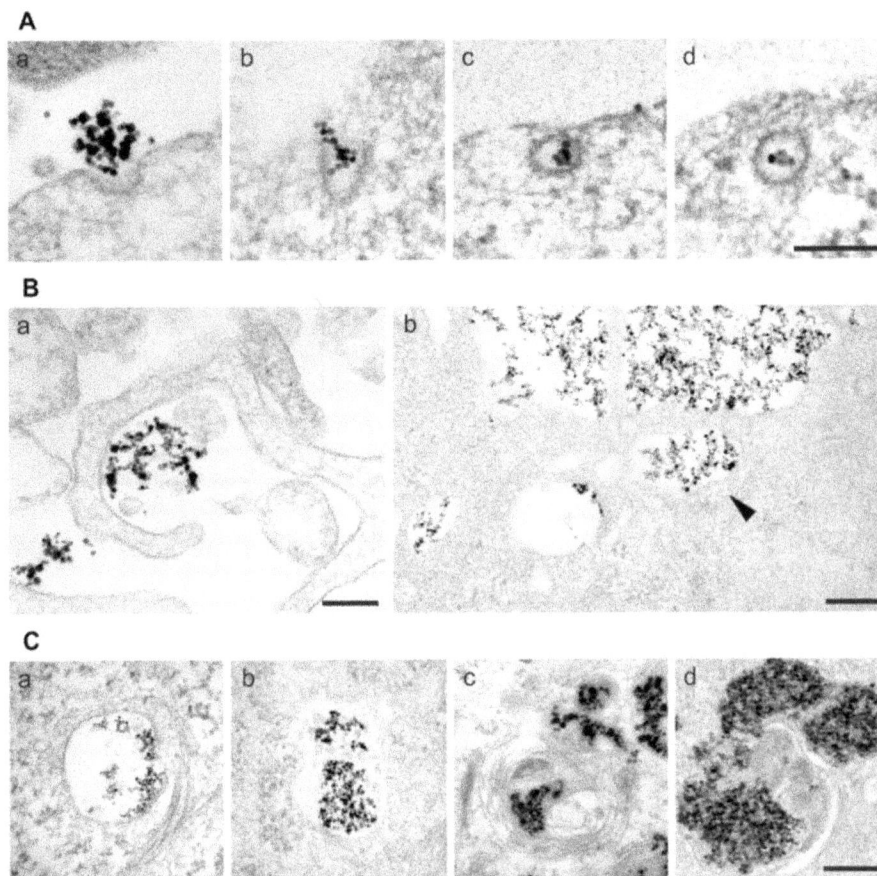

**Figure 4 Electron microscopy study of SPION interaction and uptake. (A)** Electron microscopy images of thin sections of cells interacting with DMSA-SPION by clathrin mediated uptake (<200 nm in diameter aggregates). Scale bar represents 200 nm. **(B)** Two images by electron microscopy of thin sections of cells showing typical images of macropinocytosis for DMSA-SPION uptake (>200 nm in diameter aggregates). Scale bars represent 200 nm. **(C)** Electron microscopy images of different types of endosomes containing SPION aggregates: (a) Early endosome. (b) Multivesicular body containing intraluminal vesicles. (c) Late endosome characterized by a multilamellar morphology. (d) Late endosomes and lysosomes with multivesicular structure and large electron-dense areas. Scale bar represents 200 nm.

showed that incorporation of DMSA-SPION and their intracellular trafficking feature the same overall characteristics in the case of the non-cancerous breast epithelial cells (see Additional file 1).

### Intracellular persistence of SPION

Other important questions related to the incorporation of nanoparticles into cells are to establish how long they remain inside cells and to disclose their eventual release mechanism. To get an insight into these questions, after 24 h incubation, nanoparticles were removed and cultures were further incubated up to 72 h at 37°C. Samples, taken at 24, 48 and 72 h, were stained with Prussian blue and observed by bright field microscopy. Figure 5A shows that SPION remain within MCF-7 cells in vesicles up to 72 h.

To get more detailed information on the evolution of the intracellular vesicles after prolonged incubation times, a parallel analysis to that described above was carried out using electron microscopy. Cells containing DMSA-SPION evolved and divided in a similar way as control cells without DMSA-SPION. Multi-vesicular bodies and lysosomes containing nanoparticles did not change much, even after extended incubation intervals (Figure 5B a-d). SPION clusters were retained inside the vesicles and these vesicles further evolved towards late endosomal or lysosomal morphology, but neither their number nor their localization in cell cytoplasm underwent significant changes, thereby indicating that DMSA-SPION were not massively released from cells. These results suggest that, although cells keep dividing, iron oxide nanoparticles persist inside them for a long time. These qualitative results were confirmed by quantification of intracellular iron content in ferrozine-based assay (Figure 5C), which confirmed that the amount of iron remains substantially unaltered inside the cells after 48 h post-incubation interval.

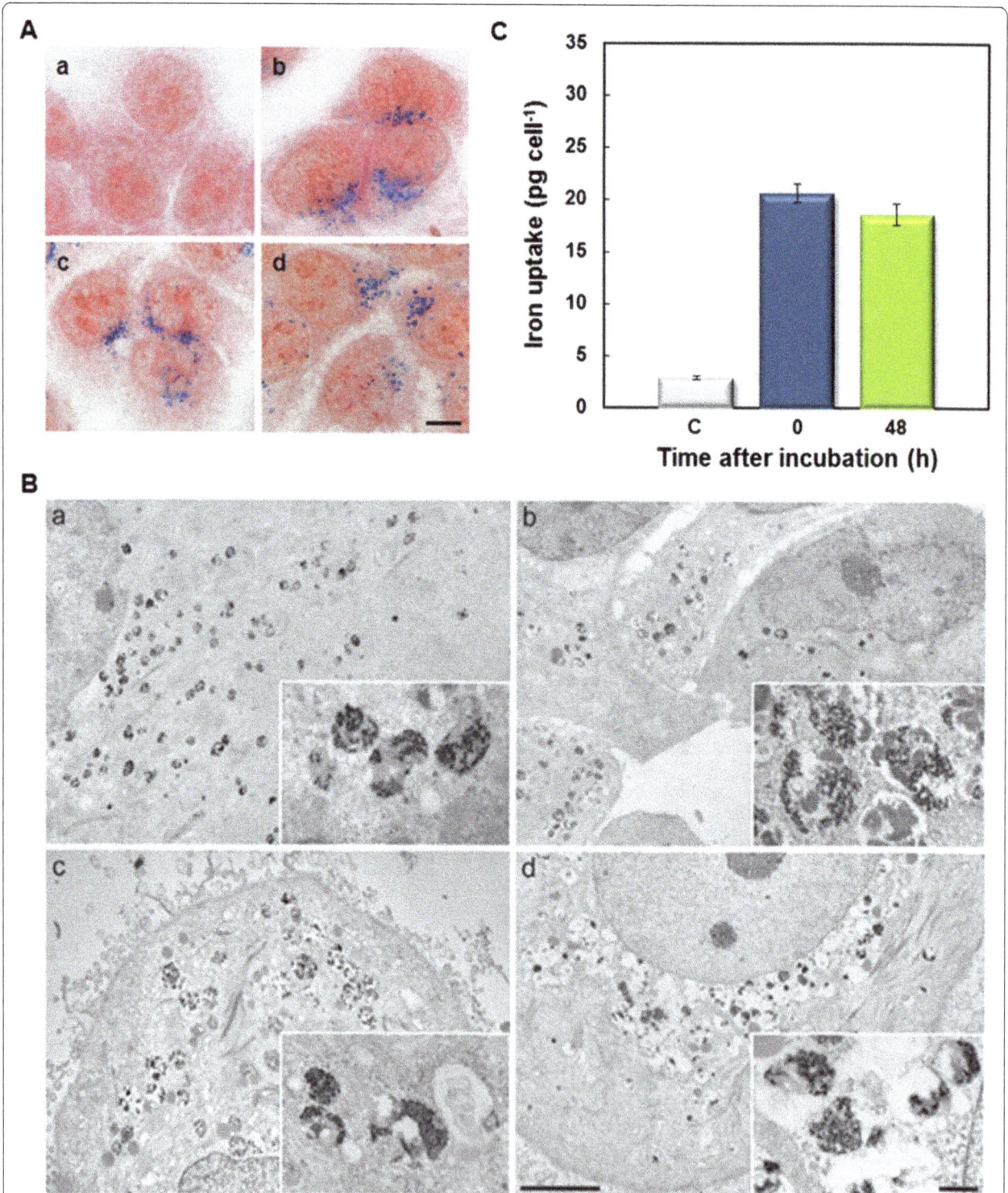

**Figure 5 Persistence of internalized DMSA-SPION. (A)** MCF-7 cells incubated with nanoparticles for 24 h, stained with Prussian blue reaction after different post-incubation times and visualized by bright field microscopy. (a) Untreated control cells. (b-d) Cells incubated for 24 h and stained 24, 48 and 72 h after incubation, respectively. Scale bar represents 10 μm. **(B)** Study of persistence by electron microscopy: (a) Cells were incubated with DMSA-SPION for 24 h. The cells were further incubated in medium without particles for additional (b) 24 h, (c) 48 h and (d) 72 h. Insets show larger magnification details of the endosomes. Scale bars represent 5 μm in overall areas and 500 nm in larger magnification insets, respectively. **(C)** Intracellular iron content quantification by ferrozine assay (expressed as weight of iron per cell) in control (non-treated) cells (c), and immediately (0) or 48 h after incubation with DMSA-SPION.

## Cytotoxicity of DMSA-SPION

Exposure to SPION has been associated with significant toxic effects due to the generation of ROS, which result in deleterious cellular consequences eventually leading to cell death [32-35]. There are contradictory results related to biocompatibility of DMSA-coated magnetic nanoparticles. Several reports have described some cytotoxicity for DMSA magnetic iron oxide nanoparticles in different cell lines [19,36]. On the contrary, little effects on cell viability, oxidative stress, cell cycle or apoptosis have been reported for these magnetic nanoparticles by other authors [17,37].

Taking into account such a contradictory background, we decided to analyze the biocompatibility of these nanoparticles using several complementary approaches, such as (i) studies of cytoskeletal components, (ii) cell morphology observations by bright field microscopy (neutral red and Hoechst-33258 staining), (iii) analysis of the cell cycle, (iv) detection of ROS generation and, (v) two alternative viability tests.

### (i) Analysis of cytoskeletal components

Two components of cytoskeleton were analyzed: microtubules (MTs) and actin filaments (F-actin). MTs are highly dynamic fibers of the cytoskeleton, with critical functions in eukaryotic cells including intracellular transport, organization of cell structural dynamics and cell division. We have evaluated the effects of nanoparticle internalization on MTs during interphase and mitosis by means of indirect immunofluorescence analysis to α-tubulin (DNA counterstained with Hoechst-33258). Figure 6A shows fluorescence images of MTs (green) and DNA (blue) for interphase and metaphase MCF-7 control cells. After 24, 48 or 72 h of incubation with nanoparticles, interphase microtubules maintain their normal morphology and distribution. In the same samples, DMSA-SPION were visualized inside the cells by bright field microscopy. Distributions of mitotic spindles and chromosomes were also similar to metaphase control cells up to 72 h after incubation.

We also investigated the effects of SPION on F-actin and vinculin, a protein implicated in cell adhesion as a focal adhesion complex component. F-actin builds the thinnest filaments of cytoskeleton in the cytoplasm of eukaryotic cells. They are involved in cell morphology, transport of vesicles and organelles, positioning of cellular components, cytokinesis, cell motion, cell-cell and cell-substrate interactions, and signal transduction. Focal adhesions are specialized sites containing a complex network of proteins, included vinculin, favoring interactions between cell and extracellular matrix through the actin cytoskeleton [38]. Figure 6B shows fluorescence images of actin microfilaments (red), vinculin protein (green) and DNA (blue) for MCF-7 control cells. Incorporation

of DMSA-SPION, followed by localization of them inside the cells by bright field microscopy, did not affect the organization of stress fibers or focal adhesions.

### (ii) Cell morphology

MCF-7 cells were exposed to 24 h incubation with DMSA-SPION and then they were stained with neutral red or Hoechst-33258 to observe cytoplasmic and nuclear morphology, respectively. Cells stained with neutral red have a similar morphology to control cells after nanoparticle incorporation in cytoplasm and, nuclei also presented the same characteristics as control cells (Figure 7A).

### (iii) Cell cycle

As shown in Figure 7B, cell cycle distribution was not affected after incubation of cells with 0.4 mg ml$^{-1}$ SPION for 24 h when compared to untreated control populations. A broad overview of the effects of magnetic and nonmagnetic nanoparticles on the cell life cycle has been recently compiled by Mahmoudi et al. [39].

### (iv) Detection of ROS generation

To analyze whether DMSA-SPION produce ROS, cells were preincubated with SPION for 24, 48 and 72 h and then treated with the fluorochrome probe DCFH-DA [40]. As shown in Figure 7C, no significant fluorescent signal was detected after 72 h incubation with SPION at 0.4 mg ml$^{-1}$. Several in vitro studies have suggested that a range of iron oxide nanoparticles with different physico-chemical characteristics induce ROS formation which can lead to cellular injury and death [32-35].

### (v) Cell viability studies

MTT assay showed that cell viability was not significantly affected by the presence of DMSA-SPION at 24 h of treatment (>96% viability in relation to the control sample), even at the highest concentration (0.4 mg ml$^{-1}$) (Figure 7D a). The results obtained using Trypan blue assay (Figure 7D b), confirmed the biocompatibility of DMSA-SPION, and cell survival was > 90% after 24 h incubation. It is important to note that Trypan blue exclusion test has been proposed as the gold standard method to validate the cell viability after magnetic nanoparticle incubation [41]. These results were further confirmed using a multiparametric High Content Screening Cytotoxicity Assay in agreement with a previously published report [42], (data not shown).

In summary, the results presented here justify a deeper research on the synthesis and biological characterization of iron oxide nanoparticles. The complementary approaches recommended for risk assessment of nanoparticles [43,44] indicate that DMSA-SPION are safe and efficient nanoparticles for possible biomedical applications. This is a crucial fact, before further functionalization of these SPION for

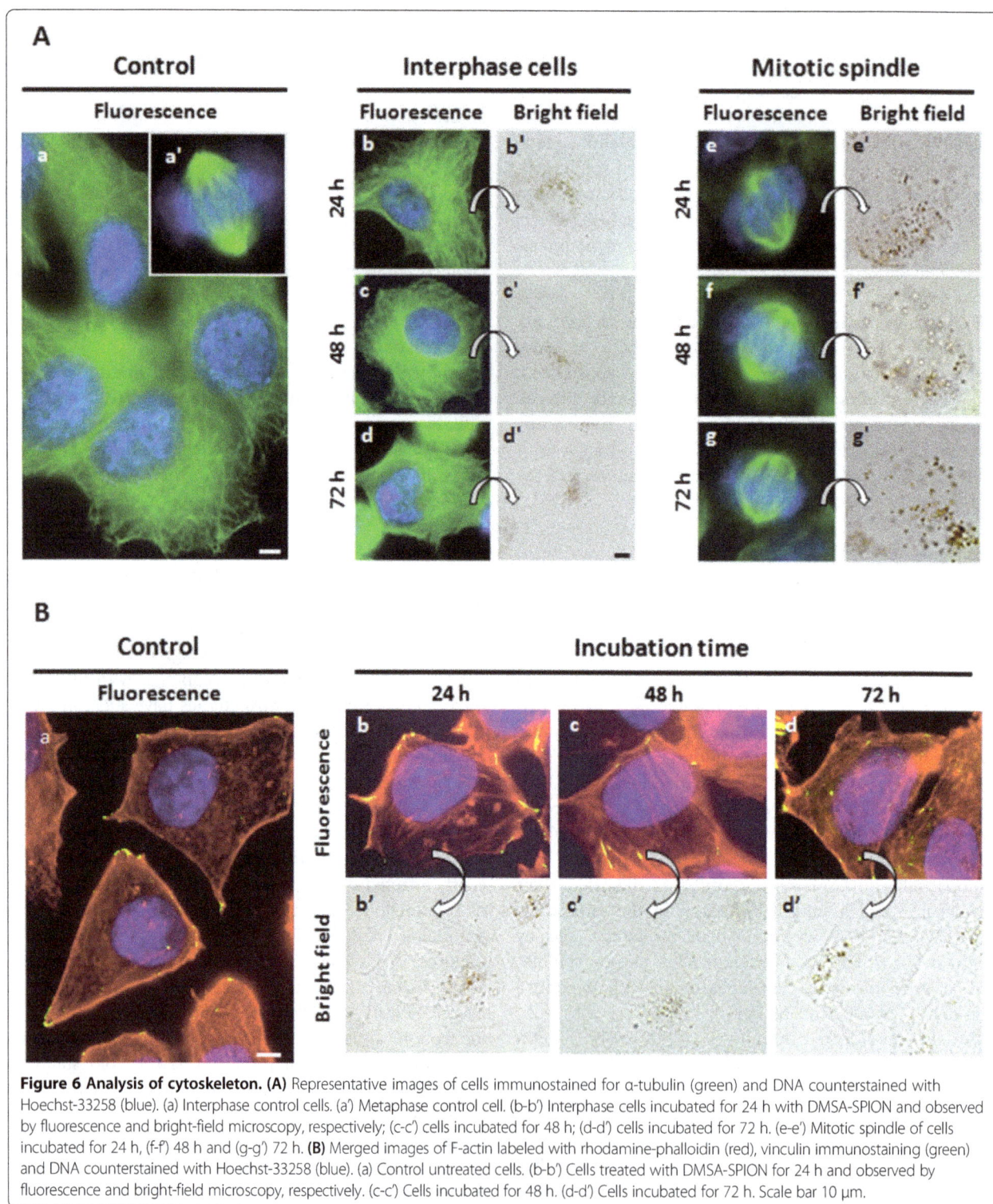

**Figure 6 Analysis of cytoskeleton. (A)** Representative images of cells immunostained for α-tubulin (green) and DNA counterstained with Hoechst-33258 (blue). (a) Interphase control cells. (a') Metaphase control cell. (b-b') Interphase cells incubated for 24 h with DMSA-SPION and observed by fluorescence and bright-field microscopy, respectively; (c-c') cells incubated for 48 h; (d-d') cells incubated for 72 h. (e-e') Mitotic spindle of cells incubated for 24 h, (f-f') 48 h and (g-g') 72 h. **(B)** Merged images of F-actin labeled with rhodamine-phalloidin (red), vinculin immunostaining (green) and DNA counterstained with Hoechst-33258 (blue). (a) Control untreated cells. (b-b') Cells treated with DMSA-SPION for 24 h and observed by fluorescence and bright-field microscopy, respectively. (c-c') Cells incubated for 48 h. (d-d') Cells incubated for 72 h. Scale bar 10 μm.

medical applications (drug delivery and/or hyperthermia), that require high levels of intracellular accumulation for effective treatment.

It is important to point out that the purpose of our study was twofold: i) to analyze the effectiveness of DMSA-SPION accumulation within tumor cells and ii)

to confirm the absence of toxicity induced by nanoparticles (non-functionalized), to ensure their biocompatibility, even if they were accumulated by non-tumor cells. This is especially important, taking into account the pressing need to identify any potential cellular damage associated with SPION [32]. In the broader context, following such

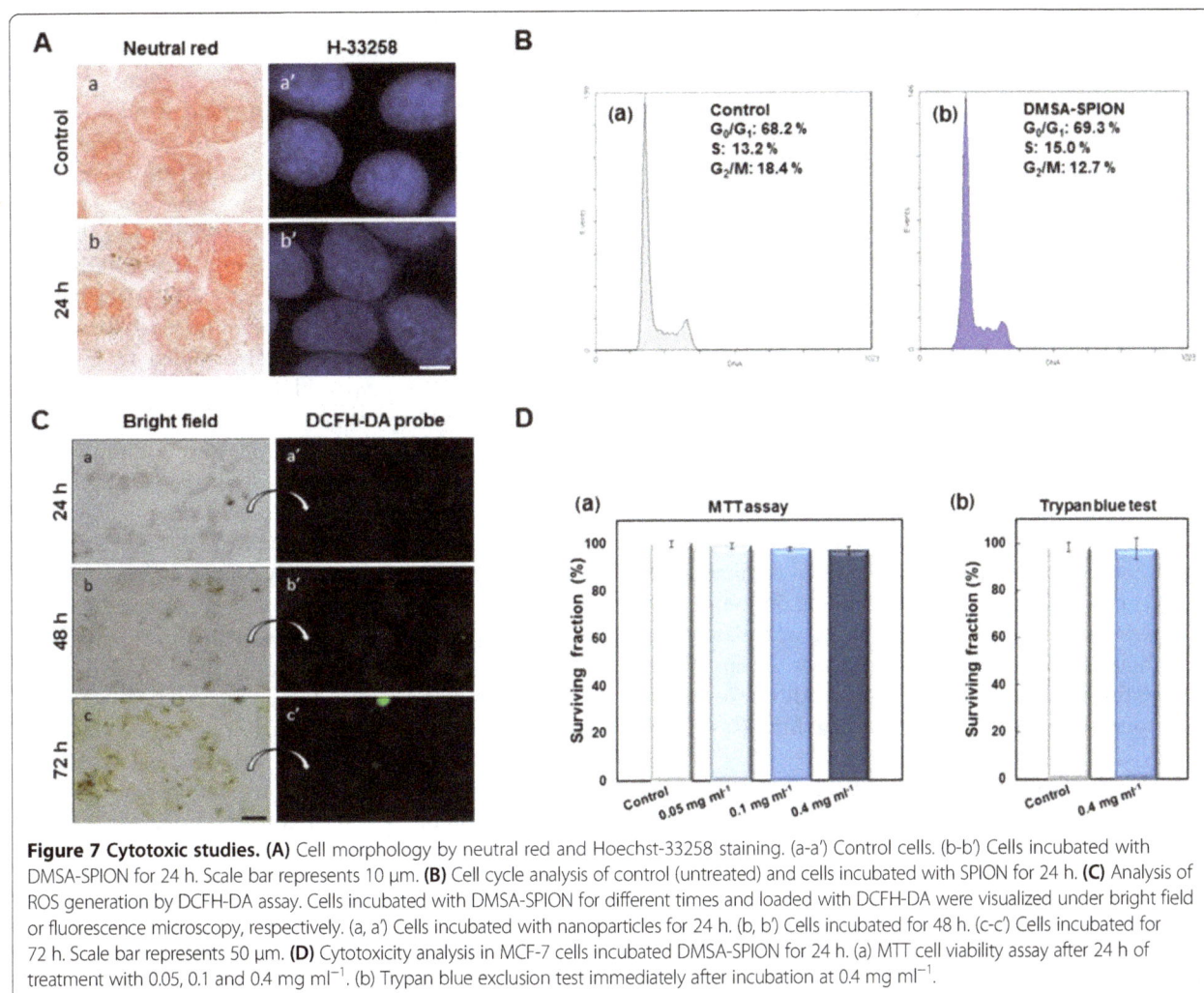

**Figure 7 Cytotoxic studies.** **(A)** Cell morphology by neutral red and Hoechst-33258 staining. (a-a') Control cells. (b-b') Cells incubated with DMSA-SPION for 24 h. Scale bar represents 10 μm. **(B)** Cell cycle analysis of control (untreated) and cells incubated with SPION for 24 h. **(C)** Analysis of ROS generation by DCFH-DA assay. Cells incubated with DMSA-SPION for different times and loaded with DCFH-DA were visualized under bright field or fluorescence microscopy, respectively. (a, a') Cells incubated with nanoparticles for 24 h. (b, b') Cells incubated for 48 h. (c-c') Cells incubated for 72 h. Scale bar represents 50 μm. **(D)** Cytotoxicity analysis in MCF-7 cells incubated DMSA-SPION for 24 h. (a) MTT cell viability assay after 24 h of treatment with 0.05, 0.1 and 0.4 mg ml$^{-1}$. (b) Trypan blue exclusion test immediately after incubation at 0.4 mg ml$^{-1}$.

work carried out these "marginally toxic nanoparticles" will be further functionalized with biologically active molecular moieties such as peptides and antibodies for breast cancer targeting. From this prospective, our study is relevant to the safe development of nanoparticles for biomedical applications, as well as to understanding their biological behavior in the "bare" or non-functionalized state, since once delivered inside the cells, nanoparticles can be processed by intracellular pathways (e.g. distinct endocytic pathways) and "stripped" or separated from the molecules they have been originally conjugated with.

## Conclusions

Dimercaptosuccinic acid surface coating of SPION enhanced their cellular uptake efficiency without inducing either cytotoxicity, alteration of the major cytoskeletal components, vinculin protein dynamics, cell cycle or ROS formation in MCF-7 breast cancer cell line. Incorporation of DMSA-SPION inside the cells followed two endocytic pathways depending on the size of the particle aggregates: smaller aggregates were incorporated using a clathrin-

dependent path, while larger aggregates were incorporated by macropinocytosis. In all cases, SPION aggregates were found surrounded by endocytotic membrane, which localized in perinuclear areas after long incubation times, but never inside the cell nucleus. Following cellular uptake, SPION showed a slow release rate and continuous persistence over extended intervals inside the cells. These characteristics are relevant for the rational design and subsequent utilization of SPION for biomedical applications, both for diagnosis by magnetic resonance imaging (MRI) and for targeted therapy of cancer by hyperthermia and releasing anti-cancer molecules with significantly reduced side effects.

## Methods

### Magnetic nanoparticles

Superparamagnetic iron oxide nanoparticles of uniform size (15 nm) were obtained by thermal decomposition of an iron oleate complex in 1-octadecene [12]. These particles, with a coating of DMSA that make them stable in aqueous buffers, were kindly provided by Dr. Puerto

Morales (ICMM-CSIC) as part of MULTFUN FP7 NMP project (see details in Additional file 2).

DMSA-SPION were sterilized by 0.22 µm pore size filtration (Millipore Corp., Bedford, USA). SPION stock at 4 mg ml$^{-1}$ was dispersed by sonication for 5 min in a 40 kHz sonicator bath (Branson 3510 ultrasonic cleaner, Thomas Scientific, Swedesboro, USA). SPION were then resuspended in complete cell culture media at a final concentration of 0.4 mg ml$^{-1}$. The mixture was then sonicated for 1 min and incubated with cells at different times.

## Cell cultures

Human breast cancer MCF-7 cells were grown as monolayer cultures in Dulbecco's modified Eagle's medium (DMEM), supplemented with 10% (v/v) fetal bovine serum (FBS), 50 units ml$^{-1}$ penicillin and 50 µg ml$^{-1}$ streptomycin. All products were purchased from Gibco (Paisley, Scotland, UK) and sterilized by means of 0.22 µm filters. Cell cultures were grown in an incubator with 5% $CO_2$ plus 95% air at 37°C. Depending on the purpose of experiment, cells were seeded on 24-well plates (with or without 10 mm square coverslips) or 25 cm$^2$ flasks. Sub-confluent cell cultures were used. All sterile plastics were sourced from Corning (Corning Inc., New York, USA).

Non-tumorigenic human breast epithelial cell line MCF-10A was used for comparison in some experiments (see Supporting Information). Cell lines used in this study were obtained from American Type Culture Collection (ATCC)®.

## DMSA-SPION internalization
### Live cell imaging

In order to analyze internalization of nanoparticles, MCF-7 cells were grown on coverslips and incubated for 24 h with DMSA-SPION. After incubation, culture medium was removed and samples were washed three times with phosphate-buffered saline (PBS, pH 7.4). Then, cells were observed immediately under bright light microscopy without being processed, to avoid potential fixation artifacts.

## Prussian blue staining

Cells preincubated with nanoparticles for different periods of time (0.5, 1, 3, 6, 12, 24, 48 or 72 h), were visualized by Prussian blue staining for iron detection [17,45]. Briefly, cells were fixed in methanol (at -20°C) for 5 min, stained with an equal volume of 4% hydrochloric acid and 4% potassium ferrocyanide trihydrate for 15 min, and counterstained with 0.5% neutral red for 2 min. Preparations were then washed with distilled water, air dried, and mounted in DePeX (Serva, Heidelberg, Germany). All other reagents were purchased from Panreac Química (Montcada i Reixac, Spain).

## Quantification of iron in cultured cells
### Colorimetric ferrozine-based method

This sensitive assay permits the quantification of iron in cultured cells [46]. In time-dependent studies, MCF-7 cells seeded in 24-well plates were incubated with DMSA-SPION at a fixed concentration of 0.5 mg ml$^{-1}$ for 24 or 48 h. For intracellular persistence studies, cells were incubated 24 h and intracellular iron content was evaluated 48 h after removing DMSA-SPION from culture media by three washes with PBS. After that, in both cases, cells in three wells were trypsinized and cell concentrations per well were determined by hemocytometer with 0.4% Trypan blue solution. Cells grown in other 24-well dishes were frozen at -20°C for 1 h and then, 500 µl of 50 nM NaOH (Panreac Química) were added to each well for 2 h in movement. Aliquots of cell lysates were then transferred to 1.5 ml eppendorf and mixed with 500 µl of 10 mM HCl, and 500 µl of iron-releasing reagent (a freshly mixed solution of equal volumes of 1.4 M HCl and 4.5% (w/v) $KMnO_4$ (Merck, Germany) in distilled $H_2O$. These mixtures were incubated for 2 h at 60°C within a fume hood, since chlorine gas is produced during the reaction. After the mixtures had cooled to room temperature, 150 µl of iron-detection reagent (6.5 mM ferrozine (Sigma-Aldrich, St Louis, USA), 6.5 mM neocuproine (Sigma-Aldrich), 2.5 M ammonium acetate (Panreac Química), and 1 M ascorbic acid (Sigma-Aldrich) dissolved in water) were added to each tube. After 30 min, 500 µl of the solution obtained in each tube was transferred into a well of a 24-well plate, and absorbance was measured at 570 nm in a SpectraFluor spectrophotometer (Tecan Group Ltd., Männedorf, Switzerland). Iron content of the sample was calculated by comparing its absorbance to that of a range of standard concentrations of equal volume, that had been prepared in a way similar to that of the sample (mixture of 100 µl of $FeCl_3$ standards (0–300 µM) in 10 mM HCl, 100 µl 50 mM NaOH, 500 µl releasing reagent, and 1500 µl detection reagent). The determined intracellular iron concentration for each well of a cell culture was normalized against number of cells per well.

### High content screening

Quantification of iron oxide content was based on automated epifluorescence images taken from stained cell monolayer cultured on slides. On average 100 cells were selected from the two cell line provided. Images were analyzed by single channel, filtered and threshold of each channel was identified. Composite rebuilt in order to identify localization of SPION against cellular staining. Filtering was applied on the red and blue filter in order to account for the SPION or the cell only.

## Endocytic mechanisms

In order to analyze the degree of involvement of the endocytic mechanisms in internalization of nanoparticles, cells were preincubated with nanoparticles for 3 h at either 4°C or 37°C, washed three times with PBS, and stained with Prussian blue technique (as described above).

## Subcellular localization of nanoparticles

To determine DMSA-SPION subcellular location inside cells, endocytic compartments of MCF-7 cells were labelled with 50 nM LysoTracker® Red DND-99 (Molecular Probes, Eugene, Oregon, USA) fluoroprobe in culture medium, at 37°C for 30 min. Cells incubated with nanoparticles for 24 h were labelled with LysoTraker Red and then coverslips were washed with PBS and cells were observed immediately under bright field and fluorescence microscopy.

## Analysis of the cytoskeleton and adhesion proteins
### Immunofluorescence staining of α-tubulin

Cells grown on glass coverslips were incubated with nanoparticles for 24, 48 and 72 h and then, immunostained for α-tubulin. Briefly, cells were fixed with cold methanol for 5 min, washed three times for 5 min with PBS, and then permeabilized with 0.5% Triton X-100 (Sigma-Aldrich) in PBS for 5 min. After Triton removal, cells were incubated with primary monoclonal mouse anti-α-tubulin antibody (Sigma-Aldrich) diluted 1:100 at 37°C in a wet chamber for 1 h. Three washings with PBS were then carried out before addiction of Triton X-100 for 5 min. Incubation of the secondary antibody (Fab specific goat anti-mouse FITC-IgG; Sigma-Aldrich) was identical to that of the first one. Then, DNA was counterstained by Hoechst-33258 (0.05 mg ml$^{-1}$ in distilled water) for 5 min. Finally, cells were washed with PBS and mounted with ProLong Gold (Molecular Probes) antifade reagent.

### Vinculin immunofluorescence and F-actin staining

For vinculin immunostaining, cells grown on coverslips were fixed with formaldehyde in PBS (1:10 v/v), for 20 min at 4°C, washed three times for 5 min with PBS and permeabilized with 0.5% Triton X-100. After incubation with a blocking solution (5% bovine serum albumin, 5% FBS, 0.02% Triton X-100 in PBS) at room temperature for 30 min, cells were incubated with 1:50 solution mouse monoclonal anti-vinculin (Sigma-Aldrich) at 37°C in a wet chamber for 1 h. Primary antibody binding was detected using Fab specific goat anti-mouse FITC-IgG diluted 1:50. F-actin was visualized in the same samples by incubation with rhodamine-labeled phalloidin (Sigma-Aldrich) diluted 1:200 at 37°C in a wet chamber for 25 min. Then, samples were washed three times with PBS, counterstained with Hoechst-33258 for 5 min, washed with PBS and mounted with Prolong Gold antifade reagent.

## Cell morphology analysis
### Neutral red staining

MCF-7 cells grown on coverslips in 24-well plates were incubated with DMSA-SPION for 24 h, fixed in methanol at –20°C for 5 min and then stained with 0.5% neutral red for 2 min. After that, samples were washed with distilled water, air dried, mounted in DePeX and visualized by light microscopy.

### Hoechst-33258 staining

Cells seeded on coverslips and treated with nanoparticles for 24 h were fixed in methanol at –20°C for 5 min and stained with Hoechst-33258 for 5 min. Samples were washed with distilled water, air dried, and mounted in DePeX for observation using fluorescence microscopy.

## Cell cycle analysis

MCF-7 cells were plated in 25-cm$^2$ flasks and incubated with DMSA-SPION for 24 h. Analysis of cell cycle was performed by flow cytometry using propidium iodide (PI) labeling of DNA cell content. Cells were trypsinized (also harvesting possible detached cells) and centrifuged at 1200 rpm for 5 min. After centrifugation, pellet was resuspended in 100 µl of culture medium without phenol red. Then, it was added 50 µl of Coulter DNA Prep Reagents Kit (Beckman-Coulter Inc, California, USA), 1 ml of PI solution with RNase and incubated for 30 min at 37°C. Both reagents were purchased from Sigma-Aldrich. Distribution of cells in different phases of cell cycle was determined using a Coulter Epics XL-MCL flow cytometer (Beckman-Coulter Inc.) with an argon laser line (488 nm), complemented with appropriate filters, and a minimum of 10$^4$ labeled cells per sample were analyzed in each experimental condition. Percent of cells in each phase of the cell cycle was compared with that of control cells (without nanoparticles incubation). At least 10000 fluorescent events were counted per sample.

## Measurement of intracellular ROS

Intracellular ROS levels were determined using 2′,7′-dichlorodihydrofluorescein diacetate (DCFH-DA) assay. Cells were seeded on coverslips and, after exposure to nanoparticles for 24, 48 and 72 h, were washed with PBS and incubated with 10 µM DCFH-DA (Sigma-Aldrich) for 30 min. Then, cells were washed with PBS again and visualized immediately by fluorescence microscopy. Bright field microscopy was also used to corroborate accumulation of nanoparticles. For control induction of oxidative stress, cells were treated with 800 µM H$_2$O$_2$ (Panreac Química) for 1 h 30 min in complete medium. ROS production was observed in cells, 1 h 30 min after that H$_2$O$_2$ was removed, with 10 µM DCFH-DA for 30 min.

## Cytotoxicity assays

### MTT test

Cytotoxicity was assessed by MTT colorimetric assay 24 after incubation with DMSA-SPION. Immediately prior to use, a stock solution of dimethylthiazolyl-diphenyl-tetrazolium bromide (MTT; Sigma-Aldrich, 1 mg ml$^{-1}$) in PBS was prepared. Five hundred microliters of this MTT solution (50 µg ml$^{-1}$ MTT in culture medium) was added to each culture dish without coverslip. Cells were incubated for 3 h, then reduced formazan was extracted with 500 µl dimethylsulfoxide and absorbance measured at 570 nm in a SpectraFluor spectrophotometer (Tecan Group Ltd, Männedorf, Switzerland). Cell survival was expressed as the percentage of absorption of treated cells in comparison with that of control cells.

### Trypan blue exclusion test

Cell viability was quantified by Trypan blue dye exclusion method. Briefly, after 24 h of incubation with DMSA-SPION, trypsin was added to control and treated cells. After cells were detached from the plate, they were resuspended in culture media. Equal volumes of each cell suspension and trypan blue solution (0.2% in PBS) were mixed and used for cell counting by hemocytometer. Blue-stained cells were counted as nonviable cells and unstained cells as viable cells.

### Bright field and fluorescence microscopy

Observation of samples processed for bright field and fluorescence microscopy were made with an Olympus BX61 epifluorescence microscope, equipped with an Olympus DP50 digital camera (Olympus, Tokyo, Japan), and processed using the Adobe Photoshop 7 software (Adobe Systems, San Jose, CA, USA). The following filters were used to visualize the fluorescence signal of probes: UV excitation light (365–390 nm) for Hoechst-33258, blue (460–490 nm) for FITC, and green (510–550 nm) for TRITC.

### Statistical analysis

Statistical analysis was performed by GraphPad Prism Software (GraphPad Inc., CA, USA) using one-way ANOVA and Tukey's test. The threshold for significance was $P = 0.05$ and $P$ values $< 0.05$ (*), $< 0.01$ (**) and $< 0.005$ (***) were considered as significant.

### Sample preparation for transmission electron microscopy

MCF-7 cells were incubated with SPION at different times, as described above, washed with PBS and treated with a mixture of 2% formaldehyde (Ultra Pure EM Grade, Polysciences Inc., Philadelphia, USA) and 2.5% glutaraldehyde (EM Grade, TAAB Laboratories Equipment Ltd., Berks, UK) in PBS for 1 h at room temperature. The cell monolayer on the coverslips was then washed with PBS

and distilled water, post-fixed for 45 minutes with 1% osmium tetroxide (TAAB Laboratories Equipment Ltd.) in PBS, washed with distilled water, treated during 45 minutes with 1% aqueous uranyl acetate (Electron Microscopy Sciences, Hatfield, USA), washed again and dehydrated with growing quantities (50%, 75%, 95% and 100%) of ethanol seccosolv (Merck KGaA, Darmstadt, Germany). The samples were maintained in coverslips throughout the process and finally embedded in epoxy resin 812 (TAAB Laboratories Equipment Ltd.) contained in gelatine capsules (Electron Microscopy Sciences). The epoxy resin was polymerized for 2 days at 60°C. Resin was detached from the coverslips by successive immersions in liquid nitrogen and hot water. Ultrathin, 70-nm-thick sections were obtained with an Ultracut UCT ultramicrotome (Leica Microsystems), transferred to 200 mesh Nickel EM grids (Gilder, Lincolnshire, UK) and stained with 3% aqueous uranyl acetate (10 minutes) and lead citrate (2 minutes) (Electron Microscopy Science). Sections were visualized on a JEOL JEM 1200 EXII electron microscope operating at 100 kV (JEOL Ltd., Tokyo, Japan).

## Additional files

> **Additional file 1:** Uptake, accumulation and cytotoxicity of DMSA-SPION into non oncogenic MCF-10A cells.
>
> **Additional file 2:** Nanoparticle concentration and stability characterization by Nanoparticle Tracking and Analysis (NTA).

### Abbreviations

SPION: Superparamagnetic iron oxide nanoparticles; DMSA: meso-2,3-dimercaptosuccinic acid; DMSA-SPION: Dimercaptosuccinic acid coated superparamagnetic iron oxide nanoparticles; MNP: Magnetic nanoparticles; NP: Nanoparticles; TEM: Transmission electron microscopy; PBS: Phosphate buffered saline buffer; FBS: Fetal bovine serum; DMEM: Dulbecco's modified Eagle's medium; HCl: Hydrochloric acid; MTs: Microtubules; F-Actin: Actin filaments; FITC-IgG: Fluorescein isothiocyanate conjugated immunoglobulin-G; ROS: Reactive oxygen species; DCFH-DA: 2′,7′-dichlorodihydrofluorescein diacetate; PI: Propidium iodide; MRI: Magnetic resonance imaging; MTT: Dimethylthiazolyl-diphenyl-tetrazolium bromide.

### Competing interests

The authors declare that they have no competing interests.

### Authors' contributions

AV and JLC conceived and designed the study and wrote the manuscript. MC (M Calero) and MCh (M Chiappi) have carried out the majority of experimental techniques and contributed equally to this paper under supervision of AV and JLC respectively. ALC have contributed to cell cycle experiments and ferrozine assay and performed statistical analysis. MJR processed the electron microscopy samples. FJC participated in microscopy and interpretation. KCS, APM and YV completed quantification by High Content Screening, measured DMSA-SPION size in water and culture medium by Nanoparticle Tracking and Analysis (NTA) and partly wrote the manuscript. All authors read and approved the final manuscript.

### Acknowledgements

The research leading to these results have received partial funding from the European Seventh Framework Programme (FP7/2007-2013) under the project MULTIFUN grant agreement no. 262943, and the project Nanofrontmag-CM (S2013/MIT-2850) from the Comunidad de Madrid. Additional grants were obtained from BFU 2011–29038 and CTQ2013-48767-C3-3-R from the Ministerio de Economia y Competitividad and S2009/Mat 1507 from the Comunidad de Madrid (to JLC), from EU FP7 project NAMDIATREAM (ref 246479) and from "la Caixa" / CNB International PhD Programme Fellowships. We acknowledge Dr. Puerto Morales and Dr. Gorka Salas for providing the SPION samples. The encouragement and continuous support of Rodolfo Miranda is deeply recognized. Authors recognize the valuable contribution of Carmen Moreno-Ortiz (Flow Cytometry, Centro Nacional de Biotecnología, Madrid).

## Author details

[1]Departamento de Biología, Universidad Autónoma de Madrid, Cantoblanco, 28049 Madrid, Spain. [2]Department of Macromolecular Structure, Centro Nacional de Biotecnología, Consejo Superior de Investigaciones Científicas, 28049 Madrid, Spain. [3]Department of Clinical Medicine, Trinity Centre for Health Science, James's Street, Dublin 8, Ireland. [4]Centre for Research on Adaptive Nanostructures and Nanodevices (CRANN), and AMBER Centre, Trinity College Dublin, College Green, Dublin 2, Ireland. [5]Instituto Madrileño de Estudios Avanzados en Nanociencia (IMDEA Nanociencia), Cantoblanco, 28049 Madrid, Spain.

## References

1. Lowe KA, Chia VM, Taylor A, O'Malley C, Kelsh M, Mohamed M, et al. An international assessment of ovarian cancer incidence and mortality. Gynecol Oncol. 2013;130:107–14.
2. Walters S, Maringe C, Butler J, Rachet B, Barrett-Lee P, Bergh J, et al. Breast cancer survival and stage at diagnosis in Australia, Canada, Denmark, Norway, Sweden and the UK, 2000–2007: a population-based study. Br J Cancer. 2013;108:1195–208.
3. Villanueva A, Canete M, Roca AG, Calero M, Veintemillas-Verdaguer S, Serna CJ, et al. The influence of surface functionalization on the enhanced internalization of magnetic nanoparticles in cancer cells. Nanotechnology. 2009;20:115103.
4. Schroeder A, Heller DA, Winslow MM, Dahlman JE, Pratt GW, Langer R, et al. Treating metastatic cancer with nanotechnology. Nat Rev Cancer. 2011;12:39–50.
5. Pollert E, Kaspar P, Zaveta K, Herynek V, Burian M, Jendelova P. Magnetic Nanoparticles for Therapy and Diagnostics. Magnetics, IEEE Transactions on. 2013;49:7–10.
6. Mahmoudi M, Sant S, Wang B, Laurent S, Sen T. Superparamagnetic iron oxide nanoparticles (SPIONs): development, surface modification and applications in chemotherapy. Adv Drug Deliv Rev. 2011;63:24–46.
7. Kralj S, Drofenik M, Makovec D. Controlled surface functionalization of silica-coated magnetic nanoparticles with terminal amino and carboxyl groups. J Nanopart Res. 2011;13:2829–41.
8. Mailander V, Landfester K. Interaction of nanoparticles with cells. Biomacromolecules. 2009;10:2379–400.
9. Huang HC, Chang PY, Chang K, Chen CY, Lin CW, Chen JH, et al. Formulation of novel lipid-coated magnetic nanoparticles as the probe for in vivo imaging. J Biomed Sci. 2009;16:86.
10. Arora S, Rajwade JM, Paknikar KM. Nanotoxicology and in vitro studies: the need of the hour. Toxicol Appl Pharmacol. 2012;258:151–65.
11. Brunner TJ, Wick P, Manser P, Spohn P, Grass RN, Limbach LK, et al. In vitro cytotoxicity of oxide nanoparticles: comparison to asbestos, silica, and the effect of particle solubility. Environ Sci Technol. 2006;40:4374–81.
12. Salas G, Casado C, Teran FJ, Miranda R, Serna CJ, Morales MP. Controlled synthesis of uniform magnetite nanocrystals with high-quality properties for biomedical applications. J Mater Chem. 2012;22:21065–75.
13. Gratton SE, Ropp PA, Pohlhaus PD, Luft JC, Madden VJ, Napier ME, et al. The effect of particle design on cellular internalization pathways. Proc Natl Acad Sci U S A. 2008;105:11613–8.
14. Rejman J, Oberle V, Zuhorn IS, Hoekstra D. Size-dependent internalization of particles via the pathways of clathrin- and caveolae-mediated endocytosis. Biochem J. 2004;377:159–69.
15. Zhu XM, Wang YX, Leung KC, Lee SF, Zhao F, Wang DW, et al. Enhanced cellular uptake of aminosilane-coated superparamagnetic iron oxide nanoparticles in mammalian cell lines. Int J Nanomedicine. 2012;7:953–64.
16. Li Y, Chen Z, Gu N. In vitro biological effects of magnetic nanoparticles. Chin Sci Bull. 2012;57:3972–8.
17. Calero M, Gutierrrez L, Salas G, Luengo Y, Lazaro A, Acedo P, et al. Efficient and safe internalization of magnetic iron oxide nanoparticles: two fundamental requirements for biomedical applications. Nanomedicine. 2014;10:733–43.
18. Liu Y, Wang J. Effects of DMSA-coated Fe3O4 nanoparticles on the transcription of genes related to iron and osmosis homeostasis. Toxicol Sci. 2013;131:521–36.
19. Pisanic 2nd TR, Blackwell JD, Shubayev VI, Finones RR, Jin S. Nanotoxicity of iron oxide nanoparticle internalization in growing neurons. Biomaterials. 2007;28:2572–81.
20. Wang Z, Cuschieri A. Tumour cell labelling by magnetic nanoparticles with determination of intracellular iron content and spatial distribution of the intracellular iron. Int J Mol Sci. 2013;14:9111–25.
21. Gu J, Xu H, Han Y, Dai W, Hao W, Wang C, et al. The internalization pathway, metabolic fate and biological effect of superparamagnetic iron oxide nanoparticles in the macrophage-like RAW264.7 cell. Sci China Life Sci. 2011;54:793–805.
22. Mahajan S, Koul V, Choudhary V, Shishodia G, Bharti AC. Preparation and in vitro evaluation of folate-receptor-targeted SPION-polymer micelle hybrids for MRI contrast enhancement in cancer imaging. Nanotechnology. 2013;24:015603.
23. Naqvi S, Samim M, Abdin M, Ahmed FJ, Maitra A, Prashant C, et al. Concentration-dependent toxicity of iron oxide nanoparticles mediated by increased oxidative stress. Int J Nanomedicine. 2010;5:983–9.
24. Chen CC, Ku MC DMJ, Lai JS, Hueng DY, Chang C. Simple SPION incubation as an efficient intracellular labeling method for tracking neural progenitor cells using MRI. PLoS One. 2013;8:e56125.
25. Kavsan VM, Iershov AV, Balynska OV. Immortalized cells and one oncogene in malignant transformation: old insights on new explanation. BMC Cell Biol. 2011;12:23.
26. Fernandez-Cobo M, Holland JF, Pogo BG. Transcription profiles of non-immortalized breast cancer cell lines. BMC Cancer. 2006;6:99.
27. Xiao Y, Forry SP, Gao X, Holbrook RD, Telford WG, Tona A. Dynamics and mechanisms of quantum dot nanoparticle cellular uptake. J Nanobiotechnology. 2010;8:13.
28. Zhang Y, Yang M, Portney NG, Cui D, Budak G, Ozbay E, et al. Zeta potential: a surface electrical characteristic to probe the interaction of nanoparticles with normal and cancer human breast epithelial cells. Biomed Microdevices. 2008;10:321–8.
29. Shang L, Nienhaus K, Nienhaus GU. Engineered nanoparticles interacting with cells: size matters. J Nanobiotechnology. 2014;12:5.
30. Canete M, Soriano J, Villanueva A, Roca AG, Veintemillas S, Serna CJ, et al. The endocytic penetration mechanism of iron oxide magnetic nanoparticles with positively charged cover: a morphological approach. Int J Mol Med. 2010;26:533–9.
31. Verma A, Stellacci F. Effect of surface properties on nanoparticle-cell interactions. Small. 2010;6:12–21.
32. Singh N, Jenkins GJ, Asadi R, Doak S. Potential toxicity of superparamagnetic iron oxide nanoparticles (SPION). Nano Rev. 2010;1:5358.
33. Shubayev VI, Pisanic 2nd TR, Jin S. Magnetic nanoparticles for theragnostics. Adv Drug Deliv Rev. 2009;61:467–77.
34. Liu Y, Li X, Bao S, Lu Z, Li Q, Li CM. Plastic protein microarray to investigate the molecular pathways of magnetic nanoparticle-induced nanotoxicity. Nanotechnology. 2013;24:175501.
35. Hanini A, Schmitt A, Kacem K, Chau F, Ammar S, Gavard J. Evaluation of iron oxide nanoparticle biocompatibility. Int J Nanomedicine. 2011;6:787–94.
36. Ge G, Wu H, Xiong F, Zhang Y, Guo Z, Bian Z, et al. The cytotoxicity evaluation of magnetic iron oxide nanoparticles on human aortic endothelial cells. Nanoscale Res Lett. 2013;8:215.
37. Mejias R, Gutierrez L, Salas G, Perez-Yague S, Zotes TM, Lazaro FJ, et al. Dimercaptosuccinic acid-coated magnetite nanoparticles for magnetically guided in vivo delivery of interferon gamma for cancer immunotherapy. Biomaterials. 2011;32:2938–52.
38. Critchley DR. Focal adhesions - the cytoskeletal connection. Curr Opin Cell Biol. 2000;12:133–9.
39. Mahmoudi M, Azadmanesh K, Shokrgozar MA, Journeay WS, Laurent S. Effect of nanoparticles on the cell life cycle. Chem Rev. 2011;111:3407–32.
40. Wang H, Joseph JA. Quantifying cellular oxidative stress by dichlorofluorescein assay using microplate reader. Free Radic Biol Med. 1999;27:612–6.
41. Hoskins C, Wang L, Cheng WP, Cuschieri A. Dilemmas in the reliable estimation of the in-vitro cell viability in magnetic nanoparticle engineering: which tests and what protocols? Nanoscale Res Lett. 2012;7:77.

42. Prina-Mello A, Crosbie-Staunton K, Salas G, del Puerto MM, Volkov Y. Multiparametric Toxicity Evaluation of SPIONs by High Content Screening Technique: Identification of Biocompatible Multifunctional Nanoparticles for Nanomedicine. Magnetics, IEEE Transactions on. 2013;49:377–82.

43. Mahmoudi M, Hofmann H, Rothen-Rutishauser B, Petri-Fink A. Assessing the in vitro and in vivo toxicity of superparamagnetic iron oxide nanoparticles. Chem Rev. 2012;112:2323–38.

44. Soenen SJ, De Cuyper M. How to assess cytotoxicity of (iron oxide-based) nanoparticles: a technical note using cationic magnetoliposomes. Contrast Media Mol Imaging. 2011;6:153–64.

45. Cengelli F, Grzyb JA, Montoro A, Hofmann H, Hanessian S, Juillerat-Jeanneret L. Surface-functionalized ultrasmall superparamagnetic nanoparticles as magnetic delivery vectors for camptothecin. ChemMedChem. 2009;4:988–97.

46. Riemer J, Hoepken HH, Czerwinska H, Robinson SR, Dringen R. Colorimetric ferrozine-based assay for the quantitation of iron in cultured cells. Anal Biochem. 2004;331:370–5.

# Permissions

# List of Contributors

**Gervais Rioux**
Department of Microbiology, Infectiology and Immunology, 'Centre de recherche en Infectiologie', Laval University, 2705 boul. Laurier, Quebec City, PQ G1V 4G2, Canada

**Claudia Mathieu**
Department of Microbiology, Infectiology and Immunology, 'Centre de recherche en Infectiologie', Laval University, 2705 boul. Laurier, Quebec City, PQ G1V 4G2, Canada

**Alexis Russell**
Department of Microbiology, Infectiology and Immunology, 'Centre de recherche en Infectiologie', Laval University, 2705 boul. Laurier, Quebec City, PQ G1V 4G2, Canada

**Marilène Bolduc**
Department of Microbiology, Infectiology and Immunology, 'Centre de recherche en Infectiologie', Laval University, 2705 boul. Laurier, Quebec City, PQ G1V 4G2, Canada

**Marie-Eve Laliberté-Gagné**
Department of Microbiology, Infectiology and Immunology, 'Centre de recherche en Infectiologie', Laval University, 2705 boul. Laurier, Quebec City, PQ G1V 4G2, Canada

**Pierre Savard**
Neurosciences, Laval University, Quebec City, PQ, Canada

**Denis Leclerc**
Department of Microbiology, Infectiology and Immunology, 'Centre de recherche en Infectiologie', Laval University, 2705 boul. Laurier, Quebec City, PQ G1V 4G2, Canada

**Sang Rye Park**
Department of Dental Hygiene, Kyungnam College of Information and Technology, Busan 617-701, Rep. Korea

**Hyun Wook Lee**
Department of Electrical Engineering, Pohang University of Science and Technology, Pohang 790-784,Rep. Korea

**Jin Woo Hong**
Department of Korean Internal Medicine, School of Korean Medicine, Pusan National University, Yangsan 626-870, Korea

**Hae June Lee**
Department of Electronics Engineering, Pusan National University, Busan 609-735, Rep. Korea

**Ji Young Kim**
Department of Dental Hygiene, Kyungnam College of Information and Technology, Busan 617-701, Rep. Korea

**Byul bo-ra Choi**
Department of Oral Anatomy, School of Dentistry, Pusan National University, Yangsan 602-739, Rep. Korea

**Gyoo Cheon Kim**
Department of Oral Anatomy, School of Dentistry, Pusan National University, Yangsan 602-739, Rep. Korea

**Young Chan Jeon**
Department of Dental Prosthetics, School of Dentistry, Pusan National University, Yangsan 602-739, Republic of Korea

**Tengfei Weng**
School of Pharmacy, Key Laboratory of Smart Drug Delivery of Ministry of Education, Fudan University, Shanghai 201203, PR China
West China School of Pharmacy, Sichuan University, Chengdu, Sichuan 610041, PR China

**Jianping Qi**
School of Pharmacy, Key Laboratory of Smart Drug Delivery of Ministry of Education, Fudan University, Shanghai 201203, PR China

**Yi Lu**
School of Pharmacy, Key Laboratory of Smart Drug Delivery of Ministry of Education, Fudan University, Shanghai 201203, PR China

**Kai Wang**
School of Pharmacy, Key Laboratory of Smart Drug Delivery of Ministry of Education, Fudan University, Shanghai 201203, PR China
West China School of Pharmacy, Sichuan University, Chengdu, Sichuan 610041, PR China

**Zhiqiang Tian**
School of Pharmacy, Key Laboratory of Smart Drug Delivery of Ministry of Education, Fudan University, Shanghai 201203, PR China

**Kaili Hu**
Murad Research Center for Modernized Chinese Medicine, Shanghai University of Traditional Chinese Medicine, Shanghai 201203, PR China

**Zongning Yi**
West China School of Pharmacy, Sichuan University, Chengdu, Sichuan 610041, PR China

**Wei Wu**
School of Pharmacy, Key Laboratory of Smart Drug Delivery of Ministry of Education, Fudan University, Shanghai 201203, PR China

**Jisha Jayadevan Pillai**
Chemical Biology, Rajiv Gandhi Centre for Biotechnology, Thiruvananthapuram-695 014, Poojappura, Kerala, India

**Arun Kumar Theralikattu Thulasidasan**
Division of Cancer Research, Rajiv Gandhi Centre for Biotechnology, Thiruvananthapuram-695 014, Poojappura, Kerala, India

**Ruby John Anto**
Division of Cancer Research, Rajiv Gandhi Centre for Biotechnology, Thiruvananthapuram-695 014, Poojappura, Kerala, India

**Devika Nandan Chithralekha**
Chemical Biology, Rajiv Gandhi Centre for Biotechnology, Thiruvananthapuram-695 014, Poojappura, Kerala, India

**Ashwanikumar Narayanan**
Chemical Biology, Rajiv Gandhi Centre for Biotechnology, Thiruvananthapuram-695 014, Poojappura, Kerala, India

**Gopalakrishnapillai Sankaramangalam Vinod Kumar**
Chemical Biology, Rajiv Gandhi Centre for Biotechnology, Thiruvananthapuram-695 014, Poojappura, Kerala, India

**Markus Schomaker**
Department of Biomedical Optics, Laser Zentrum Hannover, Hollerithallee 8, 30419 Hannover, Germany

**Dag Heinemann**
Department of Biomedical Optics, Laser Zentrum Hannover, Hollerithallee 8, 30419 Hannover, Germany

**Stefan Kalies**
Department of Biomedical Optics, Laser Zentrum Hannover, Hollerithallee 8, 30419 Hannover, Germany

**Saskia Willenbrock**
Small Animal Clinic, University of Veterinary Medicine Hannover, Bünteweg 9, 30559 Hannover, Germany

**Siegfried Wagner**
Small Animal Clinic, University of Veterinary Medicine Hannover, Bünteweg 9, 30559 Hannover, Germany

**Ingo Nolte**
Small Animal Clinic, University of Veterinary Medicine Hannover, Bünteweg 9, 30559 Hannover, Germany

**Tammo Ripken**
Department of Biomedical Optics, Laser Zentrum Hannover, Hollerithallee 8, 30419 Hannover, Germany

**Hugo Murua Escobar**
Small Animal Clinic, University of Veterinary Medicine Hannover, Bünteweg 9, 30559 Hannover, Germany
Department of Hematology, Oncology, and Palliative Medicine, University of Rostock, Ernst- Heydemann-Str. 6, 18057 Rostock, Germany

**Heiko Meyer**
Department of Biomedical Optics, Laser Zentrum Hannover, Hollerithallee 8, 30419 Hannover, Germany
Department of Cardiothoracic Transplantation and Vascular Surgery, Hannover Medical School, Carl-Neuberg-Str. 1, 30625 Hannover, Germany

**Alexander Heisterkamp**
Department of Biomedical Optics, Laser Zentrum Hannover, Hollerithallee 8, 30419 Hannover, Germany
Institut für Quantenoptik Leibniz Universität Hannover Welfengarten 1, 30167 Hannover, Germany

**Che-Chuan Yang**
MagQu Co., Ltd., Sindian Dist, New Taipei City 231, Taiwan

**Shieh-Yueh Yang**
MagQu Co., Ltd., Sindian Dist, New Taipei City 231, Taiwan

**Chia-Shin Ho**
MagQu Co., Ltd.,Sindian Dist, New Taipei City 231, Taiwan

**Jui-Feng Chang**
MagQu Co., Ltd., Sindian Dist, New Taipei City 231, Taiwan

**Bing-Hsien Liu**
MagQu Co., Ltd., Sindian Dist, New Taipei City 231, Taiwan

**Kai-Wen Huang**
Department of Surgery & Hepatitis Research Center, National Taiwan University Hospital,Taipei 100, Taiwan
Graduate Institute of Clinical Medicine, College of Medicine, National Taiwan University, Taipei 100, Taiwan

**Yijie Shi**
College of Pharmacy, Liaoning Medical University, Jinzhou 121000, P R China

**Chang Su**
College of Veterinary Medicine, Liaoning Medical University, Jinzhou 121000, P R China

**Wenyu Cui**
National Vaccine & Serum Institute, Beijing 100024, China

**Hongdan Li**
Central Laboratory of Liaoning Medical University, Jinzhou 121000, P R China

**Liwei Liu**
College of Pharmacy, Liaoning Medical University, Jinzhou 121000, P R China

**Bo Feng**
College of Pharmacy, Liaoning Medical University, Jinzhou 121000, P R China

**Ming Liu**
College of Pharmacy, Liaoning Medical University, Jinzhou 121000, P R China

**Rongjian Su**
Central Laboratory of Liaoning Medical University, Jinzhou 121000, P R China

**Liang Zhao**
College of Pharmacy, Liaoning Medical University, Jinzhou 121000, P R China

**Khushboo Singh**
Department of Genetics, M.D. University, Rohtak 124001, Haryana, India

**Manju Panghal**
Department of Genetics, M.D. University, Rohtak 124001, Haryana, India

**Sangeeta Kadyan**
Department of Genetics, M.D. University, Rohtak 124001, Haryana, India

**Uma Chaudhary**
Department of Microbiology, Pt. B.D.S Post Graduate Institute of Medical Sciences Rohtak, Rohtak 124001, Haryana, India

**Jaya Parkash Yadav**
Department of Genetics, M.D. University, Rohtak 124001, Haryana, India

**Min Jung Kim**
College of Pharmacy, Seoul National University, Seoul 151-742, South Korea

**Sabarinathan Rangasamy**
College of Pharmacy, Seoul National University, Seoul 151-742, South Korea

**Yumi Shim**
College of Pharmacy, Seoul National University, Seoul 151-742, South Korea

**Joon Myong Song**
College of Pharmacy, Seoul National University, Seoul 151-742, South Korea

**Sonia Centi**
Dipartimento di Scienze Biomediche Sperimentali e Cliniche 'Mario Serio', Università degli Studi di Firenze, Viale Pieraccini 6, 50139 Firenze, Italy

**Francesca Tatini**
Istituto di Fisica Applicata 'Nello Carrara', Consiglio Nazionale delle Ricerche, Via Madonna del Piano 10, 50019 Sesto Fiorentino, Italy

**Fulvio Ratto**
Istituto di Fisica Applicata 'Nello Carrara', Consiglio Nazionale delle Ricerche, Via Madonna del Piano 10, 50019 Sesto Fiorentino, Italy

**Alessio Gnerucci**
Dipartimento di Scienze Biomediche Sperimentali e Cliniche 'Mario Serio', Università degli Studi di Firenze, Viale Pieraccini 6, 50139 Firenze, Italy

**Raffaella Mercatelli**
Dipartimento di Chimica 'Ugo Shiff', Università degli Studi di Firenze, Via della Lastruccia 3, 50019 Sesto Fiorentino, Italy

**Giovanni Romano**
Dipartimento di Scienze Biomediche Sperimentali e Cliniche 'Mario Serio', Università degli Studi di Firenze, Viale Pieraccini 6, 50139 Firenze, Italy

**Ida Landini**
Dipartimento di Scienze della Salute, Università degli Studi di Firenze, Viale Pieraccini 6, 50139 Firenze, Italy

**Stefania Nobili**
Dipartimento di Scienze della Salute, Università degli Studi di Firenze, Viale Pieraccini 6, 50139 Firenze, Italy

**Andrea Ravalli**
Dipartimento di Chimica 'Ugo Shiff', Università degli Studi di Firenze, Via della Lastruccia 3, 50019 Sesto Fiorentino, Italy

**Giovanna Marrazz**
Dipartimento di Chimica 'Ugo Shiff', Università degli Studi di Firenze, Via della Lastruccia 3, 50019 Sesto Fiorentino, Italy

**Enrico Mini**
Dipartimento di Medicina Sperimentale e Clinica, Università degli Studi di Firenze, Largo Brambilla 3, 50134 Firenze, Italy

**Franco Fusi**
Dipartimento di Scienze Biomediche Sperimentali e Cliniche 'Mario Serio', Università degli Studi di Firenze, Viale Pieraccini 6, 50139 Firenze, Italy

**Roberto Pin**
Istituto di Fisica Applicata 'Nello Carrara', Consiglio Nazionale delle Ricerche, Via Madonna del Piano 10, 50019 Sesto Fiorentino, Italy

**Vinicius S Cardoso**
Research Center in Biodiversity and Biotechnology (Biotec), Campus Parnaíba, Federal University of Piauí, Av São Sebastian 2819, 64202-020 Parnaíba, Piauí, Brazil Physiotherapy Department, Campus Parnaíba, Federal University of Piauí, Av. São Sebastião 2819, 64202-020 Parnaíba, Piauí, Brazil

**Patrick V Quelemes**
Research Center in Biodiversity and Biotechnology (Biotec), Campus Parnaíba, Federal University of Piauí, Av São Sebastian 2819, 64202-020 Parnaíba, Piauí, Brazil

**Adriany Amorin**
Research Center in Biodiversity and Biotechnology (Biotec), Campus Parnaíba, Federal University of Piauí, Av São Sebastian 2819, 64202-020 Parnaíba, Piauí, Brazil

**Fernando Lucas Primo**
Departamento de Química, Laboratório de Fotobiologia e Fotomedicina, Faculdade de Filosofia, Ciências e Letras de Ribeirão Preto, Universidade de São Paulo, 14040-901, Ribeirão Preto, SP, Brazil

**Graciely Gomides Gobo**
Departamento de Química, Laboratório de Fotobiologia e Fotomedicina, Faculdade de Filosofia, Ciências e Letras de Ribeirão Preto, Universidade de São Paulo, 14040-901, Ribeirão Preto, SP, Brazil

**Antonio C Tedesco**
Departamento de Química, Laboratório de Fotobiologia e Fotomedicina, Faculdade de Filosofia, Ciências e Letras de Ribeirão Preto, Universidade de São Paulo, 14040-901, Ribeirão Preto, SP, Brazil

**Ana C Mafud**
Institute of Physics of São Carlos (IFSC), University of São Paulo (USP), 13566-590 São Carlos, SP, Brazil

**Yvonne P Mascarenhas**
Institute of Physics of São Carlos (IFSC), University of São Paulo (USP), 13566-590 São Carlos, SP, Brazil

**José Raimundo Corrêa**
Laboratory of Microscopy, Institute of Biology, University of Brasília, 70910900 Brasília, DF, Brazil

**Selma AS Kuckelhaus**
Area of Morphology, Faculty of Medicine, University of Brasília, Brasília 70910900DF, Brazil

**Carla Eiras**
Interdisciplinary Laboratory for Advanced Materials (LIMAV), Federal University of Piauí, 64049-550 Teresina, PI, Brazil

**José Roberto SA Leite**
Research Center in Biodiversity and Biotechnology (Biotec), Campus Parnaíba, Federal University of Piauí, Av São Sebastian 2819, 64202-020 Parnaíba, Piauí, Brazil

**Durcilene Silva**
Research Center in Biodiversity and Biotechnology (Biotec), Campus Parnaíba, Federal University of Piauí, Av São Sebastian 2819, 64202-020 Parnaíba, Piauí, Brazil

**José Ribeiro dos Santos Júnior**
Department of Chemistry, Campus Teresina, Federal University of Piauí, 64049-550 Teresina, Piauí, Brazil

**Jen-Jie Chieh**
Institute of Electro-Optical Science and Technology, National Taiwan Normal University, Taipei 116, Taiwan

**Kai-Wen Huang**
Department of Surgery and Hepatitis Research Center, National Taiwan University Hospital, Taipei 100, Taiwan Graduate Institute of Clinical Medicine, National Taiwan University, Taipei 100, Taiwan

**Yi-Yan Lee**
Institute of Electro-Optical Science and Technology, National Taiwan Normal University, Taipei 116, Taiwan

**Wen-Chun Wei**
Institute of Electro-Optical Science and Technology, National Taiwan Normal University, Taipei 116, Taiwan

**Nan Du**
The Second Department of Oncology, The First Affiliated Hospital of the General Hospital of the PLA, Beijing 100048, China

**Lin-Ping Song**
The Second Department of Oncology, The First Affiliated Hospital of the General Hospital of the PLA, Beijing 100048, China

**Xiao-Song Li**
The Second Department of Oncology, The First Affiliated Hospital of the General Hospital of the PLA, Beijing 100048, China

**Lei Wang**
Department of Medical, The First Affiliated Hospital of the General Hospital of the PLA, No. 51 Fucheng Road, Haidian District, Beijing 100048, China

**Ling Wan**
The Second Department of Oncology, The First Affiliated Hospital of the General Hospital of the PLA, Beijing 100048, China

**Hong-Ying Ma**
The Second Department of Oncology, The First Affiliated Hospital of the General Hospital of the PLA, Beijing 100048, China

**Hui Zhao**
The Second Department of Oncology, The First Affiliated Hospital of the General Hospital of the PLA, Beijing 100048, China

**Jing Zou**
Hearing and Balance Research Unit, Field of Oto-laryngology, School of Medicine, University of Tampere, Medisiinarinkatu 3, 33520 Tampere, Finland
Department of Otolaryngology-Head and Neck Surgery, Center for Otolaryngology-Head & Neck Surgery of Chinese PLA, Changhai Hospital, Second Military Medical University, Shanghai, China

**Markus Hannula**
BioMediTech and Department of Electronics and Communications Engineering, Tampere University of Technology, Tampere, Finland

**Superb Misra**
School of Geography, Earth and Environmental Sciences, University of Birmingham, Birmingham, UK
Materials Science and Engineering, Indian Institute of Technology-Gandhinagar, Ahmedabad, India

**Hao Feng**
Hearing and Balance Research Unit, Field of Oto-laryngology, School of Medicine, University of Tampere, Medisiinarinkatu 3, 33520 Tampere, Finland

**Roberto Hanoi Labrador**
Nanologica AB, Stockholm, Sweden

**Antti S Aula**
BioMediTech and Department of Electronics and Communications Engineering, Tampere University of Technology, Tampere, Finland
Department of Medical Physics, Imaging Centre, Tampere University Hospital, Tampere, Finland

**Jari Hyttinen**
BioMediTech and Department of Electronics and Communications Engineering, Tampere University of Technology, Tampere, Finland

**Ilmari Pyykkö**
Hearing and Balance Research Unit, Field of Oto-laryngology, School of Medicine, University of Tampere, Medisiinarinkatu 3, 33520 Tampere, Finland

**Guilan Quan**
School of Pharmaceutical Sciences, Sun Yat-Sen University, Guangzhou 510006, People's Republic of China

**Xin Pan**
School of Pharmaceutical Sciences, Sun Yat-Sen University, Guangzhou 510006, People's Republic of China

**Zhouhua Wang**
School of Pharmaceutical Sciences, Sun Yat-Sen University, Guangzhou 510006, People's Republic of China

**Qiaoli Wu**
School of Pharmaceutical Sciences, Sun Yat-Sen University, Guangzhou 510006, People's Republic of China

**Ge Li**
Guangzhou Neworld Pharmaceutical Ltd. Co., Guangzhou 510006, People's Republic of China

**Linghui Dian**
School of Pharmaceutical Sciences, Guangdong Medical College, Dongguan 523808, People's Republic of China

**Bao Chen**
School of Pharmaceutical Sciences, Sun Yat-Sen University, Guangzhou 510006, People's Republic of China

**Chuanbin Wu**
School of Pharmaceutical Sciences, Sun Yat-Sen University, Guangzhou 510006, People's Republic of China

**Maria Luisa Bondì**
Istituto per lo Studio dei Materiali Nanostrutturati, U.O.S. Palermo, Consiglio Nazionale delle Ricerche, Via Ugo la Malfa 153, Palermo 90146, Italy

**Antonina Azzolina**
Istituto di Biomedicina e Immunologia Molecolare "Alberto Monroy", Consiglio Nazionale delle Ricerche, Via Ugo la Malfa 153 Palermo 90146, Italy

**Emanuela Fabiola Craparo**
Lab. Of Biocompatible Polymers, Dipartimento di Scienze e Tecnologie Biologiche Chimiche e Farmaceutiche (STEBICEF), via Archirafi 32, Palermo 90123, Italy

**Chiara Botto**
Lab. Of Biocompatible Polymers, Dipartimento di Scienze e Tecnologie Biologiche Chimiche e Farmaceutiche (STEBICEF), via Archirafi 32, Palermo 90123, Italy

**Erika Amore**
Istituto per lo Studio dei Materiali Nanostrutturati, U.O.S. Palermo, Consiglio Nazionale delle Ricerche, Via Ugo la Malfa 153, Palermo 90146, Italy

**Gaetano Giammona**
Lab. Of Biocompatible Polymers, Dipartimento di Scienze e Tecnologie Biologiche Chimiche e Farmaceutiche (STEBICEF), via Archirafi 32, Palermo 90123, Italy

**Melchiorre Cervello**
Istituto di Biomedicina e Immunologia Molecolare "Alberto Monroy", Consiglio Nazionale delle Ricerche, Via Ugo la Malfa 153 Palermo 90146, Italy

**Yi Yuan**
Institute of Stomatology, Nanjing Medical University, Nanjing 210029, China

**Yaqin Zhang**
Department of Biochemistry and Molecular Biology, Nanjing Medical University, Nanjing 210029, China

**Bin Liu**
Department of Biomedical Engineering, Nanjing Medical University, Nanjing 210029, China

**Heming Wu**
Institute of Stomatology, Nanjing Medical University, Nanjing 210029, China

**Yanjun Kang**

**Ming Li**
Institute of Stomatology, Nanjing Medical University, Nanjing 210029, China

**Xin Zeng**
The State Key Laboratory of Bioelectronics, Department of Biological Science and Medical Engineering, Southeast University, Nanjing 210096, China
Maternal and Child Health Institute, Nanjing Maternity and Child Health Care Hospital, Nanjing

**Nongyue He**
The State Key Laboratory of Bioelectronics, Department of Biological Science and Medical Engineering, Southeast University, Nanjing 210096, China

**Gen Zhang**
Department of Cell Biology, Nanjing Medical University, Nanjing 210029, China
The State Key Laboratory of Bioelectronics, Department of Biological Science and Medical Engineering, Southeast University, Nanjing 210096, China

**Izzat Fahimuddin Bin Mohamed Suffian**
Department of Chemical Science and Engineering, Graduate School of Engineering, Kobe University, Kobe, Japan
Institute of Pharmaceutical Science, Faculty of Life Sciences and Medicine, King's College London, London, UK

**Yuya Nishimura**
Organization of Advanced Science and Technology, Kobe University, Kobe, Japan

**Kenta Morita**
Department of Chemical Science and Engineering, Graduate School of Engineering, Kobe University, Kobe, Japan

**Sachiko Nakamura-Tsuruta**
Department of Chemical Science and Engineering, Graduate School of Engineering, Kobe University, Kobe, Japan

**Khuloud T Al-Jamal**
Institute of Pharmaceutical Science, Faculty of Life Sciences and Medicine, King's College London, London, UK

**Jun Ishii**
Organization of Advanced Science and Technology, Kobe University, Kobe, Japan

**Chiaki Ogino**
Department of Chemical Science and Engineering, Graduate School of Engineering, Kobe University, Kobe, Japan

**Akihiko Kondo**
Department of Chemical Science and Engineering, Graduate School of Engineering, Kobe University, Kobe, Japan

**Xuan Weng**
BioNano Laboratory, School of Engineering, University of Guelph, Guelph, ON N1G 2W1, Canada

**Wenting Zhao**
Department of Industrial Engineering, South China University of Technology, Guangzhou, Guangdong 510640, China

**Suresh Neethirajan**
BioNano Laboratory, School of Engineering, University of Guelph, Guelph, ON N1G 2W1, Canada

**Todd Duffield**
Department of Population Medicine, Ontario Veterinary College, University of Guelph, Guelph, ON N1G 2W1, Canada

**Macarena Calero**
Departamento de Biología, Universidad Autónoma de Madrid, Cantoblanco, 28049 Madrid, Spain
Instituto Madrileño de Estudios Avanzados en Nanociencia (IMDEA Nanociencia), Cantoblanco, 28049 Madrid, Spain

**Michele Chiappi**
Department of Macromolecular Structure, Centro Nacional de Biotecnología, Consejo Superior de Investigaciones Científicas, 28049 Madrid, Spain

**Ana Lazaro-Carrillo**
Departamento de Biología, Universidad Autónoma de Madrid, Cantoblanco, 28049 Madrid, Spain
Instituto Madrileño de Estudios Avanzados en Nanociencia (IMDEA Nanociencia), Cantoblanco, 28049 Madrid, Spain

**María José Rodríguez**
Department of Macromolecular Structure, Centro Nacional de Biotecnología, Consejo Superior de Investigaciones Científicas, 28049 Madrid, Spain

**Francisco Javier Chichón**
Department of Macromolecular Structure, Centro Nacional de Biotecnología, Consejo Superior de Investigaciones Científicas, 28049 Madrid, Spain

**Kieran Crosbie-Staunton**
Department of Clinical Medicine, Trinity Centre for Health Science, James's Street, Dublin 8, Ireland

**Adriele Prina-Mello**
Department of Clinical Medicine, Trinity Centre for Health Science, James's Street, Dublin 8, Ireland
Centre for Research on Adaptive Nanostructures and Nanodevices (CRANN), and AMBER Centre, Trinity College Dublin, College Green, Dublin 2, Ireland

**Yuri Volkov**
Department of Clinical Medicine, Trinity Centre for Health Science, James's Street, Dublin 8, Ireland
Centre for Research on Adaptive Nanostructures and Nanodevices (CRANN), and AMBER Centre, Trinity College Dublin, College Green, Dublin 2, Ireland

**Angeles Villanueva**
Departamento de Biología, Universidad Autónoma de Madrid, Cantoblanco, 28049 Madrid, Spain
Instituto Madrileño de Estudios Avanzados en Nanociencia (IMDEA Nanociencia), Cantoblanco, 28049 Madrid, Spain

**José L Carrascosa**
Department of Macromolecular Structure, Centro Nacional de Biotecnología, Consejo Superior de Investigaciones Científicas, 28049 Madrid, Spain
Instituto Madrileño de Estudios Avanzados en Nanociencia (IMDEA Nanociencia), Cantoblanco, 28049 Madrid, Spain